MOLECULAR GENETICS OF CARDIAC ELECTROPHYSIOLOGY

Developments in Cardiovascular Medicine

205. Juan Carlos Kaski, David W. Holt (eds.): *Myocardial Damage Early Detection by Novel Biochemical Markers. 1998.* ISBN 0-7923-5140-1
207. Gary F. Baxter, Derek M. Yellon, *Delayed Preconditioning and Adaptive Cardioprotection. 1998.* ISBN 0-7923-5259-9
208. Bernard Swynghedauw, *Molecular Cardiology for the Cardiologist, Second Edition* 1998. ISBN 0-7923-8323-0
209. Geoffrey Burnstock, James G.Dobson, Jr., Bruce T. Liang, Joel Linden (eds): *Cardiovascular Biology of Purines.* 1998. ISBN: 0-7923-8334-6
210. Brian D. Hoit, Richard A. Walsh (eds): *Cardiovascular Physiology in the Genetically Engineered Mouse.* 1998. ISBN: 0-7923-8356-7
211. Peter Whittaker, George S. Abela (eds.): *Direct Myocardial Revascularization: History, Methodology, Technology* 1998. ISBN: 0-7923-8398-2
212. C.A. Nienaber, R. Fattori (eds.): Diagnosis and Treatment of Aortic Diseases. 1999. ISBN: 0-7923-5517-2
213. Juan Carlos Kaski (ed.): *Chest Pain with Normal Coronary Angiograms: Pathogenesis, Diagnosis and Management.* 1999. ISBN: 0-7923-8421-0
214. P.A. Doevendans, R.S. Reneman and M. Van Bilsen (eds): *Cardiovascular Specific Gene Expression.* 1999 ISBN:0-7923-5633-0
215. G. Pons-Lladó, F. Carreras, X. Borrás, Subirana and L.J. Jiménez-Borreguero (eds.): *Atlas of Practical Cardiac Applications of MRI.* 1999 ISBN: 0-7923-5636-5
216. L.W. Klein, J.E. Calvin, *Resource Utilization in Cardiac Disease.* 1999. ISBN:0-7923-8509-8
217. R. Gorlin, G. Dangas, P. K. Toutouzas, M.M Konstadoulakis, *Contemporary Concepts in Cardiology, Pathophysiology and Clinical Management.*1999 ISBN:0-7923-8514-4
218. S. Gupta, J. Camm (eds.): *Chronic Infection, Chlamydia and Coronary Heart Disease.* 1999. ISBN:0-7923-5797-3
219. M. Rajskina: *Ventricular Fibrillation in Sudden Coronary Death.* 1999. ISBN:0-7923-8570-5
220. Z. Abedin, R. Conner: *Interpretation of Cardiac Arrhythmias: Self Assessment Approach.* 1999. ISBN:0-7923-8576-4
221. J. E. Lock, J.F. Keane, S. B. Perry: *Diagnostic and Interventional Catheterization In Congenital Heart Disease.* 2000. ISBN: 0-7923-8597-7
222. J.S. Steinberg: *Atrial Fibrillation after Cardiac Surgery.* 2000. ISBN: 0-7923-8655-8
223. E.E. van der Wall, A. van der Laarse, B.M. Pluim, A.V.G. Bruschke: Left Ventricular Hypertrophy: Physiology versus Pathology. 2000 ISBN: 0-7923-6038-9
224. J.F. Keaney, Jr. (ed.): *Oxidative Stress and Vascular Disease.* 2000. ISBN: 0-7923-8678-7
228. B.E. Jaski: *Basics of Heart Failure.* 2000 ISBN: 0-7923-7786-9
229. H.H. Osterhues, V. Hombach, A.J. Moss (eds.): *Advances in Non-Invasive Electrocardiographic Monitoring Techniques.* 2000. ISBN: 0-7923-6214-4
230. K. Robinson (ed.): *Homocysteine and Vascular Disease.* 2000 ISBN: 0-7923-6248-9
231. C.I. Berul, J.A. Towbin (eds.): *Molecular Genetics of Cardiac Electrophysiology.* 2000. ISBN: 0-7923-7829-6

Previous volumes are still available

KLUWER ACADEMIC PUBLISHERS - DORDRECHT/BOSTON/LONDON

MOLECULAR GENETICS OF CARDIAC ELECTROPHYSIOLOGY

edited by

Charles I. Berul
Department of Cardiology, Children's Hospital, Boston
Department of Pediatrics, Harvard Medical School

and

Jeffrey A. Towbin
Departments of Pediatrics (Cardiology) and
Molecular & Human Genetics
Baylor College of Medicine, Texas Children's Hospital, Houston

KLUWER ACADEMIC PUBLISHERS
Boston / Dordrecht / London

Distributors for North, Central and South America:
Kluwer Academic Publishers
101 Philip Drive
Assinippi Park
Norwell, Massachusetts 02061 USA

Distributors for all other countries:
Kluwer Academic Publishers Group
Distribution Centre
Post Office Box 322
3300 AH Dordrecht, THE NETHERLANDS

Library of Congress Cataloging-in-Publication Data

Molecular genetics of cardiac electrophysiology / edited by Charles I. Berul, Jeffrey A. Towbin.
   p. ; cm. -- (Developments in cardiovascular medicine ; 231)
  Includes index.
  ISBN 0-7923-7829-6
   1. Congenital heart disease--Pathophysiology. 2. Arrhythmia--Pathophysiology. 3.
Arrhythmia--Genetic aspects. 4. Heart cells--Electric properties. I. Berul, Charles I. II.
Towbin, Jeffrey A. III. Developments in cardiovascular medicine ; v. 231.
   [DNLM: 1. Arrhythmia--physiopathology. 2. Arrhythmia--genetics. 3.
Electrophysiology. 4. Heart Defects, Congenital--genetics. 5. Myocardial
Diseases--genetics. WG 330 M718 2000]
  RC687.M58 2000
  616.1'2807--dc21

                                                    00-28723

Printed on acid-free paper.

Printed in the United States of America

Molecular Genetics of Cardiac Electrophysiology

TABLE OF CONTENTS

CONTRIBUTING AUTHORS

Charles Antzelevitch, Ph.D.
Masonic Medical Research Laboratory
Utica, NY 13501

Michael Apkon, M.D., Ph.D.
Section of Pediatric Critical Care
Yale University School of Medicine
New Haven, CT 06520

Craig T. Basson, M.D., Ph.D.
Cardiology Division, Department of Medicine
Department of Cell Biology
Weill Medical College of Cornell University
New York, NY 10021

Charles I. Berul, M.D.
Department of Cardiology, Children's Hospital, Boston
Department of Pediatrics, Harvard Medical School
Boston, MA 02115

Laura M. Bevilacqua, M.D.
Department of Cardiology, Children's Hospital, Boston
Department of Pediatrics, Harvard Medical School
Boston, MA 02115

Neil E. Bowles, Ph.D.
Department of Pediatrics (Cardiology)
Texas Children's Hospital, Baylor College of Medicine
Houston, TX 77030

Josep Brugada, M.D.
Cardiovascular Institute Hospital Clinic
University of Barcelona
Barcelona, SPAIN

Pedro Brugada, M.D.
Cardiovascular Center
OLV Hospital
Aalst, BELGIUM

Ramon Brugada, M.D.
Department of Cardiology
Baylor College of Medicine
Houston, TX 77030

Gerald Cox, M.D.
Division of Genetics, Department of Medicine, Children's Hospital, Boston

Department of Pediatrics, Harvard Medical School
Boston, MA 02115
Ellen R. Elias, M.D.
Director, Coordinated Care Service
Department of Medicine, Children's Hospital, Boston
Department of Pediatrics, Harvard Medical School
Boston, MA 02115

Elizabeth Goldmuntz, M.D.
Division of Cardiology, The Children's Hospital of Philadelphia
University of Pennsylvania
Philadelphia, PA 19104

Steve A.N. Goldstein, M.D., Ph.D.
Section of Pediatric Cardiology
Yale University School of Medicine
New Haven, CT 06520

Robert M. Hamilton, M.D., FRCP(C)
Division of Pediatric Cardiology
Hospital for Sick Children
Toronto, Ontario, CANADA

Cathy J. Hatcher, Ph.D.
Department of Cell Biology
Weill Medical College of Cornell University
New York, NY 10021

Mira Irons, M.D.
Division of Genetics and Metabolism
Department of Medicine, Children's Hospital, Boston
Department of Pediatrics, Harvard Medical School
Boston, MA 02115

José Jalife, M.D.
Department of Pharmacology
SUNY Health Science Center
Syracuse, NY 13210

Patrick Y. Jay, M.D., Ph.D.
Department of Cardiology, Children's Hospital, Boston
Department of Pediatrics, Harvard Medical School
Boston, MA 02115

Ronald V. Lacro, M.D.
Department of Cardiology, Children's Hospital, Boston
Department of Pediatrics, Harvard Medical School
Boston, MA 02115

Deborah L. Lerner, M.D.
Department of Pediatrics
Washington University School of Medicine
St. Louis, MO 63110

Coeli M.B. Lopes, Ph.D.
Yale University School of Medicine
New Haven, CT 06520

Frank I. Marcus, M.D.
Department of Medicine
University of Arizona Health Sciences Center
Tucson, AZ 85724

Gregory E. Morley, Ph.D.
Department of Pharmacology
SUNY Health Science Center
Syracuse, NY 13210

Koonalee Nademanee, M.D.
Department of Medicine
University of Southern California
Los Angeles, CA 90033

Peter Ott, M.D.
Department of Medicine
University of Arizona Health Sciences Center
Tucson, AZ 85724

Kristen Patton, M.D.
Department of Genetics and Medicine, Brigham & Women's Hospital
Howard Hughes Medical Institute
Harvard Medical School
Boston, MA 02115

Amit Rakhit, M.D.
Department of Cardiology, Children's Hospital, Boston
Department of Pediatrics, Harvard Medical School
Boston, MA 02115

Sita Reddy, Ph.D.
Institute for Genetic Medicine
University of Southern California School of Medicine
Los Angeles, CA 90033

Robert Roberts, M.D.
Department of Cardiology
Baylor College of Medicine
Houston, TX 77030

Dan M. Roden, M.D.
Director, Division of Clinical Pharmacology
Department of Medicine and Pharmacology
Vanderbilt University School of Medicine
Nashville, TN 37232

Jeffrey E. Saffitz, M.D., Ph.D.
Department of Pathology
Center for Cardiovascular Research
Washington University School of Medicine
St. Louis, MO 63110

Christine E. Seidman, M.D.
Department of Genetics and Medicine, Brigham & Women's Hospital
Howard Hughes Medical Institute
Harvard Medical School
Boston, MA 02115

Leslie B. Smoot, M.D.
Department of Cardiology, Children's Hospital, Boston
Department of Pediatrics, Harvard Medical School
Boston, MA 02115

Baruch S. Ticho, M.D., Ph.D.
Department of Pediatrics
Massachusetts General Hospital
Harvard Medical School
Boston, MA 02114

Katherine Timothy, B.S.
Department of Cardiology
LDS Hospital
Salt Lake City, UT 84103

Jeffrey A. Towbin, M.D.
Department of Pediatrics (Cardiology), Molecular and Human Genetics
Texas Children's Hospital, Baylor College of Medicine
Houston, TX 77030

Dhananjay Vaidya, M.B.B.S.
Department of Pharmacology
SUNY Health Science Center
Syracuse, NY 13210

Richard Van Praagh, M.D.
Departments of Cardiology and Pathology, Children's Hospital, Boston
Department of Pediatrics, Harvard Medical School
Boston, MA 02115

Dan M. Roden, M.D.
Department of Medicine and Pharmacology
Vanderbilt University School of Medicine
Nashville, TN 37232

Jeffrey E. Saffitz, M.D., Ph.D.
Department of Pathology, Center for Cardiovascular Research
Washington University School of Medicine
St. Louis, MO 63110

Christine E. Seidman, M.D.
Department of Genetics and Medicine, Brigham & Women's Hospital
Howard Hughes Medical Institute, Harvard Medical School
Boston, MA 02115

Leslie B. Smoot, M.D.
Department of Cardiology, Children's Hospital, Boston
Department of Pediatrics, Harvard Medical School
Boston, MA 02115

Baruch S. Ticho, M.D., Ph.D.
Department of Pediatrics, Massachusetts General Hospital, Harvard Medical School
Boston, MA 02114

Katherine Timothy, B.S.
Department of Cardiology, LDS Hospital
Salt Lake City, UT 84103

Jeffrey A. Towbin, M.D.
Department of Pediatrics (Cardiology), Molecular and Human Genetics
Texas Children's Hospital, Baylor College of Medicine
Houston, TX 77030

Dhananjay Vaidya, M.B.B.S.
Department of Pharmacology, SUNY Health Science Center
Syracuse, NY 13210

Richard Van Praagh, M.D.
Departments of Cardiology and Pathology, Children's Hospital, Boston
Department of Pediatrics, Harvard Medical School
Boston, MA 02115

Matteo Vatta, Ph.D.
Department of Pediatrics (Cardiology)
Texas Children's Hospital, Baylor College of Medicine
Houston, TX 77030

G. Michael Vincent, M.D.
Department of Cardiology, LDS Hospital
Salt Lake City, UT 84103

ACKNOWLEDGMENTS

We would like to thank each of the chapter contributors and their colleagues and assistants for the outstanding quality, and all of the hard work that went into the production of individual chapters for this book. We would like to thank Anna Cipollone for her wonderful cover illustration, Mary Visconti and Melba Koegele for their untiring administrative assistance. We appreciate the work of the Kluwer office, particularly Melissa Ramondetta and Laura Walsh, who allowed this book to move from conception to completion. Ultimately, we thank our families for their patience, love, and understanding in enduring our absence, preoccupation, and diversion during the production of this book.

1

OVERVIEW: GENETICS OF CARDIAC ELECTROPHYSIOLOGY

Jeffrey A. Towbin, M.D. and Charles I. Berul, M.D.

Health and well being of children and adults requires normal functioning and interaction between cardiac structure, function and electrical activity. Dysfunction or dysregulation of any of these factors can individually result in significant disease but commonly it is the disruption of integral interactions between these functions that leads to the morbidity and mortality seen with cardiac disease. In this regard, cardiac electrophysiology plays a central role in the severity of disease of any cardiac patient subgroup, whether the abnormality is primary or secondary. Up until relatively recently, the relationship between structural heart disease and cardiac electrical abnormalities were not thought to have common genetic bases. However, modern molecular and clinical genetics has demonstrated some interesting and surprising models of potential disease commonality. From molecular biology, cellular physiology, whole animal integrated physiology, to clinical genetics and medicine, innovative research has allowed for novel hypotheses-driven theories regarding the genetics of cardiac electrophysiology. In this book, a group of experts lead us through some of the up-to-date methods for studying normal and altered cardiac electrophysiology, primary disorders of cardiac conduction and electrophysiology, and many of the most important disorders in which associated rhythm abnormalities occur. In each chapter, integration of clinical and basic science features are detailed and the molecular genetic understanding of each disease at the turn of the new millennium are highlighted.

The book is divided into five sections. In Section I, experimental investigation of inherited electrophysiologic disorders are discussed. Single-cell electrophysiology in health and ion channelopathies are described by Dr. Lopes and colleagues followed by animal models of cardiac rhythm disorders, discussed by Drs. Rakhit and Berul. In the last two segments of Section I, elegant descriptions of optical mapping of arrhythmias are contributed by Dr. Morley and colleagues, followed by a thorough review of the potential roles of connexins in cardiac conduction by Drs. Lerner and Saffitz.

In Section II, the molecular genetics of supraventricular arrhythmias are covered. Drs. Jay and Berul outline the current knowledge regarding inherited supraventricular tachycardias and Drs. Brugada and Roberts beautifully provide up-to-date information on familial atrial fibrillation. The section is wrapped up by Dr. Hamilton, who establishes a molecular and genetic view of the etiologies of congenital heart block.

Section III, which attempts to unravel the genetic secrets of ventricular tachyarrhythmias, contains chapters on congenital and acquired long QT syndromes, as well as a chapter on Brugada syndrome. In the initial chapter of this section, Katherine Timothy and G. Michael Vincent detail the discoveries to date on inherited long QT syndromes, followed by Dr. Roden who discusses acquired long QT syndrome, genetic factors, and compares and contrasts acquired ventricular arrhythmias with the inherited form. Dr. Towbin and the Brugada Syndrome Working Group, complete this section with an up-to-the-minute view of Brugada syndrome and a unifying concept of cardiovascular genetics, the "final common pathway" hypothesis.

Cardiac and cardioskeletal myopathies associated with electrophysiologic disorders are discussed in Section IV. Hypertrophic and dilated cardiomyopathies are covered in the opening chapters by Drs. Bevilacqua and Berul (HCM) and Towbin and Bowles (DCM). In the next chapter, Drs. Irons and Elias thoroughly describe glycogen storage diseases, with particular emphasis on cardiac involvement, followed by a comprehensive discussion of ARVD by Dr. Marcus. The section ends with chapters on the molecular genetics of muscular dystrophies, including Duchenne and Becker muscular dystrophy (Smoot and Cox) and myotonic dystrophy (Reddy and Berul), which provide information on critical regulatory mechanisms that result in a wide spectrum of clinical disease, including frameshifting and triplet repeat abnormalities.

In the final section, congenital cardiovascular disease is covered. This section attempts to link the genetic features of both structural and electrical cardiac abnormalities in the young. The beautiful work on inherited atrial septal defects (Drs. Patton and Seidman) and Holt-Oram syndrome (Drs. Hatcher and Basson) are elegantly described in the first two chapters, followed by the intriguing discussion by Drs. Ticho and Van Praagh, who outline laterality defects. In the final chapters, Marfan syndrome and its associated cardiovascular abnormalities is outlined by Dr. Lacro and finally, Dr. Goldmuntz covers the genetics of conotruncal defects with or without associated defects of CATCH-22.

The book is an attempt to bring the reader into the 21st century with a complete understanding of the clinical and molecular genetic details of a wide spectrum of disorders associated with electrophysiologic abnormalities. Our goal is to provide a current and comprehensive resource for investigators, clinicians, and students who seek further understanding of the expanding knowledge base of the relationship between genetics and the field of cardiac electrophysiology. We hope that this book helps to bridge the gap between the research bench and the clinical bedside, allowing for a new paradigm in the care of patients with these disorders.

Jeffrey A. Towbin, M.D.
Charles I. Berul, M.D
Editors

2

SINGLE-CELL ELECTROPHYSIOLOGY AND ION CHANNELOPATHIES

Coeli M.B. Lopes, Ph.D., Steve A.N. Goldstein, M.D., Ph.D., and Michael Apkon, M.D., Ph.D.

Yale University, New Haven, CT 06520

INTRODUCTION

The electrical behavior of the heart reflects interactions among highly specialized and tightly regulated excitable cells. Control of membrane potential at rest and during the action potential organizes the rhythmic electrical activity of the pacemaker regions of the heart, thereby determining the sequence of activation through the myocardium that leads to cyclical contraction and relaxation. The electrophysiological properties of individual myocytes are determined by the properties of the myriad of ion channels and electrogenic pumps that pass current across the sarcolemma. The function of these proteins can be altered by a variety of neurotransmitters, neurohormones, and drugs. In addition, regulated changes in their surface density or functional properties can have profound effects on excitability, risk of arrhythmias, and mechanical function. Examination of cardiac ion channels and their regulation is key to understanding cardiac excitability in normal and pathological states and the mechanisms underlying drug action on the heart.

The development of techniques to voltage-clamp single cells or even small areas of cell membrane using the patch-clamp technique has revolutionized our ability to examine cardiac electrical activity. These techniques have allowed the characterization of the macroscopic currents underlying excitability as well as the properties of single ion channels. In combination with modulation of channel protein expression in native cells using antisense treatment or transgenic approaches, single cell electrophysiology has given new insight into the protein subunits contributing to ion channels and of the regulatory cascades modulating their function. Cloning of genes encoding ion channels has allowed their expression in experimental cells in normal and mutant form. This provides a means of interrogating the relationship between channel structure and function and studying the interactions between various channel proteins. In addition, coupling electrophysiological and optical methods permits studies in which ion currents and changes in intracellular Ca^{2+} levels or contraction can be assessed simultaneously in single cells.

Here we review common techniques used to study the molecular basis of excitability using single cells and give examples to show how the methods have helped to reveal the role of ion channels in normal cardiac function and arrhythmias.

METHODS

Cell Isolation

Cardiac cells are electrically connected via gap junctions and must be dissociated if a single cell is to be studied in isolation. A variety of techniques have been proposed to isolate single myocardial cells. These rely on enzymatic digestion at low ambient Ca^{2+} concentrations to disrupt intercellular connections (1). The challenge in these procedures is maintaining viable myocytes that subsequently tolerate physiological Ca^{2+} concentrations. Investigators have maximized viability by cannulating the aorta (Langendorff preparation) and perfusing the coronary vessels with an oxygenated, collagenase-containing solution. A variation on this approach relies on incubation of human myocardium obtained from surgical or post-mortem specimens in an enzyme-containing bath (2).

We routinely prepare cardiac myocytes from mice by the Langendorff perfusion method (3). Briefly, mice are anesthetized with metoxyflurane and the heart removed to ice cold buffer. The aorta is cannulated with a blunt needle connected to a syringe containing Ca-free buffer and the connection stabilized by a silk suture. Ca-free solution is perfused through the heart and rapidly clears blood from the coronary arteries. It is critical that the cannula tip be above the aortic valve and that no air is introduced into the coronary arteries during cannulation. The heart is then perfused with warm (37°C) oxygenated (100% O_2) solution. The Ca^{2+}-free solution is initially used to perfuse the heart; after a few minutes the solution is exchanged for an enzyme-containing solution in which Ca^{2+} is not buffered. The solution is recirculated for approximately 30 min at which time the heart appears soft. The tissue is then dissected into small pieces using a sharp razor blade and incubated at 37°C. Incubation in collagenase solution and gentle mechanical dissociation liberates single cells. The cells settle by gravity (or gentle centrifugation) and the cell pellet is washed through a series of solutions containing gradually higher Ca^{2+} concentrations.

Cells prepared in this manner may be maintained in tissue culture media. Coating the culture wells with extracellular matrix materials facilitates attachment of cells to the substratum. Cells are studied immediately or may be maintained in short term tissue culture. Healthy myocytes are recognized by their clear striations and bright surface (Figure 1). Ventricular myocytes are quiescent at rest but contract upon electrical stimulation.

A   B

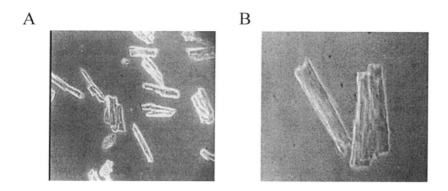

Figure 1: Isolated mouse ventricular myocytes. Digital photomicrographs recorded at
20X (A) and 40X (B) magnification.

Heterologous Expression of Channel Proteins

Examination of dissociated cardiac myocytes represents a powerful technique to
dissect the contributions of individual channels to the overall electrophysiological
characteristics of the myocyte. Although it is well suited to studying ion channels in
myocytes derived from animals, this approach is less applicable to humans because of
difficulties associated with obtaining viable samples. This limitation is particularly
marked for samples from patients with ion channel-associated disease. One solution
to this problem has been to study cloned ion channel genes in experimental cells. This
requires the characterization of the cloned channel and its successful identification as
the molecular correlate of a native ion channel. Thereafter, wild type and disease-
causing channel variants can be studied with full experimental control.

Ion channel proteins may be expressed in a variety of cell types in transient or stable
fashion. Methods used for transient expression include direct injection of cRNA, viral
transfection, RNA uptake, and electroporation. Oocytes from the frog *Xenopus laevis*
are frequently used for transient expression because they are large, readily harvested,
and are easily studied using voltage-clamp and patch-clamp techniques. Among the
advantages of heterologous expression, host cells may be selected that do not
normally express channels like those under investigation. This avoids the need to
pharmacologically inhibit native channels and eliminates the potential for secondary
drug effects. It also allows evaluation of a single channel isoform even if it is
normally at low abundance in native cells. Further, heterologous expression systems
allow manipulation of channel cDNA in order to explore structure-function
relationships, important in identifying the effects of genetic mutations. This approach
can also be used to provide insight into the function of cRNA for which the
physiological function is unknown.

An important consideration when using heterologous expression systems is whether channel function in the host cell is similar to that *in vivo*. Channel function in the host cell may differ from native function for several reasons. First, protein processing or the membrane environment may differ between the host cell and the myocyte. Second, the channel protein may associate with additional subunits in native cells that are absent in host cells, or, conversely, interact with channel proteins unique to the host cell thereby altering function. Third, the host cell may have different intracellular signaling mechanisms or different concentrations of key signaling molecules compared to cardiac myocytes.

Differences have been observed between channel function measured in different host cell types. For example, kinetics and voltage-dependence of Kv 1.5 channel activation depends on whether cells express regulatory β subunits (4). So, too,   the Kv4.2 potassium channel activates and recovers from inactivation differently depending on host cell type (5). Differences in function of native cardiac IKr channels and cells expressing cloned HERG subunits were eliminated when MiRP1 and HERG subunits were co-expressed in experimental cells; this demonstrated that these two subunits associate to form the native cardiac channel complex (6).

Single Cell Electrophysiological Techniques

Conventional microelectrode recording
Membrane potential may be recorded from isolated myocytes by impaling them with sharp glass microelectrodes. These microelectrodes are fabricated by pulling heated glass capillary tubing to a fine point and filling them with a highly concentrated electrolyte solution (generally 3 M KCl). Impaling the cell with the microelectrode establishes electrical continuity between the cell and pipette. A silver/silver-chloride (Ag/AgCl) electrode on the other end of the pipette allows connection to a high impedance electrometer for measuring the membrane potential. Current can be injected through the pipette and used to depolarize the cell to trigger an action potential. Action potentials can also be stimulated by putting the cells in an electrical field between two electrodes placed some distance away in the bathing solution. These approaches have the advantage of rather simply and faithfully recording membrane voltage but suffer from the disadvantage that membrane potential may not be controlled or clamped and the cell integrity may be disrupted by electrode penetration.

Patch clamp recording
Patch clamp recording is an electrophysiological technique whereby a patch of cell membrane is electrically isolated from the rest of the cell (7). In this technique a glass pipette with a diameter significantly larger than that used in conventional microelectrode recording (~1 μM) is pressed against the membrane forming a very high resistance seal (measured in gigaohms, 10^9 Ohms) between the cell and the pipette. The pipette is filled with a suitable solution and contains an Ag/AgCl

electrode that is connected to an appropriate amplifier. The patch-clamp amplifier uses electrical feedback to inject current through the pipette in response to an error signal between the pipette potential and a command potential. Because the voltage drop across the pipette is low compared to the membrane potential the membrane voltage can be precisely controlled.

After forming a seal, one can study ion channels within the patch in a 'on-cell' configuration (Figure 2A). Applying suction to the pipette ruptures the membrane patch, establishing electrical continuity with the interior of the cell. This allows study of all the ion channels in the cell ('whole cell' mode, Figure 2B). A small segment of the cytoplasmic side of the membrane can also be exposed to the bath solution by withdrawing the pipette from the cell surface before rupturing the membrane ('inside-out' mode, Figure 2C). Finally, the outside face of the membrane can be exposed by withdrawing a pipette after rupturing the membrane ('outside-out' mode, Figure 2D).

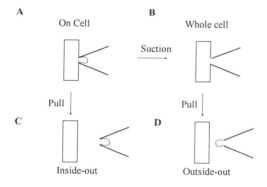

Figure 2. Configurations of patch-clamp recording showing the relationships between the cell, membrane patch, and recording electrode

Recording Membrane Potential and Whole-Cell Currents

Once the whole-cell configuration has been established, membrane potential and action potentials may be recorded in much the same manner as with conventional microelectrodes. In this recording mode, the pipette potential is allowed to vary, following the membrane potential of the cell. Action potentials are elicited by defined current injections through the pipette (Figure 3). Alternatively, whole-cell currents may be recorded under voltage-clamp conditions (Figure 4). Such measurements have been extensively used to characterize the macroscopic currents of cardiac myocytes.

One consideration in whole-cell recording is that the intracellular space is in continuity with the pipette; this allows the cell to be dialyzed by the pipette solution. This can be an advantage when control of the internal contents of the cell is required.

On the other hand, dialysis of the cellular contents may result in loss of constituents critical to ion channel function. This problem can be minimized by incorporating channel-forming antibiotics such as nystatin or amphotericin B into the pipette solution to establish electrical continuity between pipette and cell without mechanically rupturing the membrane (8). These antibiotics form channels in the membrane that allow free movement of monovalent cations but restrict movement of polyvalent cations and macromolecules.

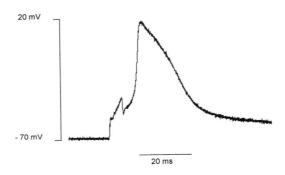

Figure 3: Action potential recorded from a mouse ventricular myocyte using the whole-cell patch-clamp technique. The initial step in potential represents an artifact of current (200 pA) injection used to evoke the action potential.

Recording the activity of single ion channels

Membrane conductance is the result of the activity of single ion channels. The macroscopic (i.e. whole-cell) current (I) contributed by a single type of ion channel depends on: the number of channels (N); the probability that a channel is open at any instant in time (P_o); the conductance of the single channel (γ); and, the electrochemical driving force for the conducting ions (defined as the difference between the membrane potential (V_m) and the equilibrium potential for the ion (E)). Thus, the macroscopic current through a particular channel type can be expressed by the equation: $I=NP_o\gamma(V_m-E)$.

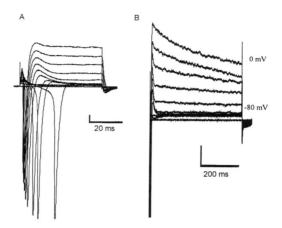

Figure 4: Whole cell measurement of voltage-activated ion currents in a single mouse ventricular myocyte at two different time scales. A) Currents evoked by 50 ms pulses from -80 mV to potentials between -70 and 0 mV in 10 mV increments. B) Currents evoked by 500 ms voltage pulses using an identical protocol as in A. Downward deflections are primarily Na^+ currents and upward are K^+ currents. The vertical scale bar represents 200 pA in both panels.

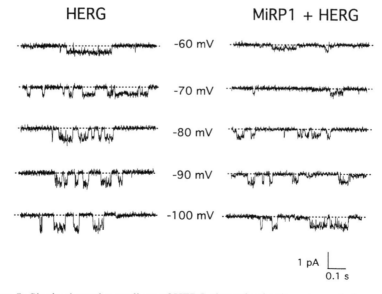

Figure 5: Single channel recordings of HERG channel subunits expressed alone or with the MinK-related protein 1 (MiRP1). Channel openings are shown as deflections below the baseline (dotted lines) (6).

When one monitors the activity of a single ion channel using one of the variations of the patch-clamp technique, it is possible to observe spontaneous transitions between non-conducting (closed) and conducting (open) states of the channel. At a given voltage, these channel openings are seen as step-wise changes in the current passed through the pipette (Figure 5). By examining the amplitude of these currents over a range of pipette potentials, it is possible to calculate the unitary conductance (γ) of the single channel as the slope of the line relating the amplitude of the current to pipette potential. The shape of the single channel current-voltage relationship is one 'fingerprint' that characterizes an ion channel.

Individual ion channels may undergo conformational changes in response to changes in membrane voltage, interactions with second messenger molecules or spontaneously over time. Each conformation (or state) may have unique open probabilities, conductances, or likelihood of transitions to other states. Interactions of drugs with ion channels can depend on the conformational state of the channel. A drug that binds to the open state of a channel can have profoundly different effects from one that binds to its closed state; this underlies the concept of use-dependent blockade (9, 10).

Measurement of Single Cell Contractions
Contractions of single myocytes can be measured whether they are spontaneous, stimulated by placing cells in an electrical field, or stimulated directly with intracellular or whole-cell microelectrodes. The later approaches allow examination of the relationship between electrical and mechanical events.
events. Individual muscle twitches may be characterized either by the force produced by the contraction or by changes in length. Force measurements have been made directly by attaching the ends of cells to glass probes connected to micro-force transducers (11). This approach allows the cell to be loaded with a defined tension at rest. Changes in length under unloaded conditions are measured optically by analysis of video images of the cell using a video edge detector (12).

PROPERTIES OF ION CHANNELS

Ion channels are classified by the type of ion that they pass, their unitary conductance, the kinetics of their conformational changes, their regulatory influences and the drugs that alter their function (13).

Ion Selectivity
The currents underling the cardiac action potential are diverse and reflect the activity of Na^+, K^+, Ca^{2+} and Cl^- selective ion channels. The ability of an ion channel to distinguish among ionic species establishes the directionality of current passing through that channel and determines whether channel opening will result in depolarization or hyperpolarization. Potassium channels, for example, are about 100

times more selective for K^+ than Na^+ (13) whereas Na^+ channels are generally 10-20 times more permeable to Na^+ than to K^+. Current through Ca^{2+} channels is predominantly carried by Ca^{2+} ions, although Ca^{2+} is outnumbered 100:1 by Na^+ in the extracellular space and 3,000:1 by K^+ in the intracellular solution. Although the ion selectivity of a channel is generally determined by its structure, selectivity may be modulated by second messenger systems (14).

Unitary Conductance
The open conformation of each ion channel has a characteristic conductance dependent on its ion selectivity and ionic environment. For some channels, conducting behavior is more complex and the open state has multiple subconductance levels. The probability of a channel being in one or another subconductance state can be influenced by the same stimuli that alter opening of channels' with a single open state current level.

Kinetics
The activation and inactivation of ion channels determines the time course of the current they pass and therefore the role they play in shaping action potentials. Channels that activate rapidly contribute more towards the early depolarizing phases of the action potential while slowly activating and inactivating channels contribute to shaping the subsequent repolarizing phases.

K^+ channel in myocardial cells can be differentiated by their activation and inactivation kinetics. Two mechanisms of inactivation are observed for the voltage-gated potassium channels, N-type and C-type (15). N-type inactivation is generally fast (ms time scale) and caused by the occlusion of inner mouth of the channel by a short segment of N-terminal residues of the channel (called the inactivation 'ball') (16). C-type inactivation involves protein conformational changes in the outer mouth of the pore (17, 18). Although, C-type inactivation can show rapid kinetics it generally occurs over a longer time scale (s) than N-type inactivation.

Voltage-gated channels have a unique transmembrane domain that allows a collection of charges to move under the influence of the membrane electric field. Movement of these charges has been associated with conformational changes in the protein that may result in either an increased or decreased probability of opening the ion conduction pathway. Voltage-dependent gating can be altered by neurotoxins, chemicals, phosphorylation, mutation and the ionic composition of the environment. Some voltage-gated channels open in response to depolarization while others respond to hyperpolarization. Voltage-dependence is one mechanism that allows channels to show rectification, that is, the ability to conduct ions preferentially in one direction across the membrane.

Inwardly rectifying potassium channels (Kir) conduct K^+ across the cell membrane more efficiently in the inward than in the outward direction. In contrast to the rectification resulting from voltage-dependent activation, the mechanism for this rectification is voltage-dependent blockade of the channel pore by intracellular Mg^{2+} and polyamines (19, 20). Inward rectifiers can be classified as strong and weak, depending on the extent to which they pass K^+ in the outward direction. Background inward-rectifiers and acetylcholine-regulated K^+ channels from heart are examples of strong inward rectifiers and ATP-sensitive K^+ channels are weak rectifiers.

Regulation and Pharmacology
A number of other factors regulate ion channel function including: phosphorylation, local ion concentration, ligand binding, and interaction with other channel subunits. In addition, diverse groups of pharmacological or toxic agents can modify channel activity. Distinct binding sites can be found on a single channel protein for drugs that alter channel function. The pharmacological sensitivity of ion channels is a valuable aid in isolating the contribution of particular channels to macroscopic currents and is the basis for many anti-arrhythmic medications.

THE ION CHANNELS IN THE HEART

Sodium Channels
The upstroke of the cardiac action potential (Figure 3) results from the influx of sodium ions through voltage-dependent Na^+ channels (Figure 4). Na^+ channels belong to a multigene family with tissue specific isoforms. Cardiac Na^+ channels are distinct in their physiological, biochemical and pharmacological properties from Na^+ channels in other tissues. Thus, cardiac Na^+ channels have a low affinity to tetrodotoxin compared to neuronal channels (21) and they are 50 to 100 times more sensitive to block by local anesthetics such as lidocaine (22). Indeed, one reason local anesthetics are effective as antiarrhythmic agents is because they block Na^+ channel activity.

Na^+ channels are subject to modulation by neurohumoral factors such as epinephrine, which decreases Na^+ conductance by shifting voltage dependent inactivation via cAMP-dependent phosphorylation (23, 24). In contrast, Na^+ channels are activated by angiotensin II (25) apparently via a shift in the voltage dependence of activation mediated by protein kinase C (PKC). This may explain why patients with chronic congestive heart failure have a reduced incidence of ventricular arrhythmia when treated with drugs that block conversion of angiotensin I to II.

Pore-forming Na^+ channel subunits have a mass of 230 to 270 kDa and four homologous domains; each domain has six proposed α-helical transmembrane segments (S1-S6) (Figure 6). The fourth segment in each domain (S4) contains positively charged amino acids and is thought to represent the voltage sensing portion of the channel. The intracellular linker between domains III and IV is critical for fast inactivation and may function as an inactivation particle similar to that involved in N-type inactivation of K^+ channels (26). Residues in the S6 region of domain IV appear to be involved in the action of some antiarrhythmic and local anesthetic drugs (27).

While the pore-forming subunit can function alone it is usually associated with a regulatory β subunit that accelerates inactivation (28).

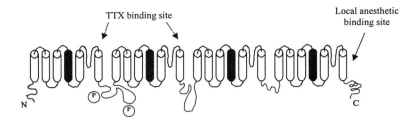

Figure 6: Proposed topology of a voltage-dependent Na+ channel demonstrating four similar domains of six helical transmembrane spanning subunit sequences. The voltage-sensing S4 segments of each domain are indicated by shading.

Calcium Channels

Voltage-gated Ca^{2+} channels play a central role in contractility and are regulated by the concentration of free cytosolic Ca^{2+} ions. Ca^{2+} channels are closed at normal resting potentials in cardiac cells. Depolarization caused by Na^+ influx during the fast upstroke of the action potential opens Ca^{2+} channels, which remain active during the plateau phase of the action potential (Figure 3). The duration of the action potential plateau depends in-part on the balance of inward current through voltage gated Ca^{2+} channels and the outward current through K^+ channels. Ca^{2+} influx induces release of intracellular Ca^{2+} store from the sarcoplasmic reticulum to initiate contraction. Dysfunction of Ca^{2+} channels has been linked to myocardial contractility increase with cardiac hypertrophy and decreased contractility in heart failure (2).

There are two main types of Ca^{2+} channels in heart: L-type and T-type. L-type channels have a *l*arge unitary conductance and contribute a long lasting current. T-type channels have a *t*iny conductance and contribute a transient current (13). L-type channels are primarily responsible for cardiac excitation-contraction coupling, while the role of T-type Ca^{2+} channels is yet uncertain. T-type channels are implicated in the early stages of cardiac development and some pathological conditions (2). Both L- and T-type channels form as a mixed complex of five subunits, a pore-forming subunit that can function independently and four regulatory subunits. Similar to the Na^+ channel, the Ca^{2+} channel pore-forming subunit is a 212 kDa protein with four homologous domains that have six proposed transmembrane domains (S1-S6) and a charge-bearing S4 domain (Figure 6).

Potassium Channels

Potassium currents in the heart are responsible for controlling action potential duration, after-hyperpolarization and regulating resting membrane potential. Cardiac potassium channels were classified initially based on analysis of whole cell currents.

Five types of currents were identified: IK1, an inwardly rectifying current; IKACh, a current activated by the muscarinic acetylcholine receptor; IKATP, a current activated when ATP levels in the cell fall; IK, a slowly activated delayed rectifier current; and I_{to}, a transient outward current.

More recently, as many as seven distinct currents have been shown to contribute to the total outward K^+ current during the action potential plateau and repolarization phases (Table1). The delayed rectifier, IK, has at least two components known as IKr (rapid) and IKs (slow) (29-31). These components can be separated based on their kinetic properties and pharmacology. The transient outward current, I_{to}, may also be composed of at least two or more subtypes based on the finding that I_{to} has different kinetics in epicardium vs. endocardium (32). In addition, a rapidly activating, extremely slowly inactivating K^+ current has also been described (IKslow) (33, 34). A depolarization-activated, non-inactivating current that activates more rapidly than IKr has also been observed and is referred to as IKsus or IKur for sustained or ultra-rapid K^+ current, respectively (33, 35). Another current, IKp, has been identified in guinea pig ventricle and termed the "plateau current" because it is active during the action potential plateau (36, 37).

Current	Activation	Inactivation
I_{to}	Fast	Fast
IKr	Moderate	Slow
IKs	Very slow	Very, very slow
IKslow	Fast	Very slow
IKp	Fast	No
IKur	Fast	No

Table 1: Voltage-gated K+ current/currents in the heart adapted from (38).

Genetic approaches have begun to reveal the molecular basis for the wide diversity of macroscopic K^+ currents. Potassium channel genes have been classified into two main groups on the basis of the structure of their pore-forming subunits. They correspond to two phenotypes: voltage-gated and inwardly rectifying K^+ currents. A third group, the 2-P domain K^+ channels, has recently been described (39). The pore-forming subunits of voltage-gated channels have six transmembrane domains (S1-S6) and a conserved pore forming (P)-domain (Figure 7). Similar to Na^+ and Ca^{2+} channels, there is a charge-bearing transmembrane domain (S4). In contrast, inwardly rectifying K^+ channel subunits contain just two hydrophobic transmembrane domains and a pore-forming P domain. Both voltage-gated and inward rectifiers channels are formed by assembly of four subunits (40, 41). The 2-P domain channel subunits of mammals contain four transmembrane domains and two P domains in each subunit and are expected to function as dimers (39).

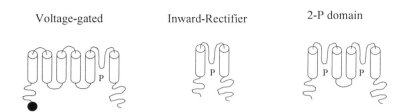

Figure 7: Proposed topology of subunits of voltage-gated, inward rectifier and mammalian 2-P domain K^+ channels adapted from (39).

Each group of channels may be further subdivided into distinct families and members of nearly every family are expressed in heart (Table 2). Voltage-gated K^+ channel subunits expressed at high levels in the heart include KvLQT1, HERG, Kv1.2, Kv1.4, Kv1.5, Kv2.1 and Kv4.2. Other voltage-gated channel subunits expressed at low levels include: Kv2.2, all members of the Kv3 and Kv4 family and Kv6.1. Voltage-gated K^+ channels are distributed throughout the heart (42, 43). Inwardly rectifying channel subunits in heart include: IRK1, Kir2.1, GIRK1, GIRK4 and Kir6.2. GIRK1 and GIRK4 subunits combine in a heteromultimeric fashion to form the cardiac isoform of the G-protein regulated KACh channel (44). In forming the KACh channel, GIRK1 is not targeted efficiently to the cell surface unless co-expressed with GIRK4 (45). At least one 2-P domain channel, OAT/TBAK, is now known to be expressed in the heart, mainly in ventricular muscle (46, 47). At physiological K^+ concentrations, this channel is a rapidly activating, non-inactivating outward rectifier and may underlie resting K^+ conductance as well as contribute to repolarization.

Diversity in K^+ channel isoform expression and the potential for heteromeric combination of pore-forming subunits is known to contribute to the wide variety of cardiac K^+ channel phenotypes. Diversity can also originate through combinations of K^+ channel complexes with modulatory proteins. Thus, heterologously expressed members of the voltage-gated family exhibit different phenotypes when coexpressed with cytoplasmic soluble β subunits (48-50).

The pore-forming HERG and KvLQT1 subunits are obligated to interact with single transmembrane MinK-related peptides (MiRPs) in order to form channels with native characteristics. These subunits influence the unitary conductance, ion selectivity, pharmacology and gating kinetics, thereby producing IKr and IKs currents (6, 52). The cardiac KATP current is similarly formed by the association of two proteins: Kir6.2 and a large integral-membrane protein, the sulfonylurea-receptor subtype SUR2A (53). Kir 6.2 subunits form the pore and the sulfonylurea-receptor is required for normal activation and regulation by ATP (54, 55).

Family	Subunit	Activation	Inactivation	Endogenous Current
Kv	Kv1.2	Fast	Very Slow	IKslow?
	Kv1.4	Fast	Fast	?
	Kv1.5	Fast	Very Slow	IKur
	Kv2.1	Slow	Very Slow	?
	Kv4.2	Fast	Fast	Ito
	Kv4.3	Fast	Fast	Ito
Eag	HERG + MiRP1	Fast	Fast	IKs
KCNQ	KvLQT1 + MinK	Moderate	Slow	IKr
2-P domain	OAT	Fast	No	IKp?

Table 2: Voltage activated myocardial K+ currents/channels adapted from (38) with (6, 47, 51).

The physiological function of many cloned ion channel subunits is still not known (Table 2). In principle, correlation of cloned channel subunits with endogenous currents can be accomplished by expressing a clone and comparing its function and pharmacology to an endogenous current. Given the great diversity of endogenous channel subunits and regulatory proteins, electrophysiological techniques have been combined with in situ hybridization, immunohistochemistry, antisense, knockout and transgenic approaches in efforts to identify the subunits in native channels. Antisense techniques have suggested that Kir 2.1 subunits are essential in the genesis of IK1 (56) and Kv1.5 subunits to formation of the ultrarapid delayed rectifier K^+ current (57). A variety of molecular techniques, including knockout mice, support the idea that Kv4.3/Kv4.2 contribute I_{to} (58-60).

CARDIAC ION CHANNELS AND DISEASE

Dysfunction of ion channels leading to disease (ion channelopathies) can result from inherited abnormalities in ion channel genes or be acquired. In both cases, diseases can be divided into those resulting from increased channel activity and those secondary to diminished function (61). Examples of inherited gain of function disorders include Liddle's syndrome (62) and paramyotonia congenita (63) in which mutations in sodium channel genes produce channels that open too often or close too slowly. Poisons and toxins that inhibit acetyl cholinesterase and produce excessive activity of normal acetylcholine receptor channels exemplify acquired gain of function disease (64). Inherited diseases associated with loss of channel function include cystic fibrosis where mutations have been shown to result in low levels of channel protein expression (65) or decreased single channel current (66). Myasthenia gravis is an example of an acquired disease where function is diminished due to autoimmune degradation of ion channels (67).

The molecular basis for one cardiac rhythm disorder, the long QT syndrome (LQTS), has recently been demonstrated to include examples of both gain and loss of function ion channelopathies. LQTS predisposes patients to torsades de pointe and the lethal cardiac arrhythmia ventricular fibrillation. The QT interval on a surface electrocardiogram reflects the period of the cardiac action potential during which the ventricular myocardium is depolarized (Figure 3). Ion channels that contribute to orderly excitation and contraction of the heart include some that depolarize the muscle (such as, voltage-gated Na^+ channels) and others that repolarize the heart to end each beat (for example, IKr and IKs)(Figure 4). Thus, Na^+ channels that initiate the cardiac action potential can carry mutations that impair their inactivation; this gain of function leads to sustained Na^+ currents and prolongation of the QT interval due to increased channel activity (Figure 8).

Loss of function associated with decreased K^+ channel activity prolongs the QT interval and has been associated with inherited mutations in HERG, MiRP1, KvLQT1 and MinK subunits. In each case, mutations lead to decreased outward K^+ currents through IKr or IKs channels due to impaired surface expression, decreased single channel current or decreased open probability (6, 51, 69). LQTS can also be acquired in patients with normal channel genes if they receive drugs that block K^+ channels such as Class III antiarrhythmics, antidepressants and antimicrobials (70, 71). Recently, an inherited mutation in MiRP1 was shown to be associated with a borderline increase in QT interval at baseline but increased affinity of the patients' IKr channels for the antibiotic clarithromycin; administration of the drug was associated with a significantly prolonged QT and ventricular fibrillation requiring cardioversion (6). Acquired LQTS has also been seen in humans in association with congestive heart failure where it appears that I_{to} function is decreased due to transcriptional downregulation of the Kv4.3 channel protein (72). In mice, transgenic expression of a non-channel transport protein, a developmentally early α-isoform of the Na-K-ATPase, has also been associated with LQTS (73).

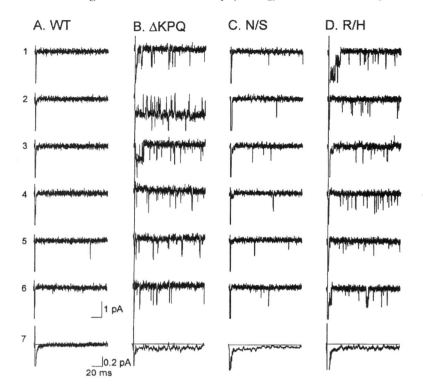

Figure 8: Single channel activity of wild-type (A) and three long QT syndrome mutant Na+ channels (B-D). Rows 1-6 represent sample currents evoked by identical depolarizations. Row 7 represents an 'ensemble' average of multiple evoked current; reproduced by permission (68). All three mutations interfere with inactivation and result in a persistent inward (depolarizing) current.

SUMMARY

Tools to examine the electrical properties and ion channels function combine with molecular biological approaches in understanding normal cardiac function and disease. These tools are crucial to the functional evaluation of identified genetic mutations and for the development and testing of rational therapeutic strategies including drug design and gene therapy.

ACKNOWLEDGMENTS

This work was supported by grants from the NIH to S.A.N.G. and M.A.

REFERENCES

1. Mitra R, Morad M. A uniform enzymatic method for dissociation of myocytes from hearts and stomachs of vertebrates. *Am J Physiol 249*, H1056 (1985).
2. Richard S, Leclercq F, Lemaire S, Piot C, Nargeot J. Ca2+ currents in compensated hypertrophy and heart failure. *Cardiovasc Res 37*, 300 (1998).
3. Wolska B, Solaro R. Method for isolation of adult mouse cardiac myocytes for studies of contraction and microfluorimetry. *Am J Physiol 271*, H1250 (1996).
4. Uebele VN, England SK, Chaudhary A, Tamkun MM, Snyders DJ. Functional differences in Kv1.5 currents expressed in mammalian cell lines are due to the presence of endogenous Kv beta 2.1 subunits. *J Biol Chem 271*, 2406 (1996).
5. Petersen KR, Nerbonne JM. Expression environment determines K+ current properties: Kv1 and Kv4 alpha-subunit-induced K+ currents in mammalian cell lines and cardiac myocytes. *Pflugers Archiv 437*, 381 (1999).
6. Abbott GW, Sesti F, Splawski I, et al. MiRP1 forms IKr potassium channels with HERG and is associated with cardiac arrhythmia. *Cell 97*, 175 (1999).
7. Hamill OP, Marty A, Neher E, Sakmann B, Sigworth FJ. Improved patch-clamp techniques for high-resolution current recording from cells and cell-free membrane patches. *Pflugers Arch 391*, 85 (1981).
8. Horn R, Marty A. Muscarinic activation of ionic currents measured by a new whole-cell recording method. *J Gen Physiol 92*, 145 (1988).
9. Davis J, Matsubara T, Scheinman MM, Katzung B, Hondeghem LH. Use-dependent effects of lidocaine on conduction in canine myocardium. *Circulation 74*, 205 (1986).
10. Starmer CF. Theoretical characterization of ion channel blockade: ligand binding to periodically accessible receptors. *J Theoret Biol 119*, 235 (1986).
11. McDonald K, Field L, Parmacek M, Soonpaa M, Leiden J, Moss R. Length dependence of Ca2+ sensitivity of tension in mouse cardiac myocytes expressing skeletal muscle troponin C *J Physiol 483*, 131 (1995).
12. Steadman B, Moore K, Spitzer K, Bridge J. A video system for measuring motion in contracting heart cells. *IEEE Trans Biomed Eng 35*, 264 (1988).
13. Hille B. Ionic Channels of Excitable Membranes. *Sinauer, Sunderland, MA*. (1992).
14. Santana LF, Gomez AM, Lederer WJ. Ca2+ flux through promiscuous cardiac Na+ channels: slip-mode conductance. *Science 279*, 1027 (1998).
15. Rasmusson RL, Morales MJ, Wang S, et al. Inactivation of voltage-gated cardiac K+ channels. *Circ Res 82*, 739 (1998).
16. Hoshi T, Zagotta WN, Aldrich RW. Biophysical and molecular mechanisms of Shaker potassium channel inactivation. *Science 250*, 533 (1990).
17. Liu Y, Jurman ME, Yellen G. Dynamic rearrangement of the outer mouth of a K+ channel during gating. *Neuron 16*, 859 (1996).
18. Yellen G, Sodickson D, Chen TY, Jurman ME. An engineered cysteine in the external mouth of a K+ channel allows inactivation to be modulated by metal binding. *Biophys J 66*, 1068 (1994).
19. Matsuda H, Saigusa A, Irisawa H. Ohmic conductance through the inwardly rectifying K channel and blocking by internal Mg^{2+}. *Nature 325*, 156 (1987).
20. Vandenberg CA. Inward rectification of a potassium channel in cardiac ventricular cells depends on internal magnesium ions. *Proc Nat Acad Sci USA 84*, 2560 (1987).
21. Baer M, Best PM, Reuter H. Voltage-dependent action of tetrodotoxin in mammalian cardiac muscle. *Nature 263*, 344 (1976).
22. Bean BP, Cohen CJ, Tsien RW. Lidocaine block of cardiac sodium channels. *J Gen Physiol 81*, 613 (1983).
23. Arita M, Kiyosue T, Aomine M, Imanishi S. Nature of "residual fast channel" dependent action potentials and slow conduction in guinea pig ventricular muscle and its modification by isoproterenol. *Am J Cardiol 51*, 1433 (1983).
24. Hisatome I, Kiyosue T, Imanishi S, Arita M. Isoproterenol inhibits residual fast channel via stimulation of β-adrenoceptors in guinea-pig ventricular muscle. *J Molec Cell Cardiol 17*, 657 (1985).

25. Moorman JR, Kirsch GE, Lacerda AE, Brown AM. Angiotensin II modulates cardiac Na+ channels in neonatal rat. *Circ Res 65*, 1804 (1989).

26. Kellenberger S, Scheuer T, Catterall WA. Movement of the Na^+ channel inactivation gate during inactivation. *J Biol Chem 271*, 30971 (1996).

27. Ragsdale DS, McPhee JC, Scheuer T, Catterall WA. Molecular determinants of state-dependent block of Na^+ channels by local anesthetics. *Science 265*, 1724 (1994).

28. McCormick KA, Isom LL, Ragsdale D, et al. Molecular determinants of Na^+ channel function in the extracellular domain of the beta1 subunit. *J Biol Chem 273*, 3954 (1998).

29. Sanguinetti MC, Jurkiewicz NK. Role of external Ca^{2+} and K^+ in gating of cardiac delayed rectifier K^+ currents. *Pflugers Archiv 420*, 180 (1992).

30. Sanguinetti MC, Jurkiewicz NK. Delayed rectifier outward K^+ current is composed of two currents in guinea pig atrial cells. *Am J Physiol 260*, H393 (1991).

31. Sanguinetti MC, Jurkiewicz NK. Two components of cardiac delayed rectifier K^+ current. *J Gen Physiol 96*, 195 (1990).

32. Brahmajothi MV, Campbell DL, Rasmusson RL, et al. Distinct transient outward potassium current (I_{to}) phenotypes and distribution of fast-inactivating potassium channel alpha subunits in ferret left ventricular myocytes. *J Gen Physiol 113*, 581 (1999).

33. Boyle WA, Nerbonne JM. A novel type of depolarization-activated K^+ current in isolated adult rat atrial myocytes. *Am J Physiol 260*, H1236 (1991).

34. Van Wagoner DR, Kirian M, Lamorgese M. Phenylephrine suppresses outward K^+ currents in rat atrial myocytes. *Am J Physiol 271*, H937 (1996).

35. Boyle WA, Nerbonne JM. Two functionally distinct 4-aminopyridine-sensitive outward K^+ currents in rat atrial myocytes. *J Gen Physiol 100*, 1041 (1992).

36. Yue DT, Marban E. A novel cardiac potassium channel that is active and conductive at depolarized potentials. *Pflugers Archiv 413*, 127 (1988).

37. Backx PH, Marban E. Background potassium current active during the plateau of the action potential in guinea pig ventricular myocytes. *Circ Res 72*, 890 (1993).

38. Nerbonne JM. Regulation of voltage-gated K^+ channel expression in the developing mammalian myocardium. *J Neurobiol 37*, 37 (1998).

39. Goldstein SA, Wang KW, Ilan N, Pausch MH. Sequence and function of the two P domain potassium channels: implications of an emerging superfamily. *J Molec Medic 76*, 13 (1998).

40. MacKinnon R. Determination of the subunit stoichiometry of a voltage-activated K^+ channel. *Nature 350*, 232 (1991).

41. Corey S, Krapivinsky G, Krapivinsky L, Clapham DE. Number and stoichiometry of subunits in the native atrial G-protein-gated K^+ channel, I_{KACh}. *J Biol Chem 273*, 5271 (1998).

42. Brahmajothi MV, Morales MJ, Liu S, et al. In situ hybridization reveals extensive diversity of K^+ channel mRNA in isolated ferret cardiac myocytes. *Circ Res 78*, 1083 (1996).

43. Dixon JE, McKinnon D. Quantitative analysis of potassium channel mRNA expression in atrial and ventricular muscle of rats. *Circ Res 75*, 252 (1994).

44. Krapivinsky G, Gordon EA, Wickman K, et al. The G-protein-gated atrial K^+ channel I_{KACh} is a heteromultimer of two inwardly rectifying K^+-channel proteins. *Nature 374*, 135 (1995).

45. Kennedy ME, Nemec J, Corey S, Wickman K, Clapham DE. GIRK4 confers appropriate processing and cell surface localization to G-protein-gated potassium channels. *J Biol Chem 274*, 2571 (1999).

46. Kim D, Fujita A, Horio Y, Kurachi Y. Cloning and functional expression of a novel cardiac two-pore background K^+ channel (cTBAK-1). *Circ Res 82*, 513 (1998).

47. Lopes C, Gallagher P, Wong C, Buck M, Goldstein S. OATs: open, acid-sensitive, two P domain K^+ channels from mouse hearts. *Biophys J 74*, A44 (1998).

48. Majumder K, De Biasi M, Wang Z, Wible BA. Molecular cloning and functional expression of a novel potassium channel beta-subunit from human atrium. *FEBS Letters, 361*, 13 (1995).

49. Castellino RC, Morales MJ, Strauss HC, Rasmusson RL. Time- and voltage-dependent modulation of a Kv1.4 channel by a beta-subunit (Kv beta 3) cloned from ferret ventricle *Am J Physiol 269*, H385 (1995).

50. Sasaki Y, Ishii K, Nunoki K, Yamagishi T, Taira N. The voltage-dependent K^+ channel (Kv1.5) cloned from rabbit heart and facilitation of inactivation of the delayed rectifier current by the rat β-subunit. *FEBS Letters, 372*, 20 (1995).

51.   Sesti F, Goldstein SA. Single-channel characteristics of wild-type IKs channels and channels formed with two minK mutants that cause long QT syndrome. *J Gen Physiol 112*, 651 (1998).

52.   Sanguinetti MC, Curran ME, Zou A, et al. Coassembly ofK(V)LQT1 and minK (IsK) proteins to form cardiac I(Ks) potassium channel. *Nature, 384*, 80 (1996).

53.   Chutkow WA, Simon MC, Le Beau MM, Burant CF. Cloning, tissue expression, and chromosomal localization of SUR2, the putative drug-binding subunit of cardiac, skeletal muscle, and vascular K_{ATP} channels. *Diabetes 45*, 1439 (1996).

54.   Sakura H, Ammala C, Smith PA, Gribble F, Ashcroft FM. Cloning and functional expression of the cDNA encoding a novel ATP-sensitive potassium channel subunit expressed in pancreatic beta-cells, brain, heart and skeletal muscle. *FEBS Letters, 377*, 338 (1995).

55.   Inagaki N, Gonoi T, Clement JP, et al. A family of sulfonylurea receptors determines the pharmacological properties of ATP-sensitive K^+ channels. *Neuron 16*, 1011 (1996).

56.   Nakamura TY, Artman M, Rudy B, Coetzee WA. Inhibition of rat ventricular IK1 with antisense oligonucleotides targeted to Kir2.1 mRNA. *Am J Physiol 274*, H892 (1998).

57.   Feng J, Wible B, Li GR, Wang Z, Nattel S. Antisense oligodeoxynucleotides directed against Kv1.5 mRNA specifically inhibit ultrarapid delayed rectifier K^+ current in cultured adult human atrial myocytes. *Circ Res 80*, 572 (1997).

58.   Dixon JE, Shi W, Wang HS, et al. Role of the Kv4.3 K^+ channel in ventricular muscle. A molecular correlate for the transient outward current. *Circ Res 79*, 659 (1996).

59.   Barry DM, Xu H, Schuessler RB, Nerbonne JM. Functional knockout of the transient outward current, long-QT syndrome, and cardiac remodeling in mice expressing a dominant-negative Kv4 alpha subunit. *Circ Res 83*, 560 (1998).

60.   Fiset C, Clark RB, Shimoni Y, Giles WR. Shal-type channels contribute to the Ca^{2+}-independent transient outward K^+ current in rat ventricle. *J of Physiol 500*, 51 (1997).

61.   Goldstein SA. Ion channels: structural basis for function and disease. *Sem Perin 20*, 520 (1996).

62.   Shimkets RA, Warnock DG, Bositis CM, et al. Liddle's syndrome: heritable human hypertension caused by mutations in the beta subunit of the epithelial sodium channel. *Cell 79*, 407 (1994).

63.   Yang N, Ji S, Zhou M, et al. Sodium channel mutations in paramyotonia congenita exhibit similar biophysical phenotypes in vitro. *Proc Nat Acad Sci USA 91*, 12785 (1994).

64.   Millard CB, Broomfield CA. Anticholinesterases: medical applications of neurochemical principles. *J Neurochem 64*, 1909 (1995).

65.   Denning GM, Anderson MP, Amara JF, et al. Processing of mutant cystic fibrosis transmembrane conductance regulator is temperature-sensitive. *Nature 358*, 761 (1992).

66.   Sheppard DN, Rich DP, Ostedgaard LS, et al. Mutations in CFTR associated with mild-disease-form Cl⁻ channels with altered pore properties [see comments]. *Nature 362*, 160 (1993).

67.   Zisman E, Katz-Levy Y, Dayan M, et al. Peptide analogs to pathogenic epitopes of the human acetylcholine receptor alpha subunit as potential modulators of myasthenia gravis. *Proc Nat Acad Sci USA 93*, 4492 (1996).

68.   Dumaine R, Wang Q, Keating MT, et al. Multiple mechanisms of Na^+ channel-linked long-QT syndrome. *Circ Res 78*, 916 (1996).

69.   Sanguinetti MC, Curran ME, Spector PS, Keating MT. Spectrum of HERG K+-channel dysfunction in an inherited cardiac arrhythmia [published erratum appears in *Proc Natl Acad Sci USA* 1996;93:8796]. *Proc Natl Acad Sci USA 93*, 2208 (1996).

70.   Roden DM, Lazzara R, Rosen M, Schwartz PJ, Towbin J, Vincent GM. Multiple mechanisms in the long-QT syndrome. Current knowledge, gaps, and future directions. *Circulation 94*, 1996 (1996).

71.   Sanguinetti MC, Spector PS. Potassium channelopathies. *Neuropharmacology 36*, 755 (1997).

72.   Kaab S, Dixon J, Duc J, et al. Molecular basis of transient outward potassium current downregulation in human heart failure. *Circulation, 98*, 1383 (1998).

73.   O'Brien S, Apkon M, Berul CI, Patel H, Zahler R. Electrocardiographic phenotype of LQTS in transgenic mice expressing human alpha3 Na,K-ATPase isoform in heart. *Circulation 96*, I (1997).

3

ANIMAL MODELS OF INHERITED ELECTROPHYSIOLOGIC DISEASES

Amit Rakhit, M.D. and Charles I. Berul, M.D.

Department of Cardiology, Children's Hospital • Boston
Department of Pediatrics, Harvard Medical School, Boston, MA 02115

INTRODUCTION

Animal models of cardiac arrhythmias are an increasingly important source of understanding for the mechanisms associated with human disease. In the study of future potential therapies for cardiac arrhythmias, the most appropriate animal models need to be identified in order to have clinical significance in treating human electrophysiologic disorders (1). With appropriate models, there is a logical progression from preclinical experimental research to clinically relevant human protocols. There have been many useful animal models in the study of human cardiovascular disease. Cardiac hemodynamics have long been studied using animal models, and recently there have been many new models of cardiovascular electrophysiology emerging in the research arena. Examples of large-animal (dog, sheep, goat) and small-animal (mouse, rabbit) models of cardiac electrophysiologic abnormalities have become well documented in the medical literature. With the recent advances in genetic and molecular biological techniques, genetically manipulated animals have become increasingly relevant models for human cardiovascular disease (2, 3).

In this chapter, we will review different animal models in common use for basic and applied laboratory electrophysiological studies today, including pertinent examples, with advantages and limitations of these models. Particular emphasis is placed on newer models and novel techniques, major advances now being offered by direct transgenic and genetically manipulated models, and the approaches and techniques involved in studying specific arrhythmia problems with these animal models.

Large-Animal Models
Despite the recent advances in pharmacological and electrophysiological modes of human clinical therapy, sudden death continues to be a significant cause of mortality. Death is usually attributable to ventricular arrhythmias, either fibrillation or tachycardia. Large animal models of cardiac arrhythmias have primarily included

dog, sheep, and goat models of tachyarrhythmias, and several recent mapping innovations have resulted from initial large-animal studies. Large-animal models have often held favor with the cardiovascular research community because they provide a closer approximation to human physiology than their small-animal counterparts, and it is technically easier to access their cardiac structures.

Ventricular Tachyarrhythmias

Experimental models of ventricular tachycardia and sudden death have focused mainly on myocardial infarction and ischemia, and few large animal genetic models of VT and sudden death exist (4). A colony of German shepherd dogs with inherited spontaneous cardiac arrhythmias and associated sudden death were well characterized by Moise (5). These animals had otherwise normal cardiac anatomy and function, though were predisposed to sudden cardiac death from ventricular arrhythmia. This colony of inbred dogs displayed frequent spontaneous, bradycardia-dependent ventricular ectopic activity. The incidence and severity of ventricular ectopy was studied noninvasively using 24-hour ambulatory electrocardiographic (ECG) recordings performed every 2 weeks from 2 months of age to the completion of the study (Figure 1). The dogs were also administered phenylephrine in order to produce reflex sinus bradycardia, and thus more easily precipitate ventricular ectopy. Ventricular tachycardia was demonstrated in the majority of the study group with exacerbation of malignant ventricular rhythms using drug provocation.

In addition to noninvasive monitoring studies, Purkinje fibers were obtained from 3 groups of dogs. The first group consisted of unaffected animals that had rare or no ventricular ectopy on ECG at baseline or after phenylephrine challenge. The second group included those dogs with frequent, nonsustained ventricular tachycardia on their 24-hour ECG recording at baseline as well as after phenylephrine challenge. The third group consisted of dogs that had initially displayed ventricular ectopy, ranging from isolated premature ventricular contractions to nonsustained ventricular tachycardia, but who did not have ectopy at the time of study. The Purkinje fibers were placed in an electrolyte-rich solution, and transmembrane recordings were obtained. Fibers were allowed to discharge spontaneously and also underwent overdrive pacing in order to determine the site of earliest triggered activity. Recordings were obtained from all regions of the fiber until the site of earliest activation was identified. The Purkinje fibers were then perfused systematically with phenylephrine, norepinephrine, epinephrine, and isoproterenol in order to determine the effects of alpha- and beta-adrenergic receptor agonists and antagonists on the early afterdepolarization development. Early afterdepolarization development was assessed by quantifying the frequency of early afterdepolarizations elicited by 10 spontaneous action potentials before the drug was administered compared with 5 seconds after drug administration. The spontaneous cycle length was measured as the interval between maximal diastolic membrane potential after the spontaneous action potential to the onset of the next triggered action potential (5).

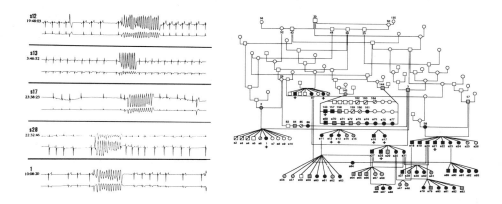

Figure 1. Electrocardiographic ambulatory recordings and pedigree chart from German shepherd dogs with propensity to ventricular arrhythmias and sudden death. The left panel illustrates examples from 5 inbred dogs. Each had many runs of ventricular tachycardia (> 480 beats/minute), and all subsequently died suddenly. The pedigree illustrates that all of the dogs had a common ancestor. Males are represented by squares and females by circles. Solid symbols are dogs with VT, and / or + sign represents dogs with sudden death. (Adapted with permission of the American College of Cardiology from Moise, et al., J Am Coll Cardiol 1994;24:233-43)

This elegant series of studies showed that early afterdepolarization-induced triggered activity in Purkinje fibers is responsible for the initiation of ventricular arrhythmias in this canine model (6). The presence of early afterdepolarizations was confirmed with electrical mapping of fibers for precise determination of the earliest impulse initiation. These animals have also been demonstrated to have abnormal heterogeneous sympathetic innervation that may contribute to their tendency for tachyarrhythmias (4). Phenylephrine potentiated the development of early afterdepolarizations in this model, whereas isoproterenol suppressed early triggered activity, perhaps by homogenization of sympathetic receptor activation. Of note, the QT intervals as measured on standard ECG for these dogs were normal. The study suggests that small regions of the ventricle whose repolarization characteristics do not significantly contribute to the composite QT interval may play a significant role in initiating ventricular arrhythmias. Heterogeneity of ventricular activation and repolarization appeared to increase vulnerability to malignant ventricular arrhythmias. This same group of German shepherd dogs was also determined to have cardiac arrhythmias occurring primarily during REM sleep or after exercise. A subsequent study evaluated the sympathetic innervation of the heart in these animals (4). The sympathetic nervous system is known to play a role in the generation of ventricular arrhythmias (7). Catecholamines can increase automaticity, induce triggered activity, and create spatial and temporal dispersion of refractoriness. Using intravenous radiolabeled MIBG, which is taken up by sympathetic nerve endings and thus provides a picture of sympathetic nerve density, the function and anatomical location of the cardiac sympathetic nerve system were studied in these animals. With immunocytochemical and histological analysis of these hearts, it was found that sympathetic innervation was regionally abnormal and markedly decreased overall in otherwise structurally normal hearts. This difference in sympathetic innervation was not seen in control German shepherd dogs. This naturally occurring large-animal model of sudden death provides yet another model for studying hypotheses thought to contribute to arrhythmogenesis.

Mapping studies of intact as well as infarcted canine hearts have also provided information about cardiac arrhythmias. Sustained reentrant ventricular tachycardias with different QRS morphologies have been shown to occur spontaneously in 25-40% of human patients with sustained VT following myocardial infarction caused by a reentrant mechanism and ischemic heart disease (8). Reentrant VT with multiple morphologies induced in infarcted canine hearts have implicated that the abnormal rhythm most commonly arises from reentrant circuits in the same region as the infarct, suggesting that most often only one region has the necessary properties to sustain reentry (9). The mechanisms that cause multiple morphology ventricular tachycardia are yet unclear. Possible explanations include that the tachycardias with multiple morphologies arise from different reentrant circuits located in separate anatomical areas. Another explanation may be that the multiple morphologies are caused by different exit routes from a single reentrant circuit. Mapping of multiple morphology ventricular tachycardia has been performed in a canine model. Adult mongrel dogs underwent a two-stage ligation of the left anterior descending (LAD) coronary artery to induce a transmural anterior septal myocardial infarction. They then underwent an open-chest electrophysiological study in which an epicardial lead was sutured over the infarcted area with the margins extending to the uninfarcted area. Multiple bipolar electrodes recorded electrophysiologic data as well as surface ECG and blood pressure measurements. Ventricular tachycardia was triggered with programmed single or double extrastimuli during pacing at various cycle lengths or by rapid overdrive ventricular pacing. The QRS morphologies were examined qualitatively to determine the existence of multiple morphology ventricular tachycardia. In approximately one-half of the cases studied, multiple morphology ventricular tachycardia was observed. There was a low incidence of reentrant sites at separate sites causing sustained tachycardia; most cases had reentrant circuits limited over the epicardial border zone that had the conduction properties necessary to maintain reentry. The exit routes were found most commonly at the LAD or the lateral apical margins (9), consistent with arrhythmia mechanisms regarding zones of slow conduction.

Recently, the association of torsades de pointes with ventricular hypertrophy was explored in dogs with chronic complete AV block (10). Atrioventricular block was created by implanting an epicardial electrode into the left ventricular apex and then injecting formaldehyde into the AV node. Electrophysiologic properties were obtained immediately after creation of AV block (acute) and then after a period of 6 weeks (chronic). Important findings of this study included the presence of biventricular hypertrophy, although LV function was similar in both the acute and chronic models. Electrophysiologic findings included prolongation of the LV and RV action potential durations; however, there was a greater increase in the LV action potential duration than the RV. This difference in action potential duration was ascribed to ventricular electrical heterogeneity, associated with the development of arrhythmias, especially torsades de pointes type VT (10).

Newer techniques have been recently developed that describe a three-dimensional, high-resolution endocardial electrophysiologic image using multielectrode probes (11). Mongrel dogs were anesthetized, intubated, and ventilated. A median sternotomy was performed and then a custom-made cylindrical probe containing 128 electrodes on its surface was inserted into the left ventricular cavitary through the left ventricular apex. Using echocardiography and epicardial electrodes as well as the endocardial electrodes, a three-dimensional image was obtained of cavitary geometry. Electrophysiological pacing studies were then performed that studied normal sinus beats, paced beats, and premature ventricular contractions. The data was then processed to give a three-dimensional view of electrical activation sequences within the left ventricle in this in vivo canine model (11).

Other studies involving reentrant wave fronts in open-chest dogs with ventricular fibrillation have shown that pharmacologic intervention with antiarrhythmic drugs can decrease ventricular fibrillation by preventing spontaneous activation wave breaks (12). Computerized mapping studies were performed in dogs with and without subendocardial ablations before and after procainamide administration. Dogs were anesthetized, intubated, and ventilated. The right ventricular subendocardial tissue was ablated in order to produce a fixed scar and a corridor zone of slow conduction, which promotes an increase in the incidence of reentry. Baseline unipolar (S1) cathode pacing was used and the tightly coupled programmed premature stimulus (S2) was delivered to induce ventricular fibrillation. The patterns of ventricular electrical activation were recorded for computer analysis, and then the dog was rescued with defibrillation shocks. The dogs were then given procainamide and the dogs underwent repeat pacing studies. An important, clinically-relevant finding of the study was that procainamide could prevent the number of spontaneous wave breaks in fibrillation and thus demonstrated a mechanism for significant antiarrhythmic effects.

A recent study demonstrated how low-energy chest wall impact could cause sudden death in a novel intact pig model (13). Sudden cardiac death among sports participants struck in the chest by a blunt object is known as commotio cordis and has gained recent media attention. The mechanism of cardiac arrest in these healthy young athletes is unknown and resuscitation efforts are usually unsuccessful. In this animal model, domesticated pigs, whose anatomy is similar to human cardiovascular anatomy, underwent low-energy blunt projectile impacts to the chest at specific stages of the cardiac cycle, to simulate being struck by a ball. Pigs were anesthetized, intubated, and ventilated. Baseline nuclear images as well as ventriculography, coronary angiography, and echocardiography were obtained. The impacts were timed and gated with the electrocardiographic R waves from the pigs and the accuracy of impact time to cardiac cycle was approximately five milliseconds. After each impact, angiography followed by echocardiography was performed along with continuous ECG and left ventricular pressure recording (Figure 2). This model revealed a high incidence of ventricular fibrillation, complete heart block, and ST-segment elevation after low-energy blows to the chest. The chest wall impact-induced arrhythmias were only statistically significant when the impact occurred during a certain period of cardiac repolarization immediately before the peak of the T wave. Ventricular fibrillation was consistently produced immediately when the impact occurred during this critical window. Chest wall trauma at other points of the cardiac cycle produced either transient complete heart block with ST elevation or bundle branch block (13). This study demonstrated that timing in relation to cardiac cycle is critical in commotio cordis type of sudden arrhythmic death, and sheds new light on the mechanism of impact-related sudden cardiac death.

These animal models provide novel approaches in understanding cardiovascular pathophysiology and provide models that are clinically relevant to human disease. Ventricular tachyarrhythmias are a frequent clinical problem in ischemic or hypertrophic hearts, after myocardial infarction, congenital heart disease, and surgical myocardial scarring. Commotio cordis mechanism of sudden death by low-impact chest trauma is rare, but of specific concern in young patients participating in various sporting events such as baseball. Research using these large-animal models provides important information useful in better understanding and treating ventricular arrhythmias and human cardiovascular pathophysiology.

Atrial tachyarrhythmias

Atrial fibrillation (AF) remains one of the most commonly encountered arrhythmias in the clinical setting; however, the mechanisms that precipitate this arrhythmia are not yet fully understood. Atrial fibrillation is a major cardiovascular cause of morbidity and mortality, but there are no completely satisfactory treatment options currently available. Atrial tachyarrhythmias (mostly atrial fibrillation) have been

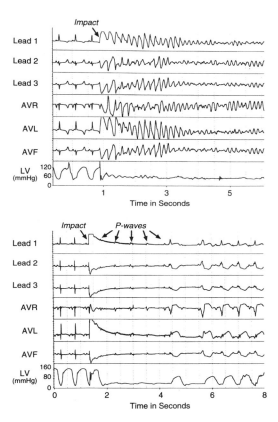

Figure 2. Results of blunt chest wall impact in a pig model of commotio cordis. The experimental design has an anesthetized pig in a sling for chest-wall impact precisely gated to the ECG and a projectile released by a computer-driven electrophysiological stimulator. The top panel illustrates an example of a T-wave impact during the vulnerable relative refractory period of repolarization. The surface ECG shows immediate ventricular fibrillation following impact, with associated loss of left ventricular pressure. The lower panel demonstrates the response to an impact gated during the QRS complex, which results in transient complete heart block, followed by left bundle branch block with ST-segment elevation. (Adapted with permission from Link, et al. N Engl J Med, © 1998 Massachusetts Medical Society. All rights reserved.)

reproduced in large-animal models, though the major limitation has been the difficulty in sustaining AF over prolonged periods. Animal models of sustained AF have been difficult to maintain, usually necessitating pharmacologic or electrical stimulation. Most recently, creation of mitral regurgitation along with rapid atrial pacing has resulted in chronic atrial fibrillation models in the canine heart, while chronic atrial pacing has yielded a similar model of AF in the goat.

Chronic AF in goats has been well described by Wijffels (14). In this series of experiments, goats were instrumented with multiple unipolar pacing electrodes sutured to the epicardial surface of the right and left atria. Approximately 2-3 weeks after surgery, the animals were connected to an automatic AF pacemaker that continuously sensed the intrinsic atrial rhythm and reinduced AF by automatic delivery of a 1-second burst stimuli as soon as sinus rhythm resumed. Because of the continuous maintenance of AF by the pacemaker, the duration of AF progressively increased and became sustained (duration >24 hours) after approximately 1 week. The sustained AF led to structural changes in the atrial myocytes seen on light and electron microscopy with lysosomal degeneration, alterations in myofilaments, mitochondria, and sarcoplasmic reticulum. Chronic hibernating myocardium, a condition that can occur in patients with low-flow ischemia caused by coronary artery stenosis for example (15), displays similar changes in ventricular myocytes as seen in atrial myocytes subjected to chronic AF. The goat chronic AF model may provide an animal model to mimic chronic hibernating myocardium in the human (16). Chronic AF in a goat model has also been shown to alter connexin isoform distribution in the atria, without changing the actual connexin levels. These inhomogeneities in cardiac gap junction proteins may also promote atrial electrical remodeling and micro-reentry circuits (17).

Canine models of sustained AF have been induced with rapid atrial pacing leading to biatrial myopathy and changes in atrial vulnerability to fibrillation (18). In one experimental example, mongrel dogs were anesthetized, intubated, and ventilated. An initial baseline electrophysiologic study was performed which particularly evaluated atrial effective refractory period (ERP), defined as the longest S1-S2 period that failed to produce atrial depolarization, and atrial vulnerability, defined as the ability to induce sustained atrial repetitive responses during programmed stimulation. After the baseline study was completed, the dogs had a pacing electrode placed into the right atrial appendage and attached to a subcutaneously-placed pacemaker. The pacemaker was programmed to 400 beats per minute for six weeks. The dogs underwent a restudy of electrophysiological parameters, which revealed a decrease in right atrial ERP and increases in p-wave duration and PA interval, parameters of intra-atrial conduction. Sustained atrial fibrillation could be induced in more than three-quarters of the dogs studied. Histological analysis was performed which revealed microscopic changes of cellular disarray and focal area of hypertrophy (18). This model is highly reproducible and provides a large animal model where sustained atrial fibrillation without valvular disease can be maintained for prolonged periods.

A similar protocol involving dogs that were atrial-paced for up to six weeks further evaluated the electrophysiological characteristics of atrial fibrillation in these animals (19). The time course of changes that occur in atrial fibrillation was studied and showed that chronic atrial tachycardia produces progressive decreases in atrial

ERP along with progressive increases in the ability to induce fibrillation with single atrial extrasystoles. The study showed that atrial fibrillation has the potential to alter atrial electrophysiology, and altered atrial conduction and refractoriness has the potential to promote atrial fibrillation.

Large animals have been useful in catheter-based electrical mapping of arrhythmias in juvenile sheep using a multielectrode basket catheter in the right atrium and right ventricle (20). The multielectrode basket catheter provided rapid endocardial mapping of activation sequences in the RA and RV and may provide a useful tool in human tachycardia evaluation. The techniques described are invaluable for computer-based precision arrhythmia characterization. Other models have used atrial pacing along with the creation of mitral regurgitation to induce AF. Mitral regurgitation has been shown to favor atrial fibrillation secondary to left atrial volume and pressure overload, reduced atrial effective refractory period, inhomogeneous atrial conduction, and increased left atrial surface area. Studies have demonstrated that susceptibility to sustained AF can be reduced by long linear atrial ablations created either surgically or with specially designed multiple-coil, temperature-feedback ablation catheters (21). As this "catheter maze procedure" is an investigational study currently being conducted in humans, the canine model can provide important information regarding complications, morbidity, and experimental variables determining which lesions are most efficacious.

Small-animal models

Molecular biological advances have led to the development of new models and approaches in identifying the genetic basis of electrophysiologic disorders. Several small-animal models of electrophysiologic and cardiovascular disease have been identified. Isolated-heart perfusion techniques have long been used to study cardiovascular hemodynamics since the technique was first described by Langendorff in 1895. Rabbit models have provided the closest approximation for hemodynamic studies using the Langendorff technique, though other models using sheep, guinea pigs, and mice have also been described. The mouse has become the principal mammalian species for transgenic studies and several mouse models for cardiac electrophysiological diseases have now been developed. Transgenic murine models have been developed as models for familial hypertrophic cardiomyopathy (22), long QT syndrome (23, 24, 25), and myotonic dystrophy (26). Other pertinent models are being engineered, including mice with defects in genes regulating cardiac connexin proteins, ion channels, G-proteins, and other proteins critical in intracellular and intercellular electrical signaling processes. These murine models display particular electrophysiologic abnormalities that can be characterized using ex vivo and in vivo techniques.

Langendorff isolated –heart techniques

The Langendorff perfused whole-heart technique was first described in 1895 as a means to study cardiovascular hemodynamics in an ex vivo setting. In the present day electrophysiological techniques using this method, the study involves removing a whole heart rapidly through a thoracotomy and connecting it to an apparatus that maintains the perfusion to the heart via the coronary arteries. An electrolyte-rich solution (Tyrode's solution, Krebs-Henseleit solution) saturated with oxygen and minimal carbon dioxide is perfused with constant perfusion pressure (i.e. 75mmHg) through a cannula in the aortic root and thus to the coronary arteries. The coronary artery flow is kept between 130 to 160 ml/minute with a temperature between 36°- 38° Celsius. The solution composition simulates serum electrolyte concentrations and contains sodium, potassium, calcium, magnesium, chloride, bicarbonate, phosphate, and glucose. The heart can then be immersed in a beaker filled with this electrolyte solution and then two electrodes can be placed within the beaker on either side of the intact heart to monitor a summation single lead ECG. Endocardial and epicardial electrodes can also be placed in multiple sites to monitor action potentials and activation mapping through vector analysis (27).

Isolated heart techniques can also be used for detailed optical mapping of action potentials (28). Light from a high intensity light source, such as tungsten-halogen, is passed through a heat filter and an interference filter. Excitation light is then shined on the epicardial surface of the vertically hanging heart. Epicardial and endocardial mapping can be performed depending on which surface is facing the light source. A lens is then used to collect the emitted light and then transferred to an emission filter, which is coupled to a video camera that records all the images. A computer then processes the multiple high-density optical images. Background fluorescence is subtracted from each frame to reveal the actual signal. Beat to beat changes in wave propagation patterns as well as patterns of excitation can then be studied.

Recently, isolated rabbit heart studies have been performed which evaluated the effects of calcium and potassium ion channel blockade on atrial conduction (29). Isolated rabbit hearts were perfused using the Langendorff technique and then recordings were obtained from twelve epicardial atrial sites. These electrodes were used to determine activation time, ERP, action potential duration, and conduction time both before and after undergoing two hours of rapid atrial pacing. Action potential duration was found to be shortened after rapid atrial pacing. This "remodeling" of the atrial conduction system in response to rapid pacing appears to be related to calcium ion channels. Furthermore, verapamil, a calcium channel blocker, prevented the decrease in action potential duration. In addition, the study demonstrated that even short periods of rapid atrial rhythms can alter atrial conduction properties. Larger animals have also been used in the Langendorff technique, most often sheep hearts. The effects of atrial fibrillation and the effects of atrial defibrillatory shocks on the activation sequences of the ventricles were studied using this method (30). Sheep hearts were isolated and perfuse as in the Langendorff technique. High-resolution optical mapping was then performed to map repolarization and depolarization of the heart (Figure 3). The effects of atrial defibrillation shocks was then studied and revealed that shocks excited the ventricles through local activation near the base of the ventricles. Appropriate timing of the shock in the vulnerable period of relative refractoriness could also induce ventricular fibrillation.

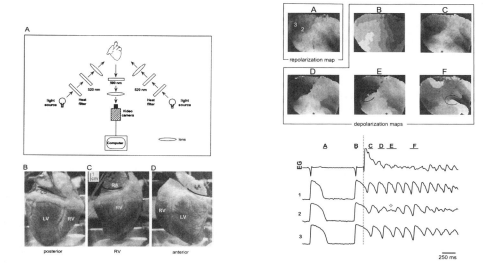

Figure 3. Experimental setup and optical mapping from sheep Langendorff-perfused heart video imaging model. Fig. 3A. Experimental design at the top (A), consisting of a perfused heart, light sources, lenses, a video camera, computer, excitation and emission filters. The lower panels illustrate views of the isolated heart from posterior side (B) with the left ventricle (LV), right ventricle (RV), and coronary sinus (CS) marked. The middle figure (C) shows the right atrium (RA) and RV, and the rightward figure (D) is the anterior surface of the isolated heart, exposing the left atrium (LA) and both ventricles. The isolated heart may be rotated to obtain serial images for activation and repolarization mapping. Fig. 3B. Optical maps obtained during induction of reentry, depicting repolarization (A) and depolarization patterns (B-F) during delivery of a critically-timed shock to induce ventricular fibrillation. The repolarization map shows the beat preceding the shock, with heterogeneous recovery. The activation maps demonstrate the site of shock as earliest activation and wavefront propagation, with a zone of slow conduction and heterogeneity during reentry tachycardia. (Adapted from Gray, et al., Circulation, © 1998 American Heart Association.)

Whole-animal experiments

Although extraneous variables, such as autonomic influences, are mostly eliminated, an obvious limitation in ex vivo studies is the lack of an intact animal model of disease. In addition, extended periods of exposure in an ex vivo artificial environment may possibly alter results, hemodynamic properties, tissue electrolyte balance, metabolic variables, and cardiac electrophysiological properties. These limitations have encouraged other researchers to establish viable small-mammal in vivo models of cardiac disease.

Mouse EP Study and Techniques

Small animal models can provide much information about specific mutations causing abnormal electrophysiologic phenotypes. An *in vivo* mouse cardiac electrophysiology study measuring ECG and electrophysiological data similar to those collected in a routine human EPS has been developed (31). In earlier reported experiments, mice were anesthetized, intubated, and mechanically ventilated.

Epicardial electrodes were placed on the surfaces of the right ventricle, left ventricle, and right atrium (Figure 4A) and a 12-lead electrocardiogram and all electrophysiologic parameters from atrial and ventricular pacing were recorded. Programmed stimulation was performed to assess the conduction characteristics and arrhythmia inducibility in an in vivo mouse model. The difficulty in this model was the necessity for an open-chest procedure and the alterations in hemodynamics and conduction associated with the intervention.

Recent advances have allowed for an endocardial approach to the murine EPS with pacing, pharmacologic intervention, blood sampling, and pressure transduction. Venous access is obtained under microscopic guidance via a right jugular vein cutdown approach (Figure 4B). An octapolar electrode catheter specifically designed for simultaneous atrial and ventricular endocardial recording and pacing is used (3). By this approach, measurement of surface ECG and simultaneous electrophysiological parameters can be obtained by pacing and recording directly from the endocardium of an intact closed-chest mouse.

Methods for studying conscious, freely moving mice with implanted telemetry devices have also been developed that can accurately measure normal electrocardiographic intervals (3, 32). Using sterile technique, mice are anesthetized and an incision is made on the back along the spine. A subcutaneous pocket is formed with blunt dissection. An implantable 3.5-gram radiofrequency transmitter is sutured to the muscle, with the leads directed caudally. The cathodal lead is looped forward to the scapula and anchored in place. The anodal lead is then brought near the heart apex. Electrocardiographic information from a single lead is then monitored by placing the animals on a receiver that records the transmitter signals. Using this telemetric technology, research on conscious untethered mice can include many ECG parameters such as heart rate and QT interval variability and other pertinent electrocardiographic changes in transgenic animal models with ion channel defects or electrophysiologic phenotypes.

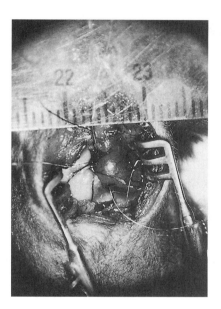 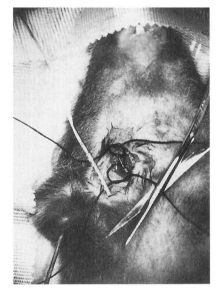

Figure 4. Depiction of the mouse electrophysiology (EP) study illustrating both the epicardial and endocardial methods. On the left is a photograph taken through an operating microscope of an epicardial approach. A midline sternotomy is performed on an anesthetized mouse. Pacing wires are sutured on to the left ventricular, right ventricular, and atrial epicardial surfaces in a bipolar fashion for stimulation and electrogram recording. On the right, an octapolar mouse EP catheter (NuMed, Inc.) is placed into the right heart via a right jugular vein cutdown. The catheter is positioned with the tip in the right ventricle so that 1 pair of electrodes can pace the RV, a pair to record the RV electrogram, 1 pair to pace the right atrium, and a pair to record the RA electrogram. A central lumen is utilized for administration of medications during the EP procedure. (Adapted from Berul, et al., Circulation, © 1996 American Heart Association, and Berul, et al., J Intervent Cardiac Electrophysiol 1998)

Genetically-Engineered Animal Techniques

An exciting approach to the study of cardiovascular diseases is the development of transgenic and other genetically-manipulated animal models. An animal that gains new genetic information from the addition of foreign DNA is said to be transgenic. Human DNA encodes for thousands of genes, all of which comprises less than 10 percent of the whole DNA. Each gene has the required sequence for the production of a specific protein that is responsible for particular functions in the cell (33).

Changes in genomic architecture of normal DNA form the basis of molecular biology techniques involved in creating transgenic models of human disease. With the identification of the multitude of genes involved in causing human disease, animal models are being developed to simulate specific human disease phenotypes. Rapid advances in technology have led to refinement of initial transgenic methods to newer and more effective solutions. Initial studies involved inserting plasmid vectors carrying the genetic material of interest into the nucleus of an oocyte or into the pronucleus of a fertilized cell. The egg would then be planted into a pseudopregnant mouse, and after birth, the recipient could be examined for expression of the foreign DNA (34).

Expression of the donor gene is variable in this model using plasmid vectors because effective expression depends on several factors: the integration site into the host DNA, number and site of promoter regions, inactivation of tandem sequences, and influences of transcription regulatory proteins. Often the plasmid vector will cause rearrangement of host cell DNA due to unregulated insertion into the chromosome, therefore leading to a non-functional cell. These difficulties in using plasmid vectors have led to newer techniques. An alternative procedure has used retroviral vectors to introduce DNA into the host cell. A retroviral vector causes minimal host DNA rearrangement. It is possible to target specific somatic mutations using this method, but it is difficult to infect the germ line; therefore, it is not possible to propagate a certain phenotype (36).

Another technique is the use of mouse embryonic stem cells, which are derived from the blastocyst stage of development that occurs shortly after fertilization yet before implantation to the uterine wall. DNA is obtained from a donor mouse or from recombinant techniques. Mouse embryonic stem cells are then transfected with this DNA by microinjection. The resulting cells are screened for adequate expression of the DNA using polymerase chain reaction (PCR), or by identifying a particular marker that has been added to the gene on the transfected cells, such as enzyme production or drug resistance (36). Once identified, the cells of interest are injected into a blastocyst, which is then implanted into the foster mother. The embryonic stem cells are then able to participate in the development of the resulting mouse. The mouse is now a chimeric animal, having tissue derived from both the implanted as well as natural stem cells. Future generations that express any transfected DNA will have been obtained from the original embryonic cell transfer.

Genes can also be "knocked out" by genetic engineering techniques by means of targeted gene disruption. A wild-type gene can be modified by interrupting a specific gene exon with a marker sequence, such as the gene neo, which confers drug resistance to G418. An exon is the portion of the gene that specifically encodes for a protein. Other parts of the gene, known as introns, comprise the regulatory portions that determine expression of the gene exon. When foreign DNA is inserted into the embryonic stem cell, it can either undergo homologous or non-homologous translocation into the cell. Homologous recombination requires that the entire gene of interest be incorporated into the chromosome with absence of the flanking regions. Cells can be screened with PCR to assess for homologous recombination in order to ascertain if the entire gene was inserted into the host cell DNA. By using gene targeting via homologous recombination in murine embryonic stem cells, a specific gene can either be ablated or modified (35). Abnormal RNA is formed, and consequently, no functional protein product will be formed. The gene will in essence be removed or "knocked out" from the genome. The resulting mouse can then be bred to obtain the homozygous form, which will display the phenotype associated with complete absence of this protein product. Genes can be removed or modified in a particular domain or even a single amino acid residue to produce new genetically manipulated animals in which the mutation can be propagated indefinitely through the germ line (36). Several transgenic and targeted disruption mouse models have been developed using these techniques, exhibiting particular cardiovascular characteristics including relevant electrophysiologic findings.

Murine Models of Electrophysiologic Diseases

There are an expanding number of interesting mouse models with electrophysiological attributes. For example, genetically manipulated mice having an α-myosin heavy chain missense mutation display a phenotype similar to familial hypertrophic cardiomyopathy in humans (22). These genetically-manipulated mice have changes characteristic of human familial hypertrophic cardiomyopathy, including alterations in myocyte and ventricular structure and a predisposition to both atrial and ventricular arrhythmias. In vivo mouse EP studies have revealed electrophysiologic abnormalities and arrhythmia inducibility (37). There were gender differences with male mice more likely to have abnormalities in sinus node function and inducibility of ventricular tachycardia (38). Heterogeneity of ventricular repolarization was demonstrated in these alpha-myosin heavy chain mutant FHC mice (39), and further studies have evaluated the response to exercise and beta-blockade. Murine models of FHC also include mutations in other sarcomeric proteins, such as cardiac troponins, tropomodulin, myosin light chain, myosin binding proteins and tropomyosin.

Recent work has demonstrated prevention of the myocardial hypertrophy by inhibiting calcineurin (40). Alterations in calcium signaling and handling, as well as other ion channel processes, will be important for determination of cardiac hypertrophy and ventricular arrhythmia vulnerability in cardiomyopathy and other cardiac pathophysiology.

Mouse models of familial dilated cardiomyopathy (FDC) have also been developed using mice lacking the gene encoding for the muscle LIM protein (MLP). FDC in humans accounts for up to 30% of all cases of idiopathic dilated cardiomyopathy (41). The majority of cases are transmitted in an autosomal dominant fashion; however, multiple modes of transmission have been described including X-linked recessive pattern, X-linked recessive with myocyte mitochondria aberration, and various linkage sites on somatic chromosomes, specifically chromosomes 3, 9, and 1 (3). These MLP-deficient mice develop a phenotype similar to FDC with disrupted cytoskeletal architecture and neonatal onset of dilated cardiomyopathy.

Tropomodulin overexpression transgenic mutations also have been utilized as murine models of dilated cardiomyopathy. Disease expression has been shown to be modulated by calcineurin signaling pathways, and dilated cardiomyopathy can be prevented with calcineurin inhibitors, such as cyclosporin (43). Electrophysiology studies can elucidate specific abnormalities in FDC mice and identify potential therapies for these disorders as the genetic basis of these diseases are discovered.

Congenital long QT syndrome (LQTS) is another example of a syndrome with transgenic animal counterparts. There is significant genetic heterogeneity, and patients having the same mutation may have varying degrees of disease severity secondary to the variable penetrance and expressivity (42). With new approaches to genetic analysis and molecular techniques, more than 30 mutations for LQTS have been described in five different sites responsible for ion channel proteins: LQT1 to chromosome 11p15.5, LQT2 to chromosome 7q35-36, LQT3 to chromosome 3p21-24, LQT4 to chromosome 4q25-27, and LQT5 to chromosome 21 (45, 46).

Genetic models of LQTS have been developed which have defects in ion channel subtypes that are important in repolarization. For example, mutations in the HERG gene have been developed by using the closely related bovine ether-a-go-go gene (BEAG). Several chimeric and mutant channels were created in Xenopus oocytes using complementary RNA/DNA constructs (43). Patch clamp studies were then performed to assess susceptibility of the mutant channels to class III antiarrhythmic drugs. The different mutants were studied to determine which specific amino acid mutation led to changes in drug binding and activity.

Murine models of long QT syndrome have also been studied. Transgenic mice with mutations in LQT1 and HERG have been developed that have overexpression of an abnormal potassium channel causing prolonged repolarization time and consequently a prolonged QT interval on surface electrocardiogram (44). Using transgene constructs with viral promoter and expression sequences, recombinant plasmid DNA was injected into fertilized oocytes derived from mice. Heterozygous and littermate control mice were studied using surface electrocardiograms to assess QT interval. Murine cardiac myocytes were then assessed for whole-cell action potential and potassium currents using patch-clamping techniques. Findings included prolongation of the QT interval as well as ion channel abnormalities that altered cardiac myocyte repolarization. Other murine models of LQTS include a mouse line with a mutation in the sodium-potassium ATPase pump (45) and acquired QT prolongation with electrolyte or metabolism perturbations.

Further studies including single-cell analysis, tissue conduction studies, and whole animal in vivo EP studies may prove useful in elucidating the mechanisms of these disease processes and the relationship of long QT syndrome to sudden death and ventricular tachyarrhythmias.

Mouse Models of Conduction Disturbances

No naturally-occurring small-animal models of inherited conduction defects have been described, but transgenic animals with specific electrical phenotypes have been engineered, which can provide a useful tool in studying cardiac conduction.

Myotonic muscular dystrophy is the most common adult-onset type of muscular dystrophy that affects all muscle types and causes varying degrees of debilitation. The cardiac system manifestations of myotonic dystrophy include AV block and bradycardia secondary to involvement of the conduction system. The disease is inherited in an autosomal dominant fashion which progressively worsens in subsequent generations secondary to a repetitive expansion of a trinucleotide repeat sequence mutation in a protein kinase gene (DMPK) on chromosome 19 (46). A murine model of DMPK deficiency has been developed which provides a relevant animal model of human myotonic dystrophy (26). We performed a full *in vivo* EP study and described the distinct electrophysiologic abnormalities of these mice that specifically affect atrioventricular (A-V) conduction properties (47). The homozygous mutant mice had more severe A-V conduction defects, yet the heterozygote DMPK +/- mice also had a characteristic milder A-V delay phenotype.

Transgenic mice with connexin protein defects may also display cardiac conduction disorders. Connexins are proteins that are responsible for inter-myocyte electrical communication and are a part of the family of gap junction proteins. Cardiac myocytes contain multiple connexin isoforms, and different parts of the myocardium display different connexin types. Disorders of gap junction proteins may lead to a variety of conduction disorders depending on the specific arrangement of the connexin protein subtypes (48). Ventricular myocytes express connexin 43 and 45; atrial myocytes express connexin 43, 45, and 40. EP studies have been reported on connexin 43 mutated mice (49) which revealed prolonged interventricular conduction delay without other electrophysiologic abnormalities. Ya and coworkers showed that major abnormalities in normal D-looping occurred in the connexin 43 deficient mice with malpositions of the atrioventricular grooves and ventricular septum with resultant right ventricular hypertrophy (50). Connexin 40-deficient mice have also been evaluated and shown to have distinct atrioventricular and distal conduction system disturbances (51), and detailed electrophysiologic studies have been recently performed.

ADVANTAGES/LIMITATIONS OF ANIMAL MODELS

Proponents of large animal cardiovascular studies have long maintained that larger animals more closely approximate human cardiovascular physiology. Schwartz reviewed a series of large animal cardiovascular studies and concluded that useful information relevant to human disease could be obtained when experiments were designed with careful attention to factors important in the clinical setting (1). Large-animal transgenic models have yet to be developed for widescale use in cardiovascular research. Recently, techniques have been developed that allow transfer of a single cell nucleus at a specific stage of development to another single, unfertilized cell without a nucleus to produce live clonal offspring (52). Cells were taken from adult lamb mammary gland, fetus, and embryo tissue and were manipulated to eventually produce live lamb offspring. Future studies using these techniques may provide for new larger animal models of disease with relevant and important cardiovascular and electrophysiologic applications.

Small genetically engineered organisms are becoming increasingly useful in the cardiovascular research arena. Because of technical and economical considerations, the mouse has become the model of choice for genetic manipulations. The development of reproducible and stable genetic mutations with identifiable phenotypes allows researchers to study phenotypic changes when the primary genetic etiology is already known. The limitations of murine cardiovascular physiology must be recognized, however. The length of the cardiac cycle is 1/10 of the human, with heart rates 500-700 beats per minute in the conscious, freely-moving mouse (3, 34). Murine models, while displaying similar phenotypes to human disease states, do not always display the full spectrum of disease found in humans. Differences in contractile proteins exist between human and mouse cardiac tissue and probably play a role in the differential responses of normal cardiac function as well as in genetically manipulated models.

Future trends in transgenic research will involve the use of larger animal models that will more closely approximate human physiology. Technology already exists for transgenic techniques in larger animals (53). The disadvantages of larger animals include higher maintenance cost, procedural complexity, and ethical issues. Ethical issues have played an important role in decisions about animal experimentation and transgenic studies, and institutions have USDA-regulated institutional animal care and use committees to monitor animal research (54).

Gene replacement therapy has been an exciting proposition in animal models of cardiovascular disease, and potential for curative therapy in human patients. Impediments to using transgenic techniques to cure genetic defects include the obstacle that transgenes must currently be inserted into the preceding generation in order to have an effect. In addition, transgene expression remains variable and not predictable. Adequate expression of a gene product may occur only in a minority of transgenic animals, and there is always the risk of overexpression of a gene product that may prove harmful.

CONCLUSIONS

With the identification of hundreds of new genes potentially modulating electrophysiological characteristics, specific genetic etiologies of cardiovascular electrical disease can be identified. In like manner, individuals with specific genetic alleles can be counseled about risk factors predisposing to certain inheritable electrophysiologic diseases. As more is learned about the molecular biology of genetic defects, emphasis will shift from diagnosis to treatment using gene therapy. Gene replacement therapy is certainly in its infancy. Although a few attempts have been made with gene therapy techniques, none have clearly proved to be curative thus far. Isolated ventricular myocytes from rabbit hearts were recently studied with gene therapy (55). These rabbits had been chronically paced in order to develop tachycardiomyopathy-induced hemodynamic failure. Their ventricular myocytes displayed down-regulation of beta-adrenergic signaling receptors (β-ARs) and upregulation of receptor inhibitors, β-adrenergic receptor kinase (βARK1). In this in vitro study, adenoviral-mediated gene transfer of human β_2-AR inhibitor, which functions as an inhibitor of the receptor kinase and thus increases activity of adrenergic receptors was achieved in isolated ventricular myocytes. The myocytes demonstrated a marked restoration of β-AR signaling. The study identified a novel strategy of gene transfer for future development in enhancing performance of heart failure either through gene transfer or through pharmacological techniques targeting this protein.

Methods of gene delivery have utilized numerous vectors: viral (retroviruses, adenoviruses), viral-conjugate vectors (adenovirus-augmented receptor-mediated vectors and hemagglutinating virus of Japan [HVJ] liposomes), and nonviral vectors (cationic liposomes, polymers, and injection of plasmid DNA) (56). The application of gene therapy to cardiovascular patients has been slow. Reasons include the fact that the risk-benefit ratio may be higher in cardiac patients than with other groups currently undergoing trials of gene therapy (cystic fibrosis, melanoma). In addition, cardiac disease tends to be multifactorial and often a single gene is not entirely responsible for a particular disease state. Gene transfer in the cardiovascular field has been useful in creating animal models of disease in which the in vivo functions of gene products (or lack of products) can be studied. As technology improves, gene-to-gene transfer and gene replacement modalities will become increasingly important areas of study and may provide rational and exciting new therapeutic approaches to human cardiovascular pathophysiology.

REFERENCES

1. Schwartz P. Do animals have clinical value? *Am J Cardiol* 1998;81:14D-20D.

2. Paigen K. A miracle enough: the power of mice. *Nat Med* 1995;1:215-220.

3. Berul CI, Mendelsohn ME. Molecular biology and genetics of cardiac disease associated with sudden death: electrophysiologic studies in mouse models of inherited diseases. In: Estes NAM, Salem DN, Wang PJ, eds. Sudden Cardiac Death in the Athlete. Armonk, NY: Futura Publishing Co, 1998, pp 465-481.

4. Dae MW, Lee RJ, Ursell PC, Chin MC, Stillson CA, Moise NS. Heterogeneous sympathetic innervation in German shepherd dogs with inherited ventricular arrhythmia and sudden cardiac death. *Circulation* 1997;96:1337-1342.

5. Moise NS, Meyers-Wallen V, Flahive WJ, Scarlett JM, Brown CA, Chavkin MJ, Dugger DA, Renaud-Farrell S, Kornreich B, Schoenborn WC, Sparks JR, Gilmour RF. Inherited ventricular arrhythmias and sudden death in German shepherd dogs. *J Am Coll Cardiol* 1994;24:233-243.

6. Gilmour RF, Moise NS. Triggered activity as a mechanism for inherited ventricular arrhythmias in German shepherd dogs. *J Am Coll Cardiol* 1996;27:1526-1533.

7. Zipes DP, Barber MJ, Takahashi N, Gilmour RF. Influences of the autonomic nervous system on the genesis of cardiac arrhythmias. *Pacing Clin Electrophysiol* 1983;6:1210-1220.

8. Wilber DJ, Davis MJ, Rosenbaum M, Ruskin JN, Garan H. Incidence and determinants of multiple morphologically distinct ventricular tachycardias. *J Am Coll Cardiol* 1987;10:583-591.

9. Constantinos C, Peters NS, Waldesker B, Ciaccio EJ, Wit AL, Coromilas J. Mechanisms causing sustained ventricular tachycardia with multiple QRS morphologies: Results of mapping studies in the infarcted canine heart. *Circulation* 1997;96:3721-3731.

10. Vos MA, de Groot SHM, Verduyn SC, der Zande J, Leunissen HDM, Cleutjens JPM, van Bilsen M, Daemen MJAP, Schreuder JJ, Allessie MA, Wellens HJJ. Enhanced susceptibility for acquired torsades de pointes arrhythmias in the dog with chronic, complete AV block is related to cardiac hypertrophy and electrical remodeling. *Circulation* 1998; 98:1125-1135.

11. Khoury DS, Berrier KL, Badruddin SM, Zoghbi WA. Three-dimensional electrophysiological imaging of the intact canine left ventricle using a noncontact multielectrode cavitary probe: study of sinus, paced, and spontaneous premature beats. *Circulation* 1998;97:399-409.

12. Kwan YY, Fan W, Hough D, Lee JJ, Fishbein MC, Karagueuzian HS, Chen PS. Effects of procainamide on wave-front dynamics during ventricular fibrillation in open-chest dogs *Circulation* 1998;97:1828-1836.

13. Link MS, Wang PJ, Pandian NG, Bharati S, Udelson JE, Lee MY, Vecchiotti MA, VanderBrink BA, Mirra G, Maron BJ, Estes NAM. An experimental model of sudden death due to low-energy chest-wall impact (commotio cordis). *New Engl J Med.* 1998;338:1805-11.

14. Wijffels MC, Kirchhof CJ, Dorland R, Allessie MA. Atrial fibrillation begets atrial fibrillation. *Circulation* 1995;92:1954-1968.

15. Rahimtoola SH. From coronary artery disease to heart failure: role of hibernating myocardium *Am J Cardiol* 1995;75:16E-22E.

16. Ausma J, Wijffels M, Thone F, Wouters L, Allessie M, Borgers M. Structural changes of atrial myocardium due to sustained atrial fibrillation in the goat. *Circulation* 1997;96:3157-3163.

17. van der Velden HMW, van Kempen MJA, Wijffels MCEF, van Zijverden M, Groenewegen WA, Allessie MA, Jongsma HJ. Altered pattern of connexin40 distribution in persistent atrial fibrillation in the goat. *J Cardiovasc Electrophysiol.* 1998;9:596-607.

18. Morillo CA, Klein GJ, Jones DL, Guiraudon CM. Chronic rapid atrial pacing: Structural, functional, and electrophysiological characteristics of a new model of sustained atrial fibrillation.*Circulation* 1995;91:1588-1595.

19. Gaspo R, Bosch RF, Talajic M, Nattel S. Functional mechanisms underlying tachycardia-induced sustained atrial fibrillation in a chronic dog model. *Circulation* 1997;96:4027-4035.

20. Triedman JK, Jenkins KJ, Colan SD, Van Praagh R, Lock JE, Walsh EP. Multipolar endocardial mapping of the right heart using a basket catheter: acute and chronic animal studies.*Pacing Clin Electrophysiol PACE* 1997;20:51-59.

21. Mitchell M, McRury I, Haines D. Linear atrial ablations in a canine model of chronic atrial fibrillation: morphologic and electrophysiologic observations. *Circulation* 1998;97:1176-1185.

22. Geisterfer-Lowrance AA, Christe M, Conner DA, Ingwall JS, Schoen FJ, Seidman CE, Seidman JG. A mouse model of familial hypertrophic cardiomyopathy. *Science* 1996;272:731-734.

23. Wang Q, Shen J, Splawski I, Atkinson D, Li Z, Robinson JL, Moss AJ, Towbin JA, Keating MT. SCN5A mutation associated with an inherited cardiac arrhythmia-long QT syndrome. *Cell* 1995;80:805-811.

24. Curran ME, Splawski I, Timothy K, Vincent GM, Green ED, Keating MT. A molecular basis of cardiac arrhythmias: HERG mutations cause long QT syndrome. *Cell* 1995;80:795-803.

25. Grace AA, Chien KR. Congenital long QT syndromes: Toward molecular dissection of arrhythmia substrates. *Circulation* 1995;92:2786-2789.

26. Reddy S, Smith DB, Rich MM, Leferovich JM, Reilly P, Davis BM, Tran K, Rayburn H, Bronson R, Cros D, Balice-Gordon RJ, Housman D. Mice lacking the myotonic dystrophy protein kinase develop a late-onset progressive myopathy. *Nat Genet* 1996;13:325-335.

27. Gottwald M, Gottwald E, Dhein S. Age-related electrophysiological and histological changes in rabbit hearts: age-related changes in electrophysiology. *Int J Cardiol* 1997;62:97-106.

28. Asano Y, Davidenko JM, Baxter WT, Gray RA, Jalife J. Optical mapping of drug-induced polymorphic arrhythmias and torsades de pointes in the isolated rabbit heart.*J Am Coll Cardiol* 1997;29:831-842.

29. Wood MA, Caponi D, Sykes AM, Wenger EJ. Atrial electrical remodeling by rapid pacing in the isolated rabbit heart: effects of Ca++ and K+ channel blockade.*J Intervent Cardiac Electrophysiol* 1998;2:15-23.

30. Gray RA, Jalife J. Effects of atrial defibrillation shocks on the ventricles in isolated sheep hearts. *Circulation* 1998;97:1613-1622.

31. Berul CI, Aronovitz MJ, Wang PJ, Mendelsohn ME. In vivo cardiac electrophysiology studies in the mouse. *Circulation* 1996;94:2641-2648.

32. Mitchell GF, Jeron A, Koren G. Measurement of heart rate and Q-T interval in the conscious mouse. *Am J Physiol* 1998; 274:H747-H751.

33. Brugada R, Roberts R. The molecular genetics of arrhythmias and sudden death.*Clin Cardiol* 1998;21:553-560.

34. Lewin B. Genes VI. Oxford: Oxford Univ. Press, 1997, pp 980-987.

35. Melton DW. Gene targeting in the mouse. *Bioessays* 1994;16:633-638.

36. James JF, Hewett TE, Robbins J. Cardiac physiology in transgenic mice. *Circ Res* 1998;82:407-415.

37. Berul CI, Christe ME, Aronovitz MA, Seidman CE, Seidman JG, Mendelsohn ME. Electrophysiological abnormalities and arrhythmias in αMHC mutant familial hypertrophic cardiomyopathy mice. *J Clin Invest* 1997;99:570-576.

38. Berul CI, Christe ME, Aronovitz MJ, Maguire CT, Seidman CE, Seidman JG, Mendelsohn ME. Familial hypertrophic cardiomyopathy mice display gender differences in electrophysiological abnormalities. *J Intervent Cardiac Electrophysiol* 1998;2:7-14.

39. Bevilacqua LM, Maguire CT, Seidman CE, Seidman JG, Berul CI.QT dispersion in αMHC familial hypertrophic cardiomyopathy mice. *Pediatr Res* 1999;45:643-647.

40. Sussman MA, Lim HW, Gude N, Taigen T, Olson EN, Robbins J, Colbert MC, Gualberto A, Wieczorek DF, Molkentin JD. Prevention of cardiac hypertrophy in mice by calcineurin inhibition. *Science* 1998;281:1690-1693.

41. Michels VV, Moll PP, Miller FA, Tajik AJ, Chu JS, Driscoll DJ, Burnett JC, Rodeheffer RJ, Chesebro JH, Tazelaar HD. The frequency of familial dilated cardiomyopathy in a series of patients with idiopathic dilated cardiomyopathy. *N Engl J Med* 1992;326:77-82.

42. Vincent GM. The molecular genetics of the long QT syndrome: genes causing fainting and sudden death. *Annu Rev Med* 1998;49:263-274.

43. Ficker E, Jarolimek W, Kiehn J, Baumann A, Brown AM. Molecular determinants of dofetilide block of HERG K+ channels. *Circ Res* 1998;82:386-395.

44. London B, Jeron A, Zhou J, Buckett P, Han X, Mitchell GF, Koren G. Long QT and ventricular arrhythmias in transgenic mice expressing the N terminus and first transmembrane segment of a voltage-gated potassium channel. *Proc Natl Acad Sci USA* 1998;95:2926-2931.

45. O'Brien SE, Apkon MA, Berul CI, Patel HT, Zahler R. Electrocardiographic phenotype of long QT syndrome in transgenic mouse model expressing human α3 Na,K-ATPase isoform in heart. *Circulation* 1997;96:I-422

46. Housman DE, Shaw DJ. Expansion of an unstable DNA region and phenotypic variation in myotonic dystrophy. *Nature* 1992;355:545-546.

47. Berul CI, Maguire CT, Aronovitz MJ, Greenwood J, Miller C, Gehrmann J, Housman D, Mendelsohn ME, Reddy S. DMPK dosage alterations result in atrioventricular conduction abnormalities in a mouse myotonic dystrophy model. *J Clin Invest* 1999;103:R1-R7.

48. Davis LM, Kanter HL, Beyer EC, Saffitz JE. Distinct gap junction protein phenotypes in cardiac tissues with disparate conduction properties. *J Am Coll Cardiol* 1994;24:1124-1132.

49. Thomas SA, Schuessler RB, Berul CI, Beardslee MA, Beyer EC, Mendelsohn ME, Saffitz JE. Disparate effects of deficient expression of connexin43 on atrial and ventricular conduction: evidence for chamber-specific molecular determinants of conduction. *Circulation* 1998;97:686-691.

50. Ya J, Erdstieck-Ernste EBHW, de Boer PAJ, van Kempen MJA, Jongsma H, Gros D, Moorman AFM, Lamers WH. Heart defects in connexin43 deficient mice. *Circ Res* 1998;82:360-366.

51. Simon AM, Goodenough DA, Paul DL. Mice lacking connexin40 have cardiac conduction abnormalities characteristic of atrioventricular block and bundle branch block. *Curr Biol* 1998;8:295-298.

52. Wilmut I, Schnieke AE, McWhir J, Kind AJ, Campbell KH. Viable offspring derived from fetal and adult mammalian cells. *Nature* 1997;385:810-813.

53. Diamond LE, McCurry KR, Martin MJ, McClellan SB, Oldham ER, Platt JL, Logan JS. Characterization of transgenic pigs expressing functionally active human CD59 on cardiac endothelium. *Transplantation* 1996;61:1241-1249.

54. Mukerjee M. Trends in animal research. *Sci Am* 1997; Feb:86-93.

55. Akhter SA, Skaer CA, Kypson AP, McDonald PH, Peppel KC, Glower DD, Lefkowitz RJ, Koch WJ. Restoration of β-adrenergic signaling in failing cardiac ventricular myocytes via adenoviral-mediated gene transfer. *Proc Natl Acad Sci USA* 1997; 94:12100-12105.

56. Nabel EG. Gene therapy for cardiovascular disease. *Circulation* 1995;91:541-548.

4

OPTICAL MAPPING OF ARRHYTHMIAS

Gregory E. Morley, Dhananjay Vaidya, and José Jalife

Dept. of Pharmacology, SUNY Health Science Center, Syracuse, NY 13210

INTRODUCTION

Optical mapping of voltage dependent fluorescence in cardiac tissue allows for the simultaneous measurement of membrane potential from many locations on the surface of the heart. The development of this technology has revolutionized the field of cardiac electrophysiology and has provided new insights into the mechanisms of initiation and maintenance of cardiac arrhythmias (1-4). Recently, we have adopted this technology to image electrical activation in the hearts of normal and transgenic mice (5-7). By combining these novel technologies we hope to learn more about the roles of specific gene products in the development of cardiac arrhythmias.

Numerous transgenic mouse models of human diseases are now available (8,9). In addition, transgenic models have also been developed to better understand the role of specific gene products (10). Transgenic mice offer a new and powerful approach to study the genetics of cardiovascular disease. Indeed, changes in the expression levels of several proteins have been linked to cardiac arrhythmias(11-13). Mutations in ion channels that lead to alteration in their kinetics have been proposed as mechanism to explain congenital long QT syndrome (14). Additionally, mutations in the coding region of the SCN5A cardiac sodium channel have been identified in families with idiopathic ventricular fibrillation (15). Changes in the expression levels of connexins proteins have also been identified in animal models of atrial fibrillation (11,12). Optical mapping provides an invaluable tool to test the organ-wide electrophysiological consequences of specific genetic manipulations. The elucidation of the disturbed electrophysiology of the transgenic substrate by optical mapping can provide a mechanistic link between molecular factors and arrhythmogenesis.

The purpose of this chapter is twofold. First we will discuss some of the technical aspects of imaging voltage dependent fluorescence in the adult mouse heart. Here we will outline some general considerations with optical mapping studies in cardiac tissue while pointing the special concerns that are unique for Langendorff perfusing and mapping the adult mouse heart. Second we will summarize some of our most recent studies where we have successfully induced and mapped ventricular arrhythmias in the normal adult mouse heart (6) and in a transgenic model of acquired cardiomyopathy (7).

METHODS

Acquisition Systems

Imaging voltage dependent fluorescence in cardiac tissue requires both high resolution and high-speed acquisition. The fluorescent signal that is recorded from each location on the surface of the heart is an optical action potential. Studies have demonstrated that the response time of these voltage dependent fluorophores is sufficient to resolve changes in membrane potential (16). Furthermore, a linear relationship has been demonstrated between the fluorescent signal and the membrane potential that is recorded with microelectrodes (16). The characteristics of the upstroke of the cardiac action potential require high-speed acquisition. Upstroke times recorded using microelectrodes indicate that the upstroke in cardiac tissue is < 1 ms. The requirement for high spatial resolution originates from the need to investigate small details of propagating waves during pacing, as well as during arrhythmias. To achieve this, there are currently two imaging strategies that are used to image voltage dependent fluorescence in cardiac tissue. One system utilizes high-speed charged coupled device (CCD) cameras (17) and the other system relies on a photodiode array (18). Today there are many commercially available CCD cameras that are capable of imaging voltage dependent fluorescence in cardiac tissue. Because of the growth in the personal computer field, improvements in the speed, number of pixels and resolution of these cameras are occurring at a rapid rate. The digital CCD cameras that are used in our laboratory are capable of acquiring a frame in 1 ms with 12-bit resolution from an array of 64×64 pixels. It should be mentioned that unlike photodiode array systems, acquisition of the signals with CCD cameras occurs throughout the sampling period (17). As a result, the fluorescent signal is integrated over the entire sampling period. The main strength of systems that used CCD cameras is the high spatial resolution that is possible.

Synchronized acquisition (stroboscopic imaging) of repetitive events

In experiments where both high temporal and spatial resolution is desired we have utilized the stroboscopic principle to improve the temporal resolution of our CCD cameras. The following is a discussion of the basis of stroboscopic imaging and how it can be utilized to improve the time resolution of CCD cameras when recording repetitive events. The stroboscopic principle owes its beginning to Roget (1825) who noticed apparent motion in the spokes of a stationary wheel as he walked along a wicket fence (19). This principle was used by Plateau and independently by Stampfer in 1832 to build devices where spatially periodic patterns (e.g., a pattern of dark and light lines) were viewed through regularly spaced holes on a spinning wheel (19). This created the illusion of moving lines that was due to the persistence of vision.

Michael Faraday in 1831 found that the principle of intermittently watching an object with temporal, but not spatial periodicity (such as a vibrating tuning fork) caused the motion of the object to be frozen, slowed down or reversed (19). This "illusion" was not merely due to the persistence of vision, but rather it was caused by the arrival of the successive viewing holes during different phases of the repetitive motion. This interesting observation is commonly used as a demonstration in high school science.

Stroboscopic Photography of Repetitive Motion

Stroboscopic photography of repetitive motion reproduces Faraday's observation, i.e., for every cycle of the repetitive motion:

(i)   If the opening/closing of the shutter is exactly in phase with the repetitive motion, the edges of the images captured on corresponding frames in every cycle will exactly coincide.

(ii)   If the opening/closing of the shutter occurs slightly earlier for each succeeding cycle (phase precession), the edges of captured images will appear to retrogress in corresponding frames of succeeding cycles.

(iii)   If the opening/closing of the shutter occurs slightly later for each succeeding cycle (phase delay), the edges of captured images will appear to progress in corresponding frames of succeeding cycles.

This observation is well known in motion pictures, where the rotation of the spokes of a wheel appears to be frozen, slowed down or reversed depending on whether the shutter closes in phase or out of phase with the revolution of the spokes (20). In cases (ii) and (iii) the intermediate positions of the trailing/leading edges seen in every cycle represent instantaneous locations of the object at the phase precession/delay. The phase precession/delay can be readily calculated if independent measures of the frame rate and frequency of the repetitive event are obtained.

Furthermore, if the experimenter uses standard electronic pulse generators to impose defined phase delays, any inaccuracies introduced by calculation of the phase delays are eliminated. This principle has been applied to the optical mapping of cardiac excitation by Wikswo et al.(3) who have introduced the term "synchronous acquisition" which is the terminology we have adopted.

Requirements for Stroboscopic Enhancement of Time Resolution (Synchronous Acquisition)

To summarize, the requirements to improve the time resolution of a camera using stroboscopic methods are:

(i)   The event to be optically recorded must be repetitive.

(ii)   The phase delay between the beginning of the event and the beginning/end of the acquisition of the frame must be accurately known. Thus the delay should be either imposed (e.g., using electronic pulse generators) or calculated from an independent measure of the frequency of the event (e.g., a volume conducted electrogram obtained at a much higher sampling frequency than the camera's frame rate).

Paced stimulation of the heart in our experimental system fulfils both of these requirements. Although there may be beat-to-beat variability, the average activation of the heart at a constant basic cycle length (BCL) is considered to be a reproducible event. The widespread use of signal averaging in cardiac (3,21,22) and neural electrophysiology (23,24), highlights this general assumption regarding the reproducibility of electrical activation of regularly paced non-arrhythmic tissue. The signal averaging of the activation process also minimizes the effect of beat-to-beat variability. This process makes the averaged record a reproducible event. Furthermore, in our optical records, signal averaging increased the signal-to-noise ratio, demonstrating that indeed a repetitive event was averaged.

We have implemented a synchronous acquisition system using a COHU CCD camera with a maximum frame rate of 240 fps. The electronic board that controls the camera (EPIX) provides a pulse at the start of every frame and this can be used to synchronize the stimulator (Frederick Haer and Co., Pulsar 6i). This stimulator allows a phase delay to be introduced with microsecond accuracy. Thus, the delay between the beginning of the frame and the stimulus is electronically controlled and accurately known.

Circuitry
A flowchart of the circuitry is shown in Figure 1. A record of several beats was taken at every delay, so that every beat in the record was stroboscopically identical (i.e., the phase delay was the same for each beat), and could thus be signal averaged. A program was written using a Digital I/O board to interface between the camera clock and the stimulator, automatically introducing phase delays at defined times.

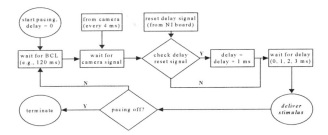

Figure 1. Flowchart of the circuitry used to implement the synchronous acquisition system.

Control I – CCD Record of Oscilloscope Sweeps

The electronics were tested using the CCD camera to record sweeps of an oscilloscope beam that were triggered by the stimulator. The oscilloscope was set to sweep at the speed of 1 division per millisecond and the frame rate of the camera was 240 fps. First, the output of the stimulator (pacing stimulus) was synchronized (delay = 0 ms) with the start of the frame (see flowchart), and a record containing several sweeps of the oscilloscope beam was taken. These movies were then signal averaged. Figure 2, panel A shows five successive frames of the signal averaged record. Each blur is the track of the oscilloscope beam during the 4 ms exposure time of each frame ("the time which the shutter was open" in terms of regular photographic terminology). Note the sharp leading edge of each blur, which represents the exact location of the oscilloscope beam at the instant that the exposure time of the corresponding frame ended.

Control II – Orderly Progression of Cardiac Activation Front (Internal Evidence)

Figure 3 shows an example of the activation sequences that were obtained from an adult mouse ventricle when paced at a BCL of 120 ms. Four frames (rows 1 – 4) from each of four averaged movies (columns I – IV) are shown in panel A. The movies I – IV were acquired with phase delays of 0, 1, 2, 3 ms, respectively. The orderly progression (indicated by the solid and dotted arrows in panel B) of the activation front between corresponding frames of the four movies shows that the average activation of the heart is indeed a repetitive process and that the synchronous acquisition system captures the this process at defined intermediate time points. Such an orderly progression was observed in all records.

Control III – Comparison with Measurements by The DALSA Camera (1484 fps)

The external control for the procedure was obtained using a DALSA camera with a frame rate of 1484 fps, where the synchronous acquisition system was not used (see (5)). Figure 4 shows the anisotropic maximum and minimum conduction velocities measured in ventricles of mice paced at a BCL of 150 ms. The measurements obtained using the the COHU camera (with synchronous acquisition, n =11) shows a statistically significant difference from the measurements obtained using the DALSA camera (without synchronous acquisition, n = 3). Please note that superimposition of the COHU and DALSA movies is not technically possible for the following reasons:

(i)   The system of synchronous acquisition can achieve offline frame rates that are integral multiples of the online frame rate of the COHU camera: i.e., for an online frame rate of 240 fps, the only achievable offline frame rates are 480 fps, 720 fps, 960 fps, etc. Images taken at any of these frame rates cannot be superimposed on images obtained with the DALSA camera (1484 fps).

(ii)   We are unable to simultaneously record fluorescent signals with both the COHU and DALSA cameras because the relatively low sensitivity of both the cameras does not allow us to divide the fluorescent signal.

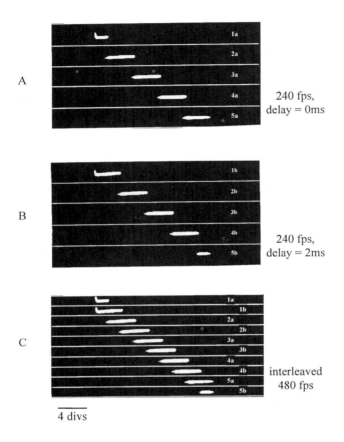

4 divs

Figure 2. CCD camera frames recording sweeps of an oscilloscope beam that were triggered by the stimulator. The oscilloscope was set to sweep speed of 1 division per millisecond and the frame rate of the camera was 240 fps. First, the output of the stimulator was synchronized (delay = 0 ms) with the start of the frame, and a record containing several sweeps of the oscilloscope beam was taken. The movies were then signal averaged. Panel A shows five successive of the signal averaged record. The track of the oscilloscope beam during the 4 ms exposure time of each frame can be seen. In panel B, the camera was set such that the start of the frame was phase delayed by 2 ms with respect to the pacing stimulus. Tracks similar to those in panel A are seen, except that the location of the leading edge is at a different position compared to the corresponding track in panel A. The corresponding frames in panels A and B are interleaved in panel C. Thus the movement of the leading edge of the beam is tracked with a 2 ms time resolution. In panel B, the camera was set such that the start of the frame was phase delayed by 2 ms with respect to the pacing stimulus. Blurs similar to those in panel A are seen, except that the location of the leading edge of each blur is at a different position compared to the corresponding blur in panel A. This is because in panel B each frame acquisition began and ended with a phase difference of exactly 2 ms compared with the corresponding frame in panel A. The corresponding frames in panels A and B are interleaved in panel C. Thus the movement of the leading edge of the beam is tracked with a 2 ms time resolution.

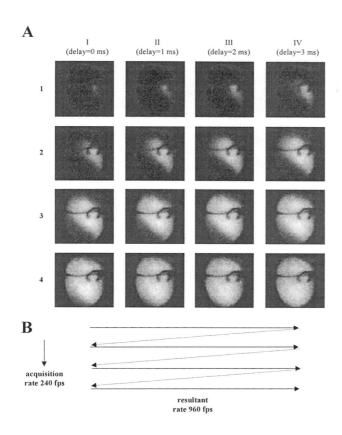

Figure 3. Activation sequences obtained from an adult mouse ventricle paced at a BCL of 120 ms. Four frames (rows 1 – 4) from each of four averaged movies (columns I – IV) are shown in panel A. The movies I – IV were acquired with phase delays of 0, 1, 2, 3 ms, respectively. Note the orderly progression of the activation front between corresponding frames of the four movies indicated by the solid and dotted arrows in panel B.

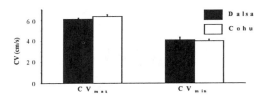

Figure 4. Comparison of maximum (CV_{max}) and minimum (CV_{min}) anisotropic conduction velocities measured on the ventricles of mice using a DALSA camera (1484 fps, no synchronous acquisition, n = 3) and a COHU camera (240 fps, with synchronous acquisition, n = 11). The ventricles were paced at 150 ms, and the velocities were measured as described in reference (5).

We have thus used the electronic capabilities of our camera and stimulator to implement a synchronous acquisition approach. Using the stroboscopic principles to increase the time resolution of our recording system allows us to increase its temporal resolution.

Langendorff Perfusion
High-resolution optical mapping studies in the adult mouse heart is relatively new (25). Therefore it may be useful to provide some details on the cannulation and perfusion techniques that we have used. The mouse heart is vulnerable to ischemic insults, therefore it is important to reestablish coronary perfusion as quickly after the heart has been excised. This is accomplished by quickly removing the heart through a thoracotomy. The heart is then briefly rinsed in warm oxygenated Tyrode's solution and transferred to a clean Petri dish. The aortic cannula is constructed from a 20g needle that is cut to approximately 3 mm. The length of the cannula is important for temperature control considerations. The cannula is placed on a 1-ml syringe and positioned such that the tip of the cannula is immersed in a bath that is filled with warm oxygenated Tyrode's solution. A small amount of solution is forced through the cannula to ensure that no air is trapped is in it. Under a dissection microscope, pericardial tissue, fat and the other great vessels are trimmed to expose the aorta. The aorta is cut approximately 2 mm above the base of the heart. Using sharp forceps, the

aorta is then cannulated. A loop of 4-0 silk is tied around the outside of the aorta approximately 1 mm above its end. A small amount of solution is forced through the cannula to test for leaks and to ensure that the heart is properly cannulated. The heart is then transferred to the Langendorff-perfusion system.

The Langendorff-perfusion system that is in place in our laboratory uses a constant pressure concept. A water-jacketed 1-liter reservoir is placed where the fluid level is 80 cm above the level of the heart. This creates 58 mmHg of constant pressure. It is our experience that under these conditions, the adult mouse heart is perfused with 2-3 ml/min, which is similar to the reported value of aortic pressure and coronary flow in the isolated mouse heart (26). Immediately before entering the aorta the solution is passed through a 5 ml water-jacketed chamber. This chamber is designed to ensure that no air enters the heart and to allow us to monitor the perfusion temperature. Once the heart is connected to the Langendorff-perfusion system the heart is immersed in a water-jacketed perfusion chamber that is constantly aerated with a 95% O_2 –5% CO_2 gas mixture. An immersion circulator maintains the temperature of the all the water-jacketed glassware at 37°C.

Once the mouse heart is connected to the Langendorff perfusion system, it is allowed to equilibrate for approximately 20 min. The heart is stained with the voltage sensitive dye di-4-ANEPPS by injecting a bolus of 25 picomoles in the 5 ml perfusion chamber. The fluorescent signal reaches a maximum in approximately 10 min.

Recording Electrograms in Mouse Heart Preparations
Filtering and sampling the electrical signal appropriately are important considerations so that the recordings are interpretable. To investigate the range of frequencies in a normal mouse electrocardiogram, a representative Lead II surface electrocardiogram is presented in panel A of figure 5. The frequency spectrum of the signal is shown in panel B. The frequencies below 290 Hz contribute 95% of the cumulative power, thus the appropriate low pass filter and sampling rates are approximately 300 Hz and 1200 samples per second. In our Langendorff-perfusion system, two electrodes are positioned on each side of the heart to record a horizontal volume-conducted electrogram. The electrodes are connected to a differential amplifier system and an analog-to-digital converter. An ECG is recorded continuously throughout the experiments.

Stimulation Protocol
To induce arrhythmias, bipolar stimulating electrodes are placed on the epicardial surface. We have tested several arrhythmia induction protocols. We have had the most success by applying trains of 10 stimuli near the 1:1 capture rate separated by approximately 1 second near the center of the anterior ventricular surface. This protocol has produced both monomorphic and polymorphic ventricular arrhythmias. It was our experience that the ability to induce arrhythmias in the mouse heart is variable and dependent on many factors including the electrode position, stimulus strength and pacing frequency. In all cases, this pacing protocol is repeated many times while changing the above variables before successfully inducing an arrhythmia.

Typically, the source of any sustained arrhythmia is located outside the field of view of the camera. Thus, to image the source of an arrhythmia the camera is repositioned.

A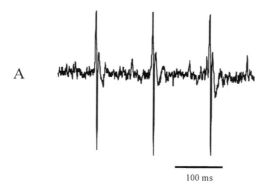

100 ms

B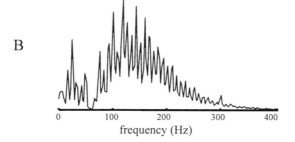

Figure 5. Panel A shows a Lead II surface electrocardiogram obtained from a conscious 4-day-old mouse. The signal was conditioned by lowpass filtering at 1 kHz and was then sampled at 5 kHz. Panel B shows a fast Fourier Transform of the signal. Note that the initial cluster of peaks (<100Hz) includes rate information, while information about the shape of the waveforms is contained above 100Hz. 95% of the cumulative power in the FFT is contributed by frequencies less than 290 Hz.

Motion Reduction

Motion reduction is an important aspect of optical mapping studies therefore to obtain high-resolution images of electrical activation we have included the excitation contraction uncoupler DAM in some studies. We have recently conducted a series of experiments were we have investigated the effects of DAM on volume conducted electrocardiograms recorded from Langendorff-perfused mouse hearts. Wildtype mouse hearts were rapidly excised, cannulated and perfused with warm (38° C) oxygenated Tyrode's solution. Hearts were then immersed in a warm temperature-controlled bath that served as a volume conductor. Following a 15-minute control period, hearts were perfused with a Tyrode's solution that contained diacetyl monoxime (DAM, 15 mM) for an additional 10 minutes. QRS durations were measured during control and while perfusing DAM. Post hoc t-test showed that no significant difference occurred between control and DAM perfusion at 37° C. However, as a positive control, changing the temperature to 27° C (see Table 1), significantly prolonged the QRS.

The QRS duration represents the time taken for ventricular excitation. Since this process involves the pattern of conduction within the His-Purkinje, as well as propagation within the ventricular myocardium, interpretation of these data are difficult. It is interesting that no significant changes in the QRS duration were due to the addition of DAM. Although this information is indirect, it suggests that DAM may not profoundly affect conduction in the ventricular myocardium or specialized conduction system.

Table 1
QRS Duration in Langendorff-Perfused Mouse Hearts

Control at 37°C	DAM at 37°C	DAM at 27°C
10.2±0.6 ms	11.7±1.6 ms	**16.2±2.1 ms***

(mean ± SEM; ANOVA – $p = 0.017$; * post hoc t-test – $p = 0.036$)

THE MOUSE HEART AS MODEL OF PROPAGATION ABNORMALITIES

Recently, we undertook the task of establishing the appropriate technology to investigate cardiac electrical properties and arrhythmias in the normal mouse heart. However, first it was necessary to describe basic electrophysiology and conduction characteristics in the normal murine heart. In recent studies, we have reported ECG parameters in both awake and anesthetized adult mice. Our results are in good agreement with those previously reported by other authors (27-30) In general, the ECG parameters reported for the mouse are variable and appear to be highly dependent on the anesthetic agent used (31,32). The heart rate of the adult mouse has been reported to be between 200-636 beats/min, with PR intervals ranging from 38 to 54 msec. QRS durations in the mouse range from 10 msec to 30 msec and QT intervals range from 59 msec to 109 msec (27,29,33-36) The shape and duration of the QRS complex represents the sum of all instantaneous vectors during ventricular activation. To study electrophysiological parameters and arrhythmias, we developed a technique that allowed for recording of electrical activity on the epicardial surface of the Langendorff-perfused adult mouse heart (7,37).

Measurements of conduction velocity (CV) and mean action potential duration (APD) were made using optical recording techniques and a voltage sensitive dye in the presence of the electromechanical uncoupler diacetyl monoxime (DAM) (7,37). As in other species (37-40), CV on the epicardial surface of the mouse ventricles was dependent on stimulation cycle length, as well as fiber orientation. Considering the wall thickness of the ventricle (< 1 mm) of the mouse and the rotational anisotropy, CV_{max} (~66 cm/s) was defined as the direction of fastest propagation and CV_{min} (~39 cm/s) as the direction of slowest propagation. Bipolar epicardial pacing of the ventricle of the mouse heart at 37° C produced elliptical isochrones with an anisotropic ratio (1.5-2) similar to that reported in larger hearts (for references see(37)). As with larger hearts, the influence of deeper layers on the epicardial electrical activity would tend to underestimate the anisotropy. In the presence of DAM, mean APD, measured at 70% repolarization (APD_{70}), did not show any cycle length dependence. However, more recent unpublished data from our lab suggest that in the absence of electromechanical uncoupling APD_{70} in the mouse heart is indeed cycle length dependent. The above measurements enabled us to calculate wavelength (WL) as the product of CV and APD. It should be noted, however, that action potentials recorded from the adult mouse heart are triangular shaped and do not have a distinct plateau phase, which complicates the estimations of WL. Both longitudinal and transverse wavelengths measured at APD_{70} were considerably larger that the long diameter of the heart (6 mm).

Sustained Reentry in the Mouse Heart
A relevant issue in this context is whether the mouse heart is an appropriate model in which to study mechanisms and dynamics of arrhythmias. In a recent study (6), burst pacing near the apex of the left ventricle (LV) induced sustained reentrant activity in a number of Langendorff-perfused adult mouse hearts. In some such hearts, sustained vortex-like activity was induced around a single core (Figure 6).

In other hearts, mirror image pairs of rotors were demonstrated. In the presence of DAM, the period of rotation of these arrhythmias ranged from 50 to 60 ms. In the absence of DAM, sustained reentry with periods as short as 28 ms were induced. Both sustained (episodes lasting >30 s) and non-sustained ventricular fibrillation were also induced in several hearts. Such data showed that the LV of the mouse heart is capable of sustaining single or pairs of viable rotors. These data challenge the critical size hypothesis (41) by demonstrating for the first time that ventricular tissue with an area of 100 mm^2 or less is capable of undergoing sustained reentrant activity. These results are unexpected in the sense that it is difficult to conceive the occurrence of fibrillation or even sustained reentry in an excitable medium whose wavelength is larger than the size of the medium. One possible explanation for this phenomenon may be found in recent computer simulations (42) that indicate that the core of a spiral wave has a strong repolarizing influence on the surrounding tissues. Under such conditions, the action potential duration of the cells near the core is shorter than the APD of cells in the periphery of the spiral wave. Such a repolarizing influence of the core was evident in the fact that the average action potential duration of the whole preparation was shorter during spiral wave activity than during external stimulation at a rate identical to that generated by the spiral wave. Similarly, preliminary measurements in the mouse heart during sustained reentrant activity show that APD may be as brief as 10 to 15 msec, compared to 40 to 50 msec during repetitive external stimulation. Thus, the above results further demonstrate that the wavelength during periodic stimulation is a poor predictor of the conditions needed for maintenance of reentry in the mouse heart.

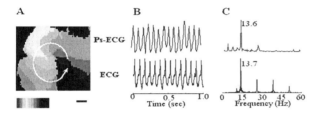

Figure 6. Sustained reentry in the mouse heart. A, Averaged isochrone map of sustained monomorphic tachycardia in the mouse heart (color scale: red = 0 ms, purple = 72 ms; bar = 1mm). B, upper trace is the horizontal pseudoelectrogram, which summarizes the whole optical record by summing signal in the right and left halves of each frame and calculating the difference signal between the two halves; the lower trace is the volume-conducted electrogram obtained during the same episode of arrhythmia. C, FFTs of both the pseudoelectrogram (upper trace) and the volume-conducted electrogram (lower trace) show a narrow peak at 13.6 and 13.7 Hz respectively, consistent with the rotor being responsible for the frequency seen in the volume-conducted electrogram. [Reprinted with permission from *Circulation Research* (Vaidya et al (6), © 1998, American Heart Association]

Arrhythmias in an Acquired Cardiomyopathy
To better understand the contribution of structural heterogeneity to acquired cardiac arrhythmogenesis, we recently characterized the electrophysiology of a mouse model that displays some of the pathological features thought to contribute to the arrhythmogenic substrate in human acquired cardiomyopathy (7). In this study, we examined whether regulated expression of a toxic gene product would result in a cardiomyopathy in which the timing and magnitude of myocardial damage could be controlled by manipulation of tetracycline treatment. It was also shown that conditional expression of the diphtheria toxin A (DTA) gene in the hearts of binary transgenic mice results in myocyte loss, interstitial fibrosis and ventricular dilatation characteristic of many forms of diseased human hearts, culminating in sudden cardiac death (see reference (7) for details). These data suggest that even in the mouse, a species considered relatively resistant to lethal arrhythmias, primary damage to the myocardium initiates a cascade of events, which result in an arrhythmogenic substrate.

Body surface electrocardiograms were recorded from anesthetized mice after withdrawal from tetracycline (7). In contrast to non-transgenic littermate control mice, transgenic mice studied displayed varying degrees of atrio-ventricular block. These observations were confirmed in conscious mice using indwelling telemetry devices implanted into the peritoneum (Figure 7). A variety of arrhythmias were observed in bigenic mice, including atrial fibrillation, pauses and complex ventricular ectopy, including runs of ventricular tachycardia. In contrast, no arrhythmias were detected in non-transgenic controls.

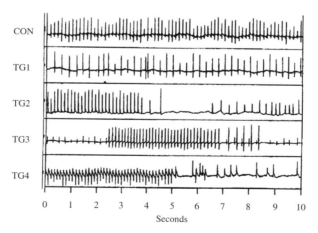

Figure 7. Representative telemetric rhythm strips from nontransgenic (control) and binary transgenic (TG1 – TG4). Abnormalities including atrial fibrillation (TG1), pauses (TG2), and runs of ventricular tachycardia (TG3 and TG4) were observed. [Reprinted with permission from *The Proceedings of the National Academy of Sciences* (Lee et al, (7)), ©1998, The National Academy of Sciences]

High resolution optical mapping of Langendorff-perfused hearts from binary transgenic mice and age-matched controls demonstrated conduction defects and arrhythmias in transgenic mice one month after withdrawal of tetracycline. Activation maps obtained from all control animals showed, propagation that proceeded smoothly from the pacing site with the expected anisotropic profile (Figure 8, panel A). Most binary transgenic hearts also showed preserved conduction maps (panel B), but several displayed markedly disturbed activation profiles, with either disorganized conduction or evidence of block during pacing (panels C - E). A premature pacing protocol in the heart showing conduction block (panel E) resulted in a reentrant arrhythmia around the region of block (panel F). All transgenic animals showed an increased susceptibility to ventricular arrhythmias compared to control hearts. Transgenic hearts displayed both spontaneous as well as inducible runs of sustained and non-sustained ventricular tachycardia.

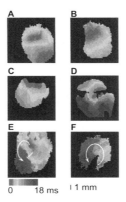

Figure 8. Representative isochrone maps showing normal anisotropic conduction observed in all control hearts (A) and most binary transgenics (B). In three transgenic mice, varying degrees of disorganised epicardial activation were observed (C – E). An area of slow conduction observed during pacing (E) served as an obstacle for inducible ventricular tachycardia (F). [Reprinted with permission from *The Proceedings of the National Academy of Sciences* (Lee et al, (7)), ©1998, The National Academy of Sciences]

CONCLUSIONS

We have presented in this chapter technical considerations concerning the optical mapping of electrical activity in the mouse heart. The mapping of arrhythmias in the normal Langendorff-perfused mouse heart gives us reason to rethink the critical mass hypothesis regarding the minimum size of a heart that may sustain reentrant arrhythmias (6). Thus many transgenic mouse models of cardiac dysfunction have thus become amenable to mechanistic investigation of arrhythmogenic potential. Indeed, as our results with the inducible model of diphtheric cardiomyopathy (7) demonstrate, bringing together the two powerful methodologies of mouse transgenesis and optical mapping can enhance our understanding of the pathogenesis of cardiac disease.

REFERENCES

1. Pertsov AM, Davidenko JM, Salomonsz R, Baxter WT, Jalife J. (1993) *Circ Res* **72**, 631-650.
2. Gray RA, Jalife J, Panfilov AV, et al. (1995) *Science* **270**, 1222-1223.
3. Wikswo JPJ, Lin SF, Abbas RA. (1995) *Biophys J* **69**, 2195-2210.
4. Pastore JM, Girouard SD, Laurita KR, Akar FG, Rosenbaum DS. (1999) *Circulation* **99**, 1385-1394.
5. Morley GE, Vaidya D, Samie FH, Lo CW, Delmar M, Jalife J. (1999) *J Cardiovasc Electrophysiol* **10**, 1361-1375.
6. Vaidya D, Morley GE, Samie FH, Jalife J. (1999) *Circ Res* **85**, 174-181.
7. Lee P, Morley G, Huang Q, et al. (1998) *Proc Natl Acad Sci USA* **95**, 11371-76.
8. Paigen K. (1995) *Nature Medicine* **1**, 215-220.
9. Lin MC, Rockman HA, Chien KR. (1995) *Nature Medicine* **1**, 749-751.
10. Yao A, Su Z, Nonaka A, et al. (1998) *Circ Res* **82**, 657-665.
11. Elvan A, Huang XD, Pressler ML, Zipes DP. (1997) *Circulation* **96**, 1675-1685.
12. van der Velden HMW, van Kempen MJ, Wijffels MC, et al. (1998) *J Cardiovasc Electrophys* **9**, 596-607.
13. Allessie MA. (1998) *J Cardiovasc Electrophys* **9**, 1378-1393.
14. London B, Jeron A, Zhou J, et al. (1998) *Proc Natl Acad Sci USA* **95**, 2926-2931.
15. Chen Q, Kirsch GE, Zhang D, et al. (1998) *Nature* **392**, 293-296.
16. Loew LM, Cohen LB, Dix J, et al. A naphthyl analog of the aminostyryl pyridinium class of potentiometric membrane dyes shows consistent sensitivity in a variety of tissue, cell and model membrane preparations. (1992) *J Membr Biol* **130**,1 –10.
17. Baxter WT, Davidenko JM, Loew LM, Wuskell JP, Jalife J. (1997) *Ann Biomed Engineer* **25**, 713-725.
18. Fast VG, Kleber AG. (1993) *Circ Res* **73**, 914-925.
19. Kivenson G. (1963) *Industrial Stroboscopy.*, Hayden Book Co., Inc.: New York
20. Chesterman WD. (1951) *The Photographic Study of Rapid Events*, Clarendon Press: Oxford
21. Gray RA, Pertsov AM, Jalife J. (1996) *Circulation* **94**, 2649-2661.
22. Ho DS, Daly M, Richards DA, Uther JB, Ross DL. (1996) *J Am Coll Cardiol* **28**, 1283-1291.
23. Bliss TV, Lomo T. (1973) *J Physiol* **232**, 331-356.
24. Noss RS, Boles CD, Yingling CD. (1996) *Electroenceph & Clin Neurophysiol* **100**, 453-461.
25. Witkowski FX, Clark RB, Larsen TS, Melnikov A, Giles WR. (1997) *Canadian Journal of Cardiology* **13**, 1077-1082.
26. Ng WA, Grupp IL, Subramaniam A, Robbins J. (1991) *Circ Res* **68**, 1742-1750.
27. Berul CI, Aronovitz MJ, Wang PJ, Mendelsohn ME. (1996) *Circulation* **94**, 2641-2648.
28. Farmer JB, Levy GP. (1968) *Br J Pharmac Chemother* **32**, 193-200.
29. Goldbarg AN, Hellerstein HK, Bruell JH, Daroczy AF. (1968) *Cardiovasc Res* **2**, 93-99.
30. Chawla KK, Harris WS. (1970) *J Electrocardiol* **3**, 317-324.
31. James JF, Hewett TE, Robbins J. (1998) *Circ Res* **82**, 407-415.
32. Christensen G, Wang Y, Chien KR. (1997) *Am J Physiol* **272**, H2513-H2524
33. Simon AM, Goodenough DA, Paul DL. (1998) *Curr Biol* **8**, 295-298.
34. Kirchhoff S, Nelles E, Hagendorff A, et al. (1998) *Curr Biol* **8**, 299-302.
35. Thomas SA, Schuessler RB, Berul CI, et al. (1998) *Circulation* **97**, 686-691.
36. Guerrero PA, Schuessler RB, Davis, LM, et al. (1997) *J Clin Invest* **99**, 1991-1998.
37. Jalife J, Gray RA, Morley GE, Davidenko J. (1998) *Chaos* **8**, 79-93.
38. Knisley SB, Hill BC. (1995) *IEEE Trans Biomed Eng* **42**, 957-966.
39. Fleet WF, Johnson TA, Cascio WE, et al. (1994) *Circulation* **90**, 3009-3017.
40. Vermeulen JT, Tan HL, Rademaker H, et al. (1996) *J Mol Cell Cardiol* **28**, 123-131.
41. Garrey WE. (1914) *Am J Physiol* **33**, 397-414.
42. Beaumont J, Davidenko N, Davidenko JM, Jalife J. (1998) *Biophys J* **75**, 1-14.

5

CONNEXINS AND CONDUCTION

Deborah L. Lerner, M.D. and Jeffrey E. Saffitz, M.D., Ph.D.

Departments of Pediatrics and Pathology, Center for Cardiovascular Research
Washington University School of Medicine, St. Louis, MO 63110

INTRODUCTION

The heart is not a true electrical syncytium. Rather, cardiac muscle is composed of individual cells each invested with an insulating lipid bilayer that would effectively prevent intercellular current flux were there not specialized cell-cell junctions to serve this purpose. In the heart, ions flow from one cell to another via gap junctions, specialized regions of the sarcolemma containing transmembrane channels that adjoin in the extracellular space to create aqueous pores that directly link the cytoplasmic compartments of neighboring cells. A gap junction consists of an array of tens to thousands of closely packed channels that permit intercellular passage of ions and small molecules up to ~1 kDa in molecular weight. Ubiquitous throughout the animal kingdom, gap junctions facilitate intercellular exchange of molecular information in virtually all multicellular tissues. They form during the earliest stages of embryonic development and are thought to play important roles in the spread of morphogens, signaling molecules and ions.

No specific genetic diseases involving gap junction proteins have yet been linked to abnormal cardiac electrophysiology. However, the cloning and sequencing of genes encoding gap junction channel proteins (connexins) has greatly advanced knowledge of the molecular structure, distribution, and potential functional specialization of gap junction channels in the heart. This chapter summarizes current understanding of the structure and function of gap junctions in the mammalian heart. It focuses primarily on the role of connexins in conduction in the normal heart, and the role of alterations in the expression, distribution and function of gap junction channel proteins in arrhythmogenesis. We also review briefly the potential roles of gap junctions in cardiac development and current knowledge about connexin gene mutations in human disease in general.

The Connexin Family of Gap Junction Proteins

Gap junction channels are formed by members of a multigene family of proteins referred to as connexins. More than a dozen unique connexins have been cloned (reviewed in 1-3). These proteins are identified using the abbreviation *Cx* for

Connexins and Conduction

connexin followed by the molecular weight of the specific protein in kiloDaltons (1). Figure 1 shows an accepted model of the structure of a gap junction, based originally on x-ray diffraction and freeze fracture electron microscopic studies of junctions isolated from hepatocyte membranes (4). An individual intercellular channel is created by stable, non-covalent interactions of two hemi-channels, referred to as connexons, each located in the plasma membrane of adjacent cells. A connexon is a multimeric structure composed of 6 integral membrane protein subunits (connexins) which surround the central aqueous pore.

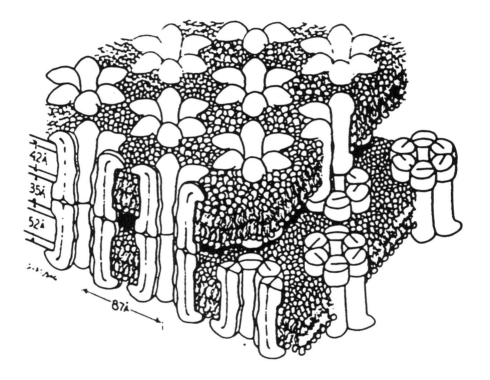

Figure 1: A model of the structure of a gap junction based on results of x-ray diffraction studies of Makowski et al. (4). Individual channels are composed of paired hexamers that traverse the membranes of adjacent cells and adjoin in the extracellular gap to form an aqueous pore that connects the cytoplasmic compartments of the two cells.

Hydropathy analysis of amino acid sequences derived from clones cDNAs combined with proteolysis studies and immunocytochemical mapping with site-specific anti-sera (5-8) have revealed the topology of connexins in the plasma membrane (Figure 2). Recently, the 3-dimensional structure of a gap junction channel formed by a specific recombinant connexin has been elucidated by electron crystallography at a resolution of 7.5Å (9). The results definitively confirm the dodecameric structure of the channel shown in Figure 1 and the connexin topology model shown in Figure 2. Based on the extent of sequence homology in critical regions within the connexin family, it is assumed that all members have 4 hydrophobic domains that span the lipid bilayer (Figure 2). The N- and C-terminal portions of the molecule and a loop connecting the second and third transmembrane domains are all hydrophilic and have been localized to the cytoplasmic side of the membrane. Two other hydrophilic regions, connecting the transmembrane domains on the extracellular face, are among the most highly conserved regions of the connexins. In contrast, the cytoplasmic loop and the C-terminal tail differ considerably among connexins in sequence and length (Figure 2). These cytoplasmic domains appear to confer specific biophysical properties on channels composed of different connexins.

Expression of Multiple Connexins in the Heart
Messenger RNAs encoding Cx37, Cx40, Cx43, Cx45, Cx46 and Cx50 have been detected in homogenates of mammalian heart muscle (10-16), but not all of these proteins are necessarily expressed by cardiac myocytes. For example, Cx37 in the heart is expressed only by coronary vascular endothelium (13). Other connexins such as Cx43 and Cx40 are expressed by both cardiac myocytes and vessel wall cells (endothelium and/or smooth muscle). The tissue distributions of Cx50 and Cx46 in the heart are poorly characterized. Cx50 has been localized to the atrioventricular valve region in the rat heart and may be expressed by an interstitial cell (14). Cx46, a protein expressed abundantly in the mammalian lens, has been detected by Northern blot analysis in homogenates of adult rat heart (15). Recent evidence suggests that this connexin may be expressed in certain specialized myocytes of the sinus node (16).

It has been unequivocally established that mammalian cardiac myocytes express Cx43, Cx45 and Cx40 but different patterns of these connexins are expressed in different tissues of the heart. The major cardiac gap junction protein Cx43 is expressed in atrial and ventricular myocytes and in the distal His-Purkinje system (17-19). Cx43 has been identified in the rabbit and canine sinus nodes (20,21), but not in bovine sinus or atrioventricular nodes (22,23). Although it is the most abundant cardiac connexin, Cx43 is expressed in numerous tissues including vascular endothelium, vascular and uterine smooth muscle, lens epithelium, fibroblasts, astrocytes, pancreatic islet cells, ovarian granulosa cells, and macrophages (24).

The distribution of Cx40 in the heart is more restricted than Cx43 (18,19,25-28). Cx40 is expressed by atrial myocytes and by the His-Purkinje fibers of the atrioventricular conduction system but not by adult ventricular myocytes. It has also been localized in at least some areas within the canine sinus node (21) and in coronary vascular endothelial cells (25). Cx45 appears to be expressed in relatively low levels in atrial myocytes and the atrioventricular conduction system of mouse and rat hearts (29). Whether it is expressed to an appreciable extent in all mammalian ventricular myocytes is not clear at the present time.

Despite uncertainties about the exact patterns of connexin expression in different tissues of the heart and possible species differences in these patterns, there is no doubt that individual cardiac myocytes express multiple proteins. For example, individual atrial myocytes and specialized myocytes in the His-Purkinje system express three gap junction channel proteins: Cx43, Cx40 and Cx45. Multilabel confocal microscopy and immuno-electron microscopy have shown that multiple connexins colocalize within gap junctions (12). Individual connexins are apparently not segregated into separate gap junctions or within subregions of individual junctions but little is known about the distribution or molecular composition of multiple connexins within gap junctions.

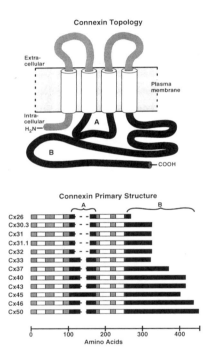

Figure 2: *Upper panel*: A model of the topology of a connexin molecule. The transmembrane domains are shown in white, the N-terminus and extracellular domains are shown in grey (hatched), and the intracellular hydrophilic loop connecting the second and third transmembrane domains (A) and the C-terminal tail (B) are shown in black. *Lower panel*: Comparison of the sequences of multiple members of the connexin family. The amino acid number begins at the N-terminus. The grey (hatched) and white segments correspond to the regions of the molecules shown in the upper panel. Divergent sequences, shown in black, are located mainly in the intracellular loop (A) and C-terminal tail (B) regions.

Heterotypic and Heteromeric Gap Junction Channels
The fact that most differentiated cells, including cardiac myocytes, express multiple connexins raises the possibility that individual channels may be composed of more than one isoform. Theoretical combinations of connexins in hybrid channels and a currently used system of nomenclature are illustrated in Figure 3. An individual connexon is referred to as homomeric if it consists of subunits of only a single type of connexin. Alternatively, a connexon composed of two or more connexin isoforms is referred to as a heteromeric connexon. The two connexons that form a single complete channel may each have an identical connexin composition and thus, create a homotypic channel. If the connexons have disparate connexin compositions, then the resultant channel is described as a heterotypic channel.

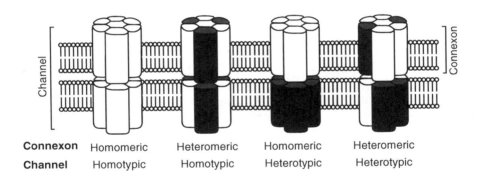

| Connexon | Homomeric | Heteromeric | Homomeric | Heteromeric |
| Channel | Homotypic | Homotypic | Heterotypic | Heterotypic |

Figure 3: Nomenclature for connexons and gap junction channels formed by 1 or more connexins. Modified from Kumar and Gilula (99).

Little is known at the present time about the natural occurrence or biological significance of hybrid channels in the heart or other differentiated tissues. It is clear, however, based largely on transfection studies in "communication deficient" cells, that various pairs of connexins can combine to form functional channels that exhibit distinct biophysical properties. With regards to potential formation of hybrid channels by connexins that are naturally expressed in the heart, it appears that homomeric Cx40 connexons cannot form functional heterotypic channels with homomeric Cx43 connexons (30-32), but Cx40 and Cx43 may form heteromeric connexons (33). Recent evidence suggests that Cx43 and Cx45 can form both heteromeric connexons and homomeric, heterotypic channels (34,35). These findings have potential implications for intercellular coupling in regions of the heart such as sinus node-atrial myocyte junctions or Purkinje fiber-ventricular myocyte junctions in which pairs of coupled cells may express different connexin phenotypes. Although the occurrence and biological significance of hybrid channels in naturally occurring tissues have not been elucidated, it is likely that hybrid channels exist in nature. Indeed, multiple connexins may have evolved to enhance fine control of intercellular communication and perhaps to establish preferential communication pathways and/or boundaries within complex multicellular structures. It should be stressed, however, that the functional significance, if any, of hybrid channels in normal cardiac physiology or pathophysiology is unknown at the present time.

Biophysical Properties of Cardiac Gap Junction Channels and Their Regulation
In general, naturally occurring gap junction channels in cardiac myocytes exhibit a range of properties that likely reflects both the diversity of single channel types and potential post-translational modifications such as connexin phosphorylation. Much of what is known about the functional properties of single gap junction channels has come from studies of homomeric, homotypic channels produced by transfection of "communication-deficient" cells. Results of these studies have demonstrated that channels formed by individual connexins exhibit distinct biophysical properties including unitary conductances, pH dependence and voltage-dependence (36). Homomeric, homomeric channels formed by the cardiac connexins are relatively non-selective. They all allow passage of ions and small molecules such as fluorescent dyes. There are differences, however, in their permeability to anions and cations, their abilities to pass fluorescent dyes of different sizes and charge densities, the degree of cytoplasmic acidification required to achieve channel closure and their sensitivity to lipophilic uncoupling agents (36).

  Cx43 channels are less sensitive to changes in transjunctional voltage than channels composed of Cx40, Cx45 or Cx37 (36,37). Main conductance states measured in Cx43 channels range from 90 to 115 pS (36-38). Mammalian Cx40 and its avian homolog, Cx42, form channels with larger conductances (150 to160 pS) than Cx43 channels (39-41), whereas Cx45 channels exhibit a considerably lower main state conductance (~25 pS) and are highly sensitive to transjunctional voltage (36,42). Studies by Delmar and colleagues have identified specific residues in Cx43 that appear to play a key role in pH gating of the channels (43,44). Results of transfection studies suggest that pH gating of Cx43 channels is mediated by a particle-receptor interaction in which the carboxy terminus acts as a gating particle that can bind non-covalently to a receptor domain, perhaps in the intracellular loop and, thereby, lead to channel closure in response to acidification (44).

Mechanisms regulating gap junctional coupling are incompletely understood but considerable attention has been focused recently on the role of connexin phosphorylation. Phosphorylation of both Cx43 and Cx45 affects channel function and possibly channel assembly in gap junctions (38,45-48). Changes in Cx43 phosphorylation have been found to affect both macroscopic junctional currents and single channel behavior in neonatal rat ventricular myocytes and other cells. Cx43 mutants with progressive deletions of the carboxy terminus form channels with different unitary conductances (49), in keeping with the hypothesis that this portion of the protein is a principal determinant of unitary conductance. However, deletion of all putative phosphorylation sites from Cx43 does not prevent formation of functional channels (50). The abundance of different phosphorylated forms of Cx43 has also been correlated with the assembly of gap junctional plaques (48). Less is known about the functional implications of different phosphorylated isoforms of Cx45. A recent study has shown, however, that mutation of specific serine residues in Cx45 has a significant impact on its turnover kinetics (51).

Changes in the intracellular milieu play an important role in regulating intercellular coupling under both physiological and pathophysiological conditions. Channel conductance properties change in response to exogenous cyclic nucleotides and other signaling molecules. The specific signal transduction pathways responsible for these changes have not been elucidated in detail. Many of these effects may ultimately be mediated by changes in phosphorylation. Gap junction channels close in response to increasing levels of intracellular Ca^{2+} and H^+ which act synergistically to promote uncoupling (52,53). Intracellular concentrations of these ions required to fully uncouple cells are probably achieved only under conditions of severe injury. Gap junction channel function is also modulated by fatty acids and lipid metabolites of ischemia which may contribute to uncoupling during early stages of myocardial infarction (54-56).

Rapid Turnover of Connexins in the Heart
Both Cx43 and Cx45 turn over rapidly ($t_{1/2}$ ~2-3 hours) in cultured neonatal rat ventricular myocytes (46,57). Recent work has demonstrated that Cx43 also turns over rapidly ($t_{1/2}$ ~1.3 hours) in isolated, perfused adult rat hearts analyzed as determined in metabolic labeling and pulse-chase experiments (58). Rapid turnover of protein in junctions may provide a mechanism by which cells adjust their levels of intercellular coupling. Interventions that affect connexin turnover could facilitate remodeling of conduction pathways and have significant consequences regarding the relative and total amounts of individual connexin proteins present in myocytes.

Studies of connexin degradation in cultured cells, including cardiac myocytes, have demonstrated that Cx43 is degraded by both endosomal and proteasomal proteolysis pathways (59,60). Both pathways also appear to be responsible for Cx43 degradation in the adult rat heart (58). It has been reported that inhibition of endosomal proteolysis in the rat heart leads to the accumulation of phosphorylated

Cx43, whereas inhibition of proteasomal degradation causes non-phosphorylated Cx43 to accumulate (58). These observations are consistent with previous studies suggesting that changes in connexin phosphorylation patterns play an important role in targeting proteins for degradation.

Functional Implications of Expression of Multiple Connexins in the Heart

Expression of multiple connexins by different cardiac tissues raises major questions about the specific functional roles of individual connexins in the heart and the potential biological purposes fulfilled by expression of multiple gap junction channel proteins. Insights into these questions have been revealed recently in studies of mouse models in which connexin expression has been manipulated by gene targeting strategies. In 1995, Reaume et al. (61) reported that targeted deletion of the gene encoding Cx43 results in neonatal death due to a complex malformation of the conotruncal region of the heart. Interestingly, similar malformations have been observed in transgenic mice in which cardiac neural crest cells were selectively targeted to either overexpress Cx43 or express a dominant negative Cx43 construct (62,63). Thus, disturbances in intercellular communication resulting in either gain or loss of function in critical tissues during development can lead to similar types of cardiac malformations.

Because mice with targeted deletion of Cx43 (Cx43$^{-/-}$) die as neonates, it has been difficult to analyze whole heart electrophysiology in these animals. However, heterozygotes (Cx43$^{+/-}$ mice) exhibit modest slowing of ventricular conduction, which appears to be attributable solely to diminished expression of Cx43 (64). It has also been reported that atrial conduction velocity is not slowed in Cx43$^{+/-}$ mice compared with wildtype controls even though both ventricular and atrial tissues normally express abundant Cx43 and its expression in Cx43$^{+/-}$ mice is diminished by ~50% in both tissues (65). Thus, it appears that Cx43 is a major coupling protein in ventricular but not atrial muscle. Recently, two groups have independently created mouse models with targeted deletion of the Cx40 gene (66,67). Phenotypes in Cx40$^{-/-}$ mice include sinoatrial, intra-atrial and atrioventricular conduction disturbances and increased vulnerability to induction of atrial arrhythmias (66-68). These findings suggest that Cx40 plays an important role as a coupling protein in tissues in which it is expressed. Nevertheless, there may be considerable redundancy in the specificity of functions fulfilled by different connexins. In a recent preliminary report (69), no overt abnormalities in cardiac structure or function were observed in mice in which the liver gap junction protein, Cx32, was substituted for one or both Cx43 alleles. With anticipated development and analysis of additional mouse models, the specific functional roles of individual connexins in normal cardiac physiology and arrhythmogenesis will be defined in detail.

Gap Junction Distributions in the Heart

Because intercellular current transfer is possible only at points where two cells share gap junctions, it follows that the number and spatial distribution of gap junctions must be important determinants of current spread in myocardium. This conclusion is supported by elucidation of distinct patterns of intercellular electrical connections in the left ventricle and the crista terminalis, two cardiac tissues with different conduction velocities and degrees of anisotropy. In ventricular muscle, longitudinal conduction velocities are typically 0.6 to 0.7 m/s and transverse velocities are ~0.2 m/s, yielding an anisotropy ratio of roughly 3:1 (70,71). Immunohistochemical studies of ventricular myocytes have shown that although many gap junctions are typically found at or near the ends of the cells where the largest intercalated disks are located, they may reside at various points on the cell surface. (Figure 4). The presence of junctions along the entire length of the cell provides opportunities for ventricular myocytes to be electrically coupled in complex three-dimensional patterns in which individual cells are connected to many neighbors in varying degrees of end-to-end and side-to-side apposition.

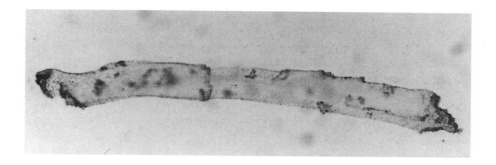

Figure 4: An isolated canine left ventricular myocyte stained with an anti-gap junction channel protein antibody to delineate the distribution of gap junctions on the cell surface. The largest gap junctions are concentrated at the ends of the cell but numerous smaller junctions arise at various points along the length of the cell. From Luke et al. (100).

Morphometric studies have revealed that an individual ventricular myocyte is interconnected to an average of 11.3 neighbors (Figure 5) (28). Approximately half of the attached neighbors are connected in a purely or predominantly side-to-side orientation (referred to as type I and type II connections, respectively, as illustrated in Figure 5) and the remaining half are connected in a purely or mainly end-to-end fashion (type III and type IV connections). This pattern of intercellular connections is consistent with the moderate degree of anisotropy typical of ventricular conduction. Activation wavefronts moving through a sheet of ventricular myocardium have numerous opportunities to propagate across intercellular junctions in both longitudinal and transverse directions. Because of the elongated shape of the cells, however, wavefronts traveling in the transverse direction must cross more intercellular junctions per unit distance traveled and, therefore, would encounter greater resistance and propagate more slowly than wavefronts traveling an equal distance in the longitudinal direction. Accordingly, anisotropy of conduction in the ventricle appears to be determined primarily by the shape of the myocytes rather than by an anisotropic distribution of intercellular junctions.

Compared with ventricular muscle, conduction in the crista terminalis, a discrete bundle of atrial myocardium that conducts impulses from the sinus node to the AV junction, is rapid (~1 m/s) and highly anisotropic. The ratio of longitudinal to transverse conduction velocity in the crista may be as high as 10:1 compared with only 3:1 in the ventricle (72). Whereas ventricular myocytes are connected on average to 11.3 neighbors, individual myocytes of the crista terminalis are connected to an average of only 6.4 neighbors (Figure 5), but the great majority of these interconnections occur between cells oriented in end-to-end apposition.

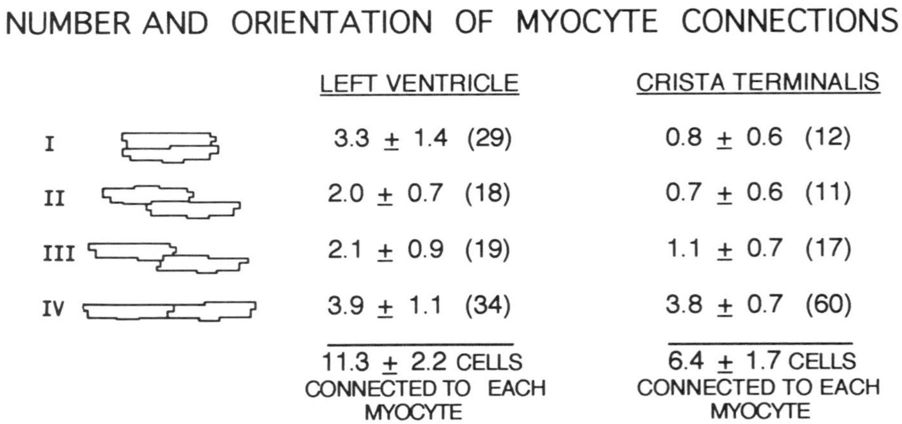

NUMBER AND ORIENTATION OF MYOCYTE CONNECTIONS

		LEFT VENTRICLE	CRISTA TERMINALIS
I		3.3 ± 1.4 (29)	0.8 ± 0.6 (12)
II		2.0 ± 0.7 (18)	0.7 ± 0.6 (11)
III		2.1 ± 0.9 (19)	1.1 ± 0.7 (17)
IV		3.9 ± 1.1 (34)	3.8 ± 0.7 (60)
		11.3 ± 2.2 CELLS CONNECTED TO EACH MYOCYTE	6.4 ± 1.7 CELLS CONNECTED TO EACH MYOCYTE

Figure 5: Diagram of the number and spatial orientation of cellular connections in canine left ventricle and crista terminalis. The numbers in parentheses indicate the percentages of each type of interconnection. Data are expressed as mean ± standard deviation, and asterisks indicate significant differences (p<0.01) between numbers of connections of each type in the ventricle and crista terminalis. From Saffitz et al. (28).

Nearly 80% of the interconnections in the crista terminalis occur between myocytes juxtaposed in a purely or mainly end-to-end orientation (type III and IV connections).

This pattern is clearly demonstrated in immunohistochemical preparations (Figure 6). Based on this morphometric analysis, it seems likely that transverse propagation in the crista terminalis would be impeded by the relative paucity of connections between cells in side-to-side apposition and the resultant increase in resistance to current propagation in the transverse direction. Highly anisotropic and rapid longitudinal conduction velocity may also be facilitated by more limited electrotonic spread (dissipation) of current in the transverse direction in the crista. Rapid conduction in the crista could also be related to the presence of high conductance Cx40 channels in atrial but not ventricular myocardium.

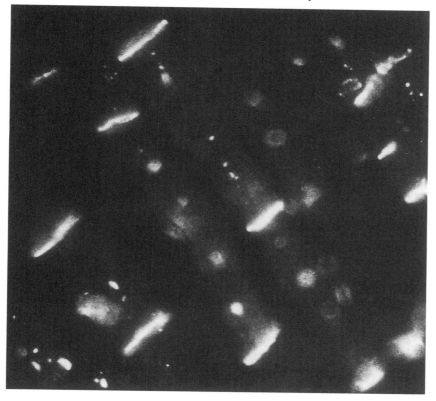

Figure 6: Section of canine crista terminalis stained with antibody against Cx43. Signal occurs almost exclusively at the end of cells. From Saffitz et al. (28).

Developmental Changes in Connexin Expression and Gap Junction Distribution
Increasing evidence, first described in Northern blot studies in the developing chick heart (10) and more recently in immunohistochemical studies in the mouse heart (73,74), suggests that cardiac connexin expression may be developmentally regulated. Both Cx40 and Cx45 are expressed during early stages of cardiac morphogenesis (8.5 dpc for Cx45 in the mouse heart) but then undergo spatiotemporal down-regulation that ultimately restricts the amount and distribution of these proteins in the adult heart (73,74). It is not known whether a similar pattern of regulation occurs in the human heart, nor are the functional consequences of this regulatory sequence apparent. It should be noted however, that Cx40-null mice exhibit no apparent cardiac malformations (66,67) whereas Cx43-null animals have defects involving cardiac neural crest derivatives (61).

In addition to potential developmental changes in the levels of connexin expression in the heart, the distribution of gap junctions in fetal and neonatal ventricular myocytes is strikingly different than that observed in myocytes of the adult ventricle (14,17,75). Neonatal ventricular myocytes are interconnected by numerous tiny, punctate gap junctions and fascia adherens junctions distributed uniformly over the cell surface. With post-natal maturation, there is progressive redistribution of both gap junctions and fascia adherens components of the intercalated disk toward the adult pattern in which large junctions at or near the ends of the cells are associated with large intercalated disks. In the human heart, this transition is not completed until approximately 6 years of age (75). A similar transition in the distribution of ventricular myocyte gap junction occurs in the rat heart (14,17).

The electrophysiological significance of different gap junction distributions at different developmental stages is unclear. Changes in gap junction distribution may help account for the observation that the interval required to depolarize the ventricles increases by only ~20% during a period of rapid growth in which heart weight increases by 16-fold (76). Redistribution of gap junctions may underlie age-related increases in conduction velocity in Purkinje fibers (77) and enhanced anisotropy in atrial muscle (78). It has also been suggested that the neonatal pattern may play a role in both hyperplastic and hypertrophic cardiac growth and help the heart maintain its overall geometry and contractile function during an interval of rapid enlargement (75).

Altered Connexin Expression and Gap Junction Distributions in Heart Disease
Alterations in connexin expression patterns, channel function and gap junction distributions probably contribute importantly to the pathogenesis of heart disease but much remains to be learned about disease mechanisms involving gap junctions. No known mutations in connexin genes have yet been identified in patients with electrophysiological abnormalities. Mutations in the gene encoding Cx43 involving putative phosphorylation sites have been reported, although not confirmed, in children with cardiac malformations characterized by disturbances in the normal

left-right asymmetry of the heart (visceroatrial heterotaxy syndromes) (79). Mutations in other connexins associated with specific non-cardiac disease states have also been delineated recently. For example, mutations in Cx32, a protein expressed in the liver but also in Schwann cells which are responsible for myelinating peripheral nerves, have been implicated in the pathogenesis of X-linked Charcot-Marie-Tooth disease (80), a form of hereditary neuropathy with demyelination. Mutations in Cx26, another protein expressed abundantly in the liver but also in other sites such as the inner ear, have been identified in kindreds affected by non-syndromic forms of hereditary deafness (81). And, mutations in the lens protein Cx50 have been implicated in the development of cataracts (82).

Although there is probably not a direct genetic basis underlying altered intercellular coupling in most forms of heart disease, both acute and chronic myocardial responses to injury may be associated with pathophysiologically relevant alterations in cell-cell communication. Changes in the amount of connexin expression and the distribution of gap junctions occur in several forms of heart disease. The functional implications of these changes have not been elucidated in detail but it is likely that these changes affect the anisotropy of conduction and potentially alter the spatial and temporal coordination of electrical activation in the heart. Altered coupling may also have important implications for cardiac metabolism and contractile function.

Studies in vitro and in vivo suggest that compensatory hypertrophic growth may be associated with increased connexin levels, increased numbers of gap junctions, and enhanced intercellular coupling. For example, long-term (24 hours) exposure of neonatal rat ventricular myocyte cultures to cAMP increases the tissue content of Cx43 by approximately 2-fold and increases the number of gap junctions interconnecting the cells (83). These changes are associated with a significant increase in conduction velocity without apparent changes in active membrane properties (83). Remodeling of conduction pathways during early, compensatory responses to increased load in vivo may also be an active process involving enhanced connexin expression and rearrangements of gap junction distributions. For example, connexin expression is enhanced during early stages of hypertrophy induced by renovascular hypertension in guinea pigs (84). Bastide et al. (25) have shown that expression of Cx40 is enhanced in Purkinje fibers of the rat when hypertrophy is induced by hypertension.

The hypertrophic response is a dynamic continuum in which progressive changes in gene expression and the structure of cells and extracellular matrix may mediate the transition from a phase of compensated structural and functional adaptation to an increasingly maladaptive state culminating in heart failure. Conduction velocity first increases in hypertrophied ventricles but then decreases as hypertrophy becomes more severe (85-87). Ventricular conduction delay, often reflected as prolongation of the QRS interval in the surface electrocardiogram, is a general feature of chronic left ventricular hypertrophy in man. Decrements in conduction velocity may be related to increases in extracellular resistance caused by interstitial fibrosis (88) and increases in intercellular resistance due to decreased connexin expression (89-92).

Recently, it has been demonstrated by immunohistochemistry that Cx43 expression is reduced in segments of "hibernating" myocardium in patients with chronic ischemic heart disease (92). Interestingly, the reduced gap junction protein expression appears to be attributable mainly to a loss of the larger gap junctions normally seen at the major intercalated disks at the ends of cells (92). These results and others suggest that reduced gap junction channel protein levels occur as a general rule in chronic myocardial disease states including healed myocardial infarction (89,90), chronic hibernation (92), end-stage disease in chronic aortic stenosis (89), and even with aging (78,88). Little is known about whether expression of multiples connexins is affected differentially in disease states. A recent study has reported, however, that Cx40 expression in the atria is selectively down-regulated in a spatially heterogeneous pattern in an experimental models of chronic, pacing-induced atrial fibrillation in goats (93).

Links Between Changes in Gap Junction Distribution and Arrhythmogenesis
The best studied disease setting in which alterations in gap junction distribution have been closely linked to reentrant arrhythmias is myocardial infarct healing. During the inflammatory and reparative phases of infarct healing, viable myocytes at the edges of the infarct scar develop complex structural alterations involving both cardiac myocytes and the extracellular matrix. A common pattern of structural alteration in peri-infarct tissue is accumulation of interstitial bundles of collagen oriented parallel to the long axis of groups of cardiac myocytes (94-96). This "substrate" has been observed in regions identified by activation mapping to be sites of slow conduction, conduction block, and complex fractionated electrograms (94-97). Ultrastructural measurements in a healed canine left ventricular infarct model have shown that epicardial border zone myocytes in bundles separated by interspersed collagen are connected by smaller gap junctions than normal myocytes (98). Furthermore, the number of cells connected to a single canine ventricular myocyte is reduced by nearly half in epicardial border zone regions but the loss of intercellular connections does not occur in a spatially uniform distribution (98). In fact, the mean number of border zone myocytes connected to one another in side-to-side configuration is reduced by 75% whereas connections between epicardial border zone cells in end-to-end orientation are reduced by only 22% (98). The predicted pathophysiological consequences of these structural alterations are consistent with observations made in both experimental animals and human arrhythmia mapping studies. Longitudinal propagation through remodeled regions would be expected to remain relatively rapid because end-to-end connections are preserved. Ventricular tachycardia is typically induced and maintained when wavefronts activate these critical regions in a direction transverse to the long myocyte axis (94-96). Macroscopic propagation in the transverse direction is likely to be impaired because side-to-side connections are selectively disrupted and wavefronts are forced to zig-zag through the tissue (96) until they reenter post-

refractory tissue and initiate the next beat of the tachycardia. The complex pathways followed by such wavefronts probably account for the slow, heterogeneous conduction properties and the presence of fractionated electrograms and late ("diastolic") potentials in border zone regions (91,94-96).

It has been clearly demonstrated that adult cardiac myocytes bordering regions of acute infarction undergo dramatic rearrangement of their gap junctions in which multiple, small junctions become uniformly dispersed over the cell surface (90,91). This pattern strikingly similar to that observed in early development (75). Thus, it appears that in response to near-lethal injury at the immediate edges of ischemic infarcts, myocytes recapitulate the fetal pattern of gap junctions, perhaps in a manner analogous to the re-expression of fetal isoforms of some contractile proteins and enzymes during induction of the hypertrophic response. The responsible mechanisms have not been defined nor have the functional consequences of this striking pattern change been elucidated directly. However, strong circumstantial evidence links this pattern to regions of abnormal conduction critical to the pathogenesis of reentrant ventricular tachycardia (91,94-96). Dynamic changes in both connexin synthesis and degradation probably play a role in this process.

REFERENCES

1. Beyer EC, Paul DL, Goodenough DA. Connexin family of gap junction proteins. *J Membr Biol* 116:187-194, 1990.

2. Willecke K, Hennemann H, Dahl E, Jungbluth S, Heynkes R. The diversity of connexin genes encoding gap junction proteins. *Eur J Cell Biol* 56:1-7, 1991.

3. Kumar NM, Gilula NB. Molecular biology and genetics of gap junction channels. *Sem Cell Biol* 3:3-16, 1992.

4. Makowski L, Caspar LDL, Phillips WC, Goodenough DA. Gap junction structures. II: Analysis of the x-ray diffraction data. *J Cell Biol* 74:629-645, 1976.

5. Beyer EC, Kistler J, Paul DL, Goodenough DA. Antisera directed against connexin43 peptides react with a 43-kD protein localized to gap junctions in myocardium and other tissues. *J Cell Biol* 108:595-605, 1989.

6. Yancey SB, John SA, Lal R, Austin BJ, Revel J-P. The 43-kD polypeptide of heart gap junctions: immunolocalization, topology, and functional domains. *J Cell Biol* 108:2241-2254, 1989.

7. Laird DW, Revel J-P. Biochemical and immunochemical analysis of the arrangement of connexin43 in rat heart gap junction membranes. *J Cell Science* 97:109-117, 1990.

8. Yeager M, Gilula NB. Membrane topology and quaternary structure of cardiac gap junction ion channels. *J Mol Biol* 223:929-948, 1992.

9. Unger VM, Kumar NM, Gilula NB, Yeager M. Three-dimensional structure of a recombinant gap junction membrane channel. *Science* 283:1176-1180, 1999.

10. Beyer EC. Molecular cloning and developmental expression of two chick embryo gap junction proteins. *J Biol Chem* 265:14439-14443, 1990.

11. Kanter HL, Saffitz JE, Beyer EC. Cardiac myocytes express multiple gap junction proteins. *Circ Res* 70:438-444, 1992.

12. Kanter HL, Laing JG, Beyer EC, Green KG, Saffitz JE. Multiple connexins colocalize in canine ventricular myocyte gap junctions. *Circ Res* 73:344-350, 1993.

13. Reed KE, Westphale EM, Larson DM, Wang HZ, Veenstra RD, Beyer EC. Molecular cloning and functional expression of human connexin37,an endothelial cell gap junction protein.*J Clin Invest* 91:997-1004, 1993.

14. Gourdie RG, Green CR, Severs NJ, Thompson RP. Immunolabeling patterns of gap junction connexins in the developing and mature rat heart. *Anat Embryol* 185:363-378, 1992.

15. Paul DL, Ebihara L, Takemoto LJ, Swenson KI, Goodenough DA. Connexin46, a novel lens gap junction protein, induces voltage-gated currents innonjunctional plasma membrane of Xenopus oocytes. J Cell Biol 115:1077-1089, 1991.

16. Verheule S. Distribution and physiology of mammalian cardiac gap junctions. Doctoral Thesis, University of Utrecht, 1999.

17. van Kempen MJ, Fromaget C, Gross D, Moorman AF, Lamers WH. Spatial distribution of connexin43, the major cardiac gap junction protein, in the developing and adult rat heart.*Circ Res* 68:1638-1651, 1991.

18. Kanter HL, Laing JG, Beau SL, Beyer EC, Saffitz JE. Distinct patterns of connexin expression in canine Purkinje fibers and ventricular muscle. *Circ Res* 72:1124-1131, 1993.

19. Davis LM, Kanter HL, Beyer EC, Saffitz JE. Distinct gap junction protein phenotypes in cardiac tissues with disparate conduction properties. *J Am Coll Cardiol* 24:1124-1132, 1994.

20. Anumonwo JMB, Wang H-Z, Trabka-Janik E, Dunham B, Veenstra RD, Delmar M, Jalife J. Gap junctional channels in adult mammalian sinus nodal cells: Immunolocalization and electrophysiology. *Circ Res* 71:229-239, 1992.

21. Kwong KF, Schuessler RB, Green KG, Boineau JP, Saffitz JE. Differential expression of gap junction proteins in the canine sinus node. *Circ Res* 82:604-612, 1998.

22. Oosthoek PW, Viragh S, Mayen AEM, van Kempen MJA, Lamers WH, Moorman AFM. Immunohistochemical delineation of the conduction system. I. The sinoatrial node. *Circ Res* 73:473-481, 1993.

23. Oosthoek PW, Viragh S, Lamers WH, Moorman AFM. Immunohistochemical delineation of the conduction system. The atrioventricular node and the Purkinje fibers. *Circ Res* 73:482-91, 1993.

24. Goodenough DA, Goliger JA, Paul DL. Connexins, connexons, and intercellular communication. *Annu Rev Biochem* 65:475-502, 1996.

25. Bastide B, Neyses L, Ganten D, Paul M, Willecke F, Traub O. Gap junction protein connexin40 is preferentially expressed in vascular endothelium and conductive bundles of rat myocardium and is increased under hypertensive conditions. *Circ Res* 73:1138-1149, 1993.

26. Gros D, Jarry-Guichard T, Ten Velde I, de Maziere A, van Kempen JA, Davoust J, Briand JP, Moorman AFM, Jongsma HJ. Restricted distribution of connexin40, a gap junctional protein, in mammalian heart. *Circ Res* 74:839-851, 1994.

27. Gourdie RG, Severs NJ, Green CR, Rothery S, Germroth P, Thompson RP. The spatial distribution and relative abundance of gap-junctional connexin40 and connexin43 correlate to functional properties of components of the cardiac atrioventricular conduction system.*J Cell Sci* 105:985-991, 1993.

28. Saffitz JE, Kanter HL, Green KG, Tolley TK, Beyer EC. Tissue-specific determinants of anisotropic conduction velocity in canine atrial and ventricular myocardium.*Circ Res* 74:1065-1070, 1994.

29. Coppen SR, Dupont E, Rothery S, Severs NJ. Connexin45 expression is preferentially associated with the ventricular conduction system in mouse and rat heart. *Circ Res* 82:232-243, 1998.

30. Bruzzone R, Haefliger JA, Gimlich RL, Paul DL. Connexin40, a component of gap junctions in vascular endothelium, is restricted in its ability to interact with other connexins.*Mol Biol Cell* 4:7-20, 1993.

31. White TW, Paul DL, Goodenough DA, Bruzzone R. Functional analysis of selective interactions among rodent connexins. *Mol Biol Cell* 6:459-470, 1995.

32. Elfgang C, Eckert R, Lichtenberg-Frate H, et al. Specific permeability and selective formation of gap junction channels in connexin-transfected HeLa cells. *J Cell Biol* 129:805-817k 1995.

33. He DS, Burt JM. Function of gap junction channels formed in cells co-expressing connexin40 and 43. In: Gap Junctions, R Werner (Ed.). Amsterdam: IOS Press, 1998, pp. 40-44.

34. Moreno AP, Fishman GI, Beyer EC, Spray DC. Voltage dependent gating and single channel analysis of heterotypic channels formed by Cx45 and Cx43. *Prog Cell Res* 4:405-408, 1995.

35. Koval M, Geist ST, Westphale EM, Kemendy EM, Civitelli R, Beyer EC, Steinberg TH. Transfected connexin45 alters gap junction permeability in cells expressing endogenous connexin43. *J Cell Biol* 130:987-995, 1944

36. Veenstra RD. Size and selectivity of gap junction channels formed from different connexins. *J Bioenerg Biomembr* 28:317-337, 1996.

37. Brink PR, Ramanan SV, Christ GJ. Human connexin43 gap junction channelgating: evidence for mode shifts and/or heterogeneity. *Am J Physiol* 271:C321-C331, 1996.

38. Moreno AP, Fishman GI, Spray DC. Phosphorylation shifts unitary conductance and modifies voltage dependent kinetics of human connexin43 gap junction channels. *Biophys J* 62:51-53, 1992.

39. Beblo DA, Wang H-Z, Beyer EC, Westphale EM, Veenstra RD. Unique conductance, gating, and selective permeability properties of gap junction channels formed by connexin40. *Circ Res* 77:813-822, 1995.

40. Bukauskas FF, Elfgang C, Willecke K, Weingart R. Biophysical properties of gap junction channels formed by mouse connexin40 in induced pairs of transfected human HeLa cells. *Biophys J* 68:2289-2298, 1995.

41. Beblo DA, Veenstra RD. Monovalent cation permeation through the connexin40 gap junction channel. Cs, Rb, K, Na, Li, TEA, TNA, TBA and effects of anions Br, Cl, F, acetate, aspartate, glutamate, and NO_3. *J Gen Physiol* 104:509-522, 1997.

42. Veenstra RD, Wang H-Z, Beyer EC, Brink PR. Selective dye and ionic permeability of gap junction channels formed by connexin45. *Circ Res* 75:483-490, 1994.

43. Ek JF, Delmar M, Perzova R, Taffet SM. Role of histidine95 on pH gating of the cardiac gap junction protein connexin43. *Circ Res* 74:1058-1064, 1994.

44. Calero G, Kanemitsu M, Taffet SM, Lair AF, Delmar M. A 17mer peptide interferes with acidification-induced uncoupling of connexin43. *Circ Res* 82:929-935, 1998.

45. Moreno AP, Sáez JC, Fishman GI, Spray DC. Human connexin43 gap junction channels - Regulation of unitary conductances by phosphorylation. *Circ Res* 74:1050-1057, 1994.

46. Laird DW, Puranam KL, Revel JP. Turnover and phosphorylation dynamics of connexin43 gap junction protein in cultured cardiac myocytes. *Biochem J* 273:67-72, 1993.

47. Lau AP, Hatch Pigott V, Crow DS. Evidence that heart connexin43 is aphosphoprotein. *J Mol Cell Cardiol* 23:659-663, 1991.

48. Musil LS, Goodenough DA. Biochemical analysis of connexin43 intracellular transport, phosphorylation, and assembly into gap junctional plaques. *J Cell Biol* 115:1357-1374, 1991.

49. Fishman GI, Moreno AP, Spray DC, Leinwand LA. Functional analysis of human cardiac gap junction channel mutants. *Proc Natl Acad Sci USA* 88:3525-3529, 1991.

50. Lash JA, Critser BS, Pressler ML. Cloning of gap junctional protein from vascular smooth muscle and expression in two-cell mouse embryos. *J Biol Chem* 265:13113-13117, 1990.

51. Hertlein B, Butterweck A, Haubrich S, Willecke K, Traub O. Phosphorylated carboxyl terminal serine residues stabilize the mouse gap junction protein connexin45 against degradation. *J Membrane Biol* 162:247-257, 1998.

52. Burt JM. Block of intercellular communication: interaction of intracellular H^+ and Ca^{2+}. *Am J Physiol* 352:C607-C612, 1987.

53. White RL, Doeller JE, Verselis VK, Wittenberg BA. Gap junctional conductance between pairs of ventricular myocytes is modulated synergistically by H^+ and Ca^{++}. *J Gen Physiol* 95:1061-1075, 1990.

54. Burt JM, Massey KD, Minnich BN. Uncoupling of cardiac cells by fatty acids: Structure-activity

relationship. *Am J Physiol* 260:C439-C448, 1991.

55.   Hirschi KK, Minnich BN, Moore LK, Burt JM. Oleic acid differentially affects gap-junction mediated communication in heart and vascular smooth muscle cells. *Am J Physiol* 265:C1517-C1526, 1993.

56.   Wu J, McHowat J, Saffitz JE, Yamada KA, Corr PB. Inhibition of gap junctional conductance by long-chain acylcarnitines and their preferential accumulation in junctional sarcolemma during hypoxia. *Circ Res* 72:879-89, 1993.

57.   Darrow BJ, Laing JG, Lampe PD, Saffitz JE, Beyer EC. Expression of multiple connexins in cultured neonatal rat ventricular myocytes. *Circ Res* 76:381-387, 1995.

58.   Beardslee MA, Laing JG, Beyer EC, Saffitz JE. Rapid turnover of connexin43 in the adult rat heart. *Circ Res* 83:629-635, 1998.

59.   Laing JG, Beyer EC. The gap junction protein connexin43 is degraded via the ubiquitin proteasome pathway. *J Biol Chem* 270:26399-26403, 1995.

60.   Laing JG, Tadros PN, Green K, Saffitz JE, Beyer EC. Proteolysis of connexin43-containing gap junctions in normal and heat-stressed cardiac myocytes. *Cardiovasc Res* 38:711-718, 1998.

61.   Reaume AG, de Sousa PA, Kulkarni S, et al. Cardiac malformation in neonatal mice lacking connexin43. *Science* 267:1831-1834, 1995.

62.   Ewart JL, Cohen MF, Meyer RA, et al. Heart and neural tube defects in transgenic mice overexpressing the Cx43 gap junction gene. *Development* 124:1281-1292, 1997.

63.   Huang GY, Wessels A, Smith BR, Linask KK, Ewart JL, Lo CW. Alteration in connexin43 gap junction gene dosage impairs conotruncal heart development. *Develop Biol* 198:32-44, 1998.

64.   Guerrero PA, Schuessler RB, Davis LM, Beyer EC, Johnson CM, Yamada KA, Saffitz JE. Slow ventricular conduction in mice heterozygous for a Cx43 null mutation. *J Clin Invest* 99:1991-1998, 1997.

65.   Thomas SA, Schuessler RB, Berul CI, Beardslee MA, Beyer EC, Mendelsohn ME, Saffitz JE. Disparate effects of deficient expression of connexin43 on atrial and ventricular conduction: Evidence for chamber-specific molecular determinants of conduction. *Circulation* 97:686-691, 1998.

66.   Kirchhoff S, Nelles E, Hagendorff A, Krüger O, Traub O, Willecke K. Reduced cardiac conduction velocity and predisposition to arrhythmias in connexin40-deficient mice. *Curr Biol* 8:299-302, 1998.

67.   Simon AM, Goodenough DA, Paul DL. Mice lacking connexin40 have cardiac conduction abnormalities characteristic of atrioventricular block and bundle branch block. *Curr Biol* 8:295-298, 1998.

68.   Hagendorff A, Schumacher B, Kirchoff S, Lüderitz B, Willecke K. Conduction disturbances and increased atrial vulnerability in connexin40-deficient mice analyzed by transesophageal stimulation. *Circulation* 99:1508-1515, 1999.

69.   Schumacher B, Hagendorff A, Plum A, Willecke K, Jung W, Lüderitz B. Electrophysiological effects of connexin43-replacement by connexin32 in transgeneous mice. *PACE* 22:858, 1999 (Abstract).

70.   Draper MH, Mya-Tu M. A comparison of the conduction velocity in cardiac tissue of various mammals. *Q J Exp Physiol* 44:91-109, 1959.

71.   Kadish AH, Shinnar M, Moore EN, Levine JH, Balke CW, Spear JF. Interaction of fiber orientation and direction of impulse propagation with anatomic barriers in anisotropic canine myocardium. *Circulation* 78:1478-1494, 1988.

72.   Spach MS, Miller WT, Geselowitz DB, Barr RC, Kootsey JM, Johnson EA. The discontinuous nature of propagation in normal canine cardiac muscle. Evidence for recurrent discontinuities of intracellular resistance that affect the membrane currents. *Circ Res* 48:39-54, 1981.

73.   Delorme B, Dahl E, Jarry-Guichard T, Briand J-P, Willecke K, Gros D, Théveniau-Ruissy M. Expression pattern of connexin gene products at the early developmental stages of the mouse cardiovascular system. *Circ Res* 81:423-437, 1997.

74. Alcoléa S, Théveniau-Ruissy M, Jarry-Guichard T, Marics I, Tzouanacou E, Chauvin J-P, Briand J-P, Moorman AFM, Lamers WH, Gros DB. Downregulation of connexin 45 gene products during mouse heart development. *Circ Res* 84:1365-1379, 1999.

75. Peters NS, Severs NJ, Rothery SM, Lincoln C, Yacoub MH, Green CR. Spatiotemporal relation between gap junctions and fascia adherens junctions during postnatal development of human ventricular myocardium. *Circulation* 90:713-725, 1994.

76. Zak R. Development and proliferative capacity of cardiac muscle cells. *Circ Res* 34(suppl II):II17-II26, 1974.

77. Rosen MR, Legato MJ, Weiss RM. Developmental changes in impulse conduction in the canine heart. *Am J Physiol* 240:H546-H554, 1981.

78. Dolber PC, Spach MS. Structure of canine Bachmann's bundle related to propagation of excitation. *Am J Physiol* 257:H1446-H1457, 1989.

79. Britz-Cunningham SH, Shah MM, Zuppan CW, Fletcher WH. Mutations of the connexin43 gap junction gene in patients with heart malformations and defects of laterality. *N Eng J Med* 332:1323-1329, 1995.

80. Bergoffen J, Scherer SS, Wang S, Scott MO, Bone LJ, Paul DL, Chen K, Lensch MW, Chance PF, Fischbeck KH. Connexin mutations in X-linked Charcot-Marie-Tooth disease. *Science* 262:2039-2042, 1993.

81. Kelsell DP, Dunlop J, Stevens HP, Lench NJ, Liang JN, Parry G, Mueller RF, Leigh IM. Connexin26 mutations in hereditary non-syndromic sensorineural deafness. *Nature* 387:80-83, 1997.

82. Shiels A, Mackay D, Ionides A, Berry V, Moore A, Bhattacharya S. A mis-sense mutation in the human connexin50 gene (GJA8) underlies autosomal dominant "Zonular Pulverulent" cataract, on chromosome 1q. *Am J Hum Genet* 62:526-532, 1998.

83. Darrow BJ, Fast VG, Kléber AG, Beyer EC, Saffitz JE. Functional and structural assessment of intercellular communication: increased conduction velocity and enhanced connexin expression in dibutyryl cAMP-treated cultured cardiac myocytes. *Circ Res* 79:174-183, 1996.

84. Peters NS, del Monte F, MacLeod KT, Green CR, Poole-Wilson PA, Severs NJ. Increased cardiac myocyte gap-junctional membrane early in renovascular hypertension. *J Am Coll Cardiol* 21:59A (abstract), 1993.

85. Winterton SJ, Turner MA, O'Gorman DJ, Flores NA, Sheridan DJ. Hypertrophy causes delayed conduction in human and guinea pig myocardium: accentuation during ischaemic perfusion. *Cardiovasc Res* 23:47-54, 1994.

86. Cooklin M, Wallis WRJ, Sheridan DJ, Fry CH. Changes in cell-to-cell electrical coupling associated with left ventricular hypertrophy. *Circ Res* 80:765-771, 1997.

87. McIntyre H, Fry CH. Abnormal action potential conduction in isolated human hypertrophied left ventricular myocardium. *J Cardiovasc Electrophysiol* 8:887-894, 1997.

88. Spach MS, Dolber PC. Relating extracellular potentials and their derivatives to anisotropic propagation at a microscopic level in human cardiac muscle. *Circ Res* 58:356-371, 1986.

89. Peters NS, Green CR, Poole-Wilson PA, Severs NJ. Reduced content of connexin43 gap junctions in ventricular myocardium from hypertrophied and ischemic human hearts. *Circulation* 88:864-875, 1993.

90. Smith JH, Green CR, Peters NS, Rothery S, Severs NJ. Altered patterns of gap junction distribution in ischemic heart disease: an immunohistochemical study of human myocardium using laser scanning confocal microscopy. *Am J Pathol* 139:801-821, 1991.

91. Peters NS, Coromilas J, Severs NJ, Wit AL. Disturbed connexin43 gap junction distribution correlates with the location of reentrant circuits in the epicardial border zone of healing canine infarcts that cause ventricular tachycardia. Circulation 95:988-996, 1997.

92. Kaprielian RR, Gunning M, Dupont E, et al. Downregulation of immunodetectable connexin43 and decreased gap junction size in the pathogenesis of chronic hibernation in the human left ventricle. *Circulation* 97:651-660, 1998.

93. van der Velden HM, van Kempen MJ, Wijffels MC, van Zijverden M, Groenewegen WA, Allessie MA, Jongsma HJ. Altered pattern of connexin40 distribution in persistent atrial fibrillation in the goat. *J Cardiovasc Electrophysiol* 9:596-607, 1998.

94. Gardner PI, Ursell PC, Fenoglio Jr JJ, Wit AL. Electrophysiologic and anatomic basis for fractionated electrograms recorded from healed myocardial infarcts. *Circulation* 72:596-611, 1985.

95. Ursell PC, Gardner PI, Albala A, Fenoglio JJ, Wit AL. Structural and electrophysiological changes in the epicardial border zone of canine myocardial infarcts during infarct healing.*Circ Res* 56:436-451, 1985.

96. Dillon SM, Allessie MA, Ursell PC, Wit AL. Influences of anisotropic tissue structure and reentrant circuits in the epicardial border zone of subacute canine infarcts.*Circ Res* 63:182-206, 1988.

97. DeBakker MJT, van Capelle FJL, Janse MJ, Tasseron S, Vermeulen JT, de Jonge N, Lahpor JR. Slow conduction in the infarcted human heart. "Zigzag" course of activation. *Circulation* 88:915-926, 1993.

98. Luke RA, Saffitz JE. Remodeling of ventricular conduction pathways in healed canine infarct border zones. *J Clin Invest* 87:1594-1602, 1991.

99. Kumar NM, Gilula NB. The gap junction communicating channel. *Cell* 84:381-388, 1996.

100. Luke RA, Beyer EC, Hoyt RH, Saffitz JE. Quantitative analysis of intercellular connections by immunohistochemistry of the cardiac gap junction protein connexin43.*Circ Res* 65;1450-1457, 1989.

6

HEREDITARY SUPRAVENTRICULAR TACHYCARDIAS

Patrick Y. Jay, M.D., Ph.D. and Charles I. Berul, M.D.

Department of Cardiology, Children's Hospital • Boston
Department of Pediatrics, Harvard Medical School, Boston, MA 02115

INTRODUCTION

The generally sporadic occurrence of Wolff-Parkinson-White (WPW) syndrome or supraventricular tachycardia (SVT) due to an accessory atrioventricular pathway does not suggest an obvious genetic basis, but several lines of evidence suggest that genetic mutations play a role in the development of this abnormality. Multiple families with supraventricular re-entrant tachycardias, either primary SVT or in association with hypertrophic cardiomyopathy, have been reported. The common occurrence of re-entrant SVT in certain forms of congenital heart disease implicates genetic mutations that disrupt normal cardiac structural and electrical system development. Finally, various rare mutations in the mitochondrial genome have been associated with WPW syndrome. This chapter reviews the evidence for the genetic and developmental basis for SVT via atrioventricular re-entry.

PRIMARY RE-ENTRANT SUPRAVENTRICULAR TACHYCARDIA

The mechanism of re-entrant SVT involves either an accessory connection between the atria and ventricles, which may be manifest or concealed on a surface electrocardiogram, or re-entry at the atrioventricular node. Wolff, Parkinson and White in 1930 first described paroxysmal SVT in patients with a short PR interval and bundle branch block pattern (1). In the following decades several reports described pedigrees with WPW syndrome in the absence of other cardiac disease (summarized in [2,3]). Vidaillet *et al* at Duke University published the largest analysis, which strongly indicated a genetic component to the development of atrioventricular accessory pathways (4). To our knowledge, there are no reports of familial primary atrioventricular nodal re-entrant tachycardia.

The Duke series demonstrated that the prevalence of pre-excitation in first-degree relatives of patients with electrophysiologically documented accessory pathways is significantly higher than that seen in the general population. The authors identified

2343 first-degree relatives of 383 patients. They examined the electrocardiograms or electrophysiologic studies of those relatives who had a history of palpitations, syncope or sudden death. Thirteen patients from ten families were identified who had one or more affected first-degree relatives. Thirteen first-degree relatives had pre-excitation, yielding a prevalence of 0.55%, significantly higher than the 0.15% found in the general population ($p<0.0001$). This figure is a conservative estimate, as five relatives who were either half-siblings or who had received their diagnosis at Duke were excluded from the calculation. Two first-degree relatives had concealed accessory pathways. Three second-degree relatives also had accessory pathways. Even more relatives, some of whom were likely carriers, had palpitations, syncope and sudden death but never had an ECG or electrophysiologic study for confirmation of diagnoses (4).

Relatives of patients with multiple accessory pathways were at even higher risk of pre-excitation compared to relatives of patients with single pathways or the general population. Of the 2106 relatives of the 339 patients with single accessory pathways, nine had pre-excitation (prevalence 0.43%). Among the 237 relatives of the 44 patients with multiple accessory pathways, four had pre-excitation (prevalence 1.7%; $p<0.05$ versus relatives of patients with single pathways and $p<0.001$ versus the general population).

Based on the ten pedigrees obtained in the Duke series, Vidaillet *et al* concluded that familial pre-excitation is transmitted as an autosomal dominant trait (4). Others who have reported and reviewed kindreds with WPW syndrome have concluded the same (2,3). There is variable penetrance of pre-excitation or symptomatic tachycardia. Not all suspected carriers of the WPW gene will show pre-excitation on an electrocardiogram. Some carriers may escape diagnosis for lack of symptomatic tachycardia, which depends on the electrophysiologic properties of the anterograde and retrograde limb of the re-entrant circuit. These properties are probably not co-inherited with the trait for pre-excitation. For instance, some of the relatives in the series had concealed accessory pathways, which is not surprising since individual patients can have intermittent pre-excitation.

In some families in the Duke series, maternal inheritance of pre-excitation cannot be excluded. Past authors who have studied familial WPW syndrome have not explicitly discussed this possibility, but WPW has been associated with Leber hereditary optic neuropathy, a mitochondrial disorder with complex penetrance patterns, as discussed below. Interestingly, Schneider described a woman and her son, both of whom had isolated WPW syndrome; two of the woman's brothers reportedly had Leber hereditary optic neuropathy (5).

No gene defect has been identified yet for familial isolated WPW syndrome. The small size of kindreds and the variable penetrance of pre-excitation or symptoms complicate the search for genetic linkage. In contrast, studies in families with hypertrophic cardiomyopathy and associated WPW syndrome have been more fruitful.

HYPERTROPHIC CARDIOMYOPATHY

Familial hypertrophic cardiomyopathy is an autosomal dominant disorder characterized by ventricular and myocyte hypertrophy, myofibril disarray, and interstitial fibrosis. Mutations that cause hypertrophic cardiomyopathy have been discovered in sarcomeric proteins such as alpha-cardiac actin (6), beta-myosin heavy chain, ventricular myosin essential and regulatory light chains, cardiac troponins T and I, alpha-tropomyosin, and cardiac myosin binding protein C (7). Accessory atrioventricular conduction was present in 5% of patients in one series (8). WPW has been reported for patients who have mutations of alpha-cardiac actin, cardiac myosin binding protein C and troponin I (6,9). Of note, the three affected members of one family, a mother, son and daughter, who carried the troponin I Gly203Ser mutation had WPW (9).

Some families with hypertrophic cardiomyopathy have an incidence of WPW greater than the 5% reported by Fananapazir *et al* (8). Three families spanning two to four generations have been reported prior to the advent of modern human molecular genetics (10-12). Echocardiography was unavailable for the earlier studies; thus, the diagnosis of hypertrophic cardiomyopathy may have potentially been missed in some relatives. The association between WPW and hypertrophic cardiomyopathy in these families may therefore be even stronger than the data indicate.

Genetic linkage has been established in two families with hypertrophic cardiomyopathy and co-inherited WPW (13,14). Some members of these families also developed atrioventricular block and intraventricular conduction delays. The affected gene maps to a locus at chromosome 7q35-7q36, but the exact gene has not yet been identified in this region, which spans 5 centimorgans.

CONGENITAL HEART DISEASE

Most patients have isolated SVT, but consideration of congenital heart defects that are associated with SVT may provide insight into the mechanism of formation of accessory atrioventricular conduction pathways. In pediatric series of WPW syndrome, 20-40% of patients have an associated congenital heart defect (15-18). The true incidence of congenital heart disease in WPW syndrome is probably overestimated in these older series because of referral bias. Nevertheless, two particular defects, Ebstein malformation of the tricuspid valve and physiologically corrected transposition of the great vessels, which is often associated with an Ebstein malformation of the left-sided tricuspid valve, are especially common in these series. Among patients with Ebstein malformation, the incidence of pre-excitation ranges from 6-30% (19-22).

In Ebstein malformation, the attachments of the posterior and septal leaflets of the tricuspid valve are displaced toward the junction of the inlet and trabecular zones of the right ventricle. The inlet portion of the right ventricle functionally becomes a part of the right atrium (23). The Ebstein malformation arises from the failure of the two leaflets to delaminate from the right ventricular myocardium during the eighth through twelfth week of embryonic development (24)[24].

The formation of an accessory atrioventricular pathway is clearly related to the development of the abnormal tricuspid valve. Intracardiac electrophysiologic study of a series of patients with Ebstein malformation and recurrent tachycardia revealed an accessory pathway in 21 of 22 patients. Eight patients had multiple pathways. All the pathways were in the right posterolateral or posteroseptal region of the atrioventricular groove, except for a left posterolateral pathway in a patient who had physiologically corrected transposition of the great arteries and thus a left-sided tricuspid valve (25). All pathways that are associated with an Ebstein malformation insert into the atrial portion of the right ventricle, as determined by intracardiac electrophysiologic study or careful histopathologic examination (25-27).

The atrioventricular pathways seen in Ebstein malformation histologically appear as either working myocardium or conduction tissue. Becker *et al* examined the accessory pathways in seven hearts. The accessory pathways in structurally normal hearts appeared similar to working myocardium regardless of the side of the pathway. In two hearts with an Ebstein malformation, one pathway looked like working myocardium. The other pathway appeared similar to conduction tissue with a node-like structure at the insertion of the atrial myocardium (26). Similar findings were made in three hearts of patients with pre-excitation, corrected transposition and Ebstein anomaly. Multiple pathways were found in two cases. In at least one of these hearts, pathways of both histologic types were found (27). Therefore, the primary mutation determines the presence of an accessory atrioventricular connection but apparently not the histologic phenotype of the tissue.

MITOCHONDRIAL DISORDERS

Mitochondria are intracellular organelles that participate in several metabolic pathways, including ATP synthesis by oxidative phosphorylation. Mitochondria are unique organelles because they contain a genome that encodes some of the polypeptides in the oxidative phosphorylation pathway and all the transfer (tRNA) and ribosomal RNA (rRNA). Nuclear genes encode the remaining mitochondrial proteins. Mitochondria self-replicate and are derived from the oocyte. Thus, mutations in the mitochondrial genome are maternally inherited (28).

Common cardiac manifestations of mitochondrial disease include conduction defects, hypertrophic cardiomyopathy, and dilated cardiomyopathy, which may in part represent progression from the hypertrophic form (29). One particular mitochondrial disorder, Leber hereditary optic neuropathy (LHON), has been associated with WPW syndrome. The primary symptom in LHON is loss of central vision due to degeneration of the retinal ganglion cells and the optic nerve axons. LHON is the first mitochondrial disorder for which a defect in the mitochondrial genome was identified (30). Three mutations at nucleotide positions 11778, 14484, and 3460 in the mitochondrial genome account for the majority of LHON cases (31). Each mutation affects a different subunit of complex I in the respiratory chain pathway.

In Finnish and Japanese families with LHON, the incidence of pre-excitation is greater than in the general population. Nikoskelainen *et al* presented nine Finnish families representing 163 persons with the LHON mitochondrial mutation. Among four families with the 11778 mutation, the incidence of WPW ranged from 0 to 21%. Two families with the 3460 mutation had incidences of 12 and 35%. The incidence varied from 0 to 8% in three families with an unknown mitochondrial mutation (32). Mashima *et al* presented their data on two Japanese families carrying the 11778 mutation. Three of 63 persons (5%) had WPW syndrome (33).

The increased incidence of WPW syndrome in LHON families has not been observed elsewhere in the world. In Tasmania and Italy, WPW has been diagnosed in LHON families, but it is unclear whether the incidences are higher than in the general population (34,35). In the United States, no ventricular pre-excitation was detected in a large LHON family (36).

Other mitochondrial mutations may increase the risk for WPW syndrome. For example, mutations in the mitochondrial gene encoding tRNA[leu(UUR)] cause several disorders in which WPW has been observed. In a review of the literature of reported cases of MELAS syndrome (myopathy, encephalopathy, lactic acidosis and stroke-like episodes), six of 43 patients (14%) had WPW (37). The incidence of WPW in the MELAS syndrome has not been addressed in other series (38,39). WPW has been described in a case of a family with a heterogeneous presentation of the tRNA[leu(UUR)] mutation. The mother had diabetes mellitus and mild neurosensory hearing loss. The first son had MELAS syndrome, recurrent pancreatitis, an abnormal glucose tolerance test, severe neurosensory hearing loss and WPW. The second son had severe neurosensory hearing loss only (40). An Italian family that carried a tRNA[leu(UUR)] mutation presented with adult-onset skeletal and cardiac myopathy; one male among 15 relatives who carried the mutation had WPW and hypertrophic cardiomyopathy (41).

Despite the high incidence of WPW in some families with LHON and the possible association with mutations of tRNA[leu(UUR)], a clear causality between mitochondrial mutations and WPW is difficult to establish. Mitochondrial diseases generally affect the nervous system, skeletal muscle and heart, but the range of signs and symptoms and the number of other affected organ systems is remarkably heterogeneous even for a specific mutation (28). Environmental and secondary genetic factors can affect clinical presentations (31). The risk of LHON, for example, may be increased by tobacco and alcohol use (42). The increased risk for males and the finding that descendents along certain matriarchal lines seem to lose their susceptibility to LHON despite carrying the primary mitochondrial mutation implicate secondary interacting genes (43). Thus, multiple variables may confound the analysis of the role of mitochondrial mutations in WPW.

DEVELOPMENTAL MECHANISMS

Present knowledge of the genetic basis of SVT via an accessory atrioventricular pathway is limited. Even when a genetic mutation has been identified, as in familial hypertrophic cardiomyopathy, the molecular mechanism that permits the accessory pathway to form remains unknown. To provide a framework for future investigation, we propose two general hypotheses based on knowledge of embryonic cardiac development. First, accessory pathways may represent the failure of regression of the continuity between the atrial and ventricular myocardium in the embryonic heart tube. Second, accessory pathways may be ectopic connections independent of the atrioventricular canal. Both hypotheses may be true. In the embryonic tube heart, the atrium is in electrical continuity with the ventricle around the circumference of the atrioventricular canal musculature. Two processes, loss of cell-to-cell contact in the atrioventricular canal and fusion of the atrioventricular sulcus and cushions tissues, separate the atrial and ventricular myocardium.

Disruption of atrioventricular continuity has been demonstrated in both chick and human hearts during development (Figure 1). Arguello *et al* have shown that in the embryonic chick heart the development of an atrioventricular delay is coincident with the dissociation of intercalated disks and desmosomes between myocytes in the atrioventricular canal and an increase in the extracellular matrix between the cells, as seen by transmission electron microscopy. These changes are not seen in the adjacent atrial or ventricular muscle (44,45). Anderson *et al* have shown that in fetal human hearts a ring of conduction tissue is present around the entire right and a portion of the left atrioventricular ring. These connections are less common in infants and are not found in normal adult hearts, indicative of regression during cardiac development (46). The ring tissue arises from the contribution of the interventricular foramen mainly to the right atrioventricular canal as the heart tube remodels to form four chambers (47,48). Defects in the process described by Arguello *et al* would lead to accessory pathways around the entire left and right atrioventricular rings, whereas persistence of the connections described by Anderson *et al* would generally lead to right-sided pathways.

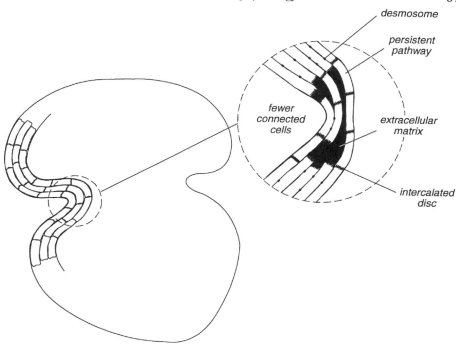

Figure 1. Electrical continuity of the atrium and ventricle in the embryonic heart tube is disrupted with the loss of intercellular contacts and an increase in the extracellular matrix in the atrioventricular canal during normal development. An accessory atrioventricular pathway, as shown, persists when this process is incomplete. Ionic coupling via gap junctions in the intercalated disks in the pathway may permit ventricular pre-excitation or atrioventricular re-entry.

Fusion of the epicardial atrioventricular sulcus tissues and endocardial cushions forms the insulating, fibrous annulus between the atrium and ventricle (49) (Figure 2). Right-sided accessory pathways generally run through defects in the fibrous ring, which are common even in normal hearts. Whether a defect in myocyte dissociation or formation of the fibrous annulus ultimately cause a particular right-sided accessory pathway to form would be difficult to determine. In contrast, the fibrous annulus around the mitral valve is generally complete. Interestingly, left-sided accessory pathways commonly skirt across the epicardial aspect of the fibrous annulus rather than through it (26). How an epicardial pathway could arise from atrioventricular canal muscle, which lies between the sulcus and cushion layers, is difficult to explain. Such pathways may be ectopic connections between the atrium and ventricle. No convincing data exist to support this hypothesis, except as inferred from the anatomic relationships of the developing fibrous annulus (49).

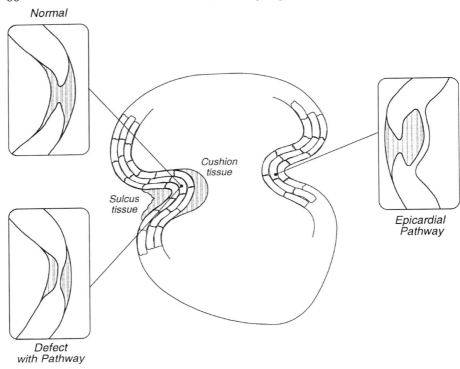

Figure 2. The fibrous annulus that separates the atrial and ventricular myocardium forms by fusion of the epicardial sulcus and endocardial cushion tissue (49). The atrioventricular canal musculature is between the two fusing tissues. There is normally complete separation, but defects are commonly found in the right atrioventricular ring in normal hearts. Accessory pathways may pass through such defects. Left-sided pathways, in contrast, often run along the epicardial aspect of the fibrous annulus, suggesting that such connections may not arise from the normal embryonic atrioventricular myocardium.

Mutations in genes that regulate or effect the normal dissociation of atrioventricular continuity during fetal development could lead to persistence of accessory pathways. For example, in hypertrophic cardiomyopathy, defects in sarcomeric proteins that diminish contractile force may stimulate hypertrophy as a compensatory mechanism (7). The signaling mechanism or hypertrophy of embryonic atrioventricular myocytes may prevent their normal dissociation. Mitochondrial disorders may increase the risk for accessory pathways by a similar signaling pathway to hypertrophy if the myocytes have decreased force production because of an energy deficit. In the Ebstein malformation, the mechanism that is defective in the process of delamination of the posterior and septal tricuspid valve leaflets from the right ventricular myocardium is likely same one involved in the dissociation of atrioventricular myocytes.

In isolated familial WPW syndrome, a gene defect could modulate atrioventricular dissociation or promote the formation of ectopic atrioventricular connections. Thus, it would be interesting to know whether the sidedness of pathways is genetically determined. For example, if left-sided pathways were an inherited trait, one might suspect a gene mutation that promoted ectopic connections.

SUMMARY

Most cases of WPW syndrome or SVT due to a concealed accessory pathway have no obvious genetic cause or familial association. Good evidence exists, however, to suggest that at least some cases, whether as a primary arrhythmia or in association with other heart disease or syndrome, have a genetic basis. In the development of the embryonic heart there exist important points where defective genes might disrupt the normal separation of atrioventricular continuity and lead to the persistence of accessory pathways. Much work lies ahead in the field, such as finding genetic linkage, identifying candidate genes, elucidating the function of these genes, and developing animal models. The genetics of SVT is in its nascency.

REFERENCES

1.   Wolff L, Parkinson J, White PD. Bundle-branch block with short P-R interval in healthy young people prone to paroxysmal tachycardia. *Am Heart J* 1930;5:685-704.

2.   Chia BL, Yew FC, Chay SO, Tan AT. Familial Wolff-Parkinson-White syndrome. *J Electrocardiol* 1982;15:195-198.

3.   Gillette PC, Freed D, McNamara DG. A proposed autosomal dominant method of inheritance of the Wolff-Parkinson-White syndrome and supraventricular tachycardia. *J Pediatr* 1978;93:257-258.

4.   Vidaillet HJJ, Pressley JC, Henke E, Harrell FEJ, German LD. Familial occurrence of accessory atrioventricular pathways (preexcitation syndrome). *N Engl J Med* 1987;317:65-69.

5.   Schneider RG. Familial occurrence of Wolff-Parkinson-White syndrome. *Am Heart J* 1969;78:34-37.

6.   Mogensen J, Klausen IC, Pedersen AK, et al. Alpha-cardiac actin is a novel disease gene in familial hypertrophic cardiomyopathy. *J Clin Invest* 1999;103:39-43.

7.   Bonne G, Carrier L, Richard P, Hainque B, Schwartz K. Familial hypertrophic cardiomyopathy: from mutations to functional defects. *Circ Res* 1998;83:580-593.

8.   Fananapazir L, Tracy CM, Leon MB, et al. Electrophysiologic abnormalities in patients with hypertrophic cardiomyopathy. *Circulation* 1989;80:1259-1268.

9.   Kimura A, Harada H, Park JE, et al. Mutations in the cardiac troponin I gene associated with hypertrophic cardiomyopathy. *Nat Genet* 1997;16:379-382.

10.   Hauser AM, Gordon S, Timmis GC. Familial hypertrophic cardiomyopathy and preexcitation. *Am Heart J* 1984;107:176-179.

11.   Massumi RA. Familial Wolff-Parkinson-White syndrome associated with cardiomyopathy *Am J Med* 1967;43:951-955.

12.   Westlake RE, Cohen W, Willis WH. Wolff-Parkinson-White syndrome and familial cardiomegaly. *Am Heart J* 1962;62:314-320.

13.   MacRae CA, Ghaisas N, Kass S, et al. Familial hypertrophic cardiomyopathy with Wolff-Parkinson-White syndrome maps to a locus on chromosome 7q3. *J Clin Invest* 1995;96:1216-1220.

14.   Mehdirad AA, Fatkin D, DiMarco JP, et al. Electrophysiologic characteristics of accessory atrioventricular connections in an inherited form of Wolff-Parkinson-White syndrome. *J Cardiovasc Electrophysiol* 1999;10:629-635.

15.   Giardina AC, Ehlers KH, Engle MA. Wolff-Parkinson-White syndrome in infants and children. A long-term follow-up study. *Br Heart J* 1972;34:839-846.

16.   Mantakas ME, McCue CM, Miller WW. Natural history of Wolff-Parkinson-White syndrome discovered in infancy. *Am J Cardiol* 1978;41:1097-1103.

17.   Perry JC, Garson AJ. Supraventricular tachycardia due to Wolff-Parkinson-White syndrome in children: early disappearance and late recurrence. *J Am Coll Cardiol* 1990;16:1215-1220.

18.   Swiderski J, Lees MH, Nadas AS. The Wolff-Parkinson-White syndrome in infancy and childhood. *Br Heart J* 1962;24:561-579.

19.   Bialostozky D, Horwitz S, Espino-Vela J. Ebstein's malformation of the tricuspid valve. A review of 65 cases. *Am J Cardiol* 1972;29:826-836.

20.   Giuliani ER, Fuster V, Brandenburg RO, Mair DD. Ebstein's anomaly: the clinical features and natural history of Ebstein's anomaly of the tricuspid valve. *Mayo Clin Proc* 1979;54:163-173.

21.   Kumar AE, Fyler DC, Miettinen OS, Nadas AS. Ebstein's anomaly. Clinical profile and natural history. *Am J Cardiol* 1971;28:84-95.

22.   Watson H. Natural history of Ebstein's anomaly of tricuspid valve in childhood and adolescence. An international co-operative study of 505 cases. *Br Heart J* 1974;36:417-427.

23.   Zuberbuhler JR, Allwork SP, Anderson RH. The spectrum of Ebstein's anomaly of the tricuspid valve. *J Thorac Cardiovasc Surg* 1979;77:202-211.

24.   Lamers WH, Viragh S, Wessels A, Moorman AF, Anderson RH. Formation of the tricuspid valve in the human heart. *Circulation* 1995;91:111-121.

25.   Smith WM, Gallagher JJ, Kerr CR, et al. The electrophysiologic basis and management of symptomatic recurrent tachycardia in patients with Ebstein's anomaly of the tricuspid valve. *Am J Cardiol* 1982;49:1223-1234.

26.   Becker AE, Anderson RH, Durrer D, Wellens HJ. The anatomical substrates of Wolff-Parkinson-White syndrome. A clinicopathologic correlation in 7 patients. *Circulation* 1978;57:870-879.

27.   Bharati S, Rosen K, Steinfield L, Miller RA, Lev M. The anatomic substrate for preexcitation in corrected transposition. *Circulation* 1980;62:831-842.

28.   Zeviani M, Tiranti V, Piantadosi C. Mitochondrial disorders. *Medicine* 1998;77:59-72.

29.   Anan R, Nakagawa M, Miyata M, et al. Cardiac involvement in mitochondrial diseases. A study on 17 patients with documented mitochondrial DNA defects. *Circulation* 1995;91:955-961.

30.   Wallace DC, Singh G, Lott MT, et al. Mitochondrial DNA mutation associated with Leber's hereditary optic neuropathy. *Science* 1988;242:1427-1430.

31.   Howell N. Leber hereditary optic neuropathy: respiratory chain dysfunction and degeneration of the optic nerve. *Vision Res* 1998;38:1495-1504.

32.   Nikoskelainen EK, Savontaus ML, Huoponen K, Antila K, Hartiala J. Pre-excitation syndrome in Leber hereditary optic neuropathy. *Lancet* 1994;344:857-8.

33.   Mashima Y, Kigasawa K, Hasegawa H, Tani M, Oguchi Y. High incidence of pre-excitation syndrome in Japanese families with Leber's hereditary optic neuropathy. *Clin Genet* 1996;50:535-537.

34.   Bower SP, Hawley I, Mackey DA. Cardiac arrhythmia and Leber's hereditary optic neuropathy. *Lancet* 1992;339:1427-1428.

35.   Federico A, Aitiani P, Lomonaco B, et al. Electrocardiographic abnormalities in Leber's hereditary optic atrophy. *J Inher Metab Dis* 1987;10 Suppl 2:256-259.

36.   Ortiz RG, Newman NJ, Manoukian SV, Diesenhouse MC, Lott MT, Wallace DC. Optic disk cupping and electrocardiographic abnormalities in an American pedigree with Leber's hereditary optic neuropathy. *Am J Ophthalmol* 1992;113:561-566.

37.   Hirano M, Ricci E, Koenigsberger MR, et al. Melas: an original case and clinical criteria for diagnosis. *Neuromuscul Disord* 1992;2:125-135.

38.   Ciafaloni E, Ricci E, Shanske S, et al. MELAS: clinical features, biochemistry, and molecular genetics. *Ann Neurol* 1992;31:391-398.

39.   Goto Y, Horai S, Matsuoka T, et al. Mitochondrial myopathy, encephalopathy, lactic acidosis, and stroke-like episodes (MELAS). *Neurology* 1992;42:545-50.

40.   Oexle K, Oberle J, Finckh B, et al. Islet cell antibodies in diabetes mellitus associated with a mitochondrial tRNA$^{(Leu(UUR))}$ gene mutation. *Exp Clin Endocrinol Diabetes* 1996;104:212-217.

41.   Zeviani M, Gellera C, Antozzi C, et al. Maternally inherited myopathy and cardiomyopathy: association with mutation in mitochondrial DNA tRNA(Leu)(UUR). *Lancet* 1991;338:143-147.

42.   Chalmers RM, Harding AE. A case-control study of Leber's hereditary optic neuropathy.*Brain* 1996;119:1481-1486.

43.   Howell N, Mackey DA. Low-penetrance branches in matrilineal pedigrees with Leber hereditary optic neuropathy. *Am J Hum Genet* 1998;63:1220-1224.

44.   Arguello C, Alanis J, Pantoja O, Valenzuela B. Electrophysiological and ultrastructural study of the atrioventricular canal during the development of the chick embryo. *J Mol Cell Cardiol* 1986;18:499-510.

45.   Arrechedera H, Strauss M, Arguello C, Ayesta C, Anselmi G. Ultrastructural study of the myocardial wall of the atrio-ventricular canal during the development of the embryonic chick heart.*J Mol Cell Cardiol* 1984;16:885-895.

46.   Anderson RH, Davies MJ, Becker AE. Atrioventricular ring specialized tissue in the normal heart. *Eur J Cardiol* 1974;2:219-230.

47.   Wessels A, Vermeulen JL, Verbeek FJ, et al. Spatial distribution of "tissue-specific" antigens in the developing human heart and skeletal muscle. III. An immunohistochemical analysis of the distribution of the neural tissue antigen G1N2 in the embryonic heart. *Anat Rec* 1992;232:97-111.

48.   Moorman AF, de Jong F, Denyn MM, Lamers WH. Development of the cardiac conduction system. *Circ Res* 1998;82:629-644.

49. Wessels A, Markman MW, Vermeulen JL, Anderson RH, Moorman AF, Lamers WH. The development of the atrioventricular junction in the human heart. *Circ Res* 1996;78:110-117.

7

FAMILIAL ATRIAL FIBRILLATION

Ramon Brugada, M.D. and Robert Roberts, M.D.

Department of Cardiology, Baylor College of Medicine, Houston, Texas

INTRODUCTION

Interest in familial or genetic heart diseases by cardiologists is often minimal because they are believed to account for only a small proportion of the diseases of the heart. However, there is a great potential to improve the diagnosis, treatment and prevention of acquired diseases from identifying the genetic defect responsible for familial diseases. This was perhaps best illustrated in the recognition and treatment of the role of cholesterol in coronary artery disease. Brown and Goldstein elucidated the receptor responsible for the uptake of cholesterol and subsequently the metabolic pathway in familial hypercholesterolemia. This familial disorder probably accounts for less than 2% of all patients with coronary artery disease. Nevertheless, these studies subsequently led to others which proved that cholesterol is a major etiological factor in acquired coronary artery disease and is now the main target of treatment for the prevention and treatment of coronary disease. Death from CAD has been reduced by 50% in the past 30 years, in large part due to the treatment of hypercholesterolemia.

The first gene responsible for a cardiomyopathy was not mapped until 1989 (1) and the gene was identified within the same year (2). Nevertheless, in less than a decade, over 40 genes have been mapped or identified to be responsible for various cardiac disorders (3) (Table 1) not including the genes for hereditary lipid disorders. In the case of atrial fibrillation, it is reasonable to expect that the genetic defect responsible for the familial form of the disease disrupts a pathway of electrical conduction throughout the atria that is also used for normal physiological atrial conduction as well as the pathway disrupted with acquired atrial fibrillation. It is well recognized that multiple currents are responsible for the generation of the action potential in the ventricle. The recent identification of several genes responsible for inherited ventricular arrhythmias, such as the long QT syndrome and Brugada syndrome, is helping to elucidate the pathways involved with ventricular arrhythmias (4;5). The identification of these genes has already improved the treatment of ventricular arrhythmias and is likely to provide the framework to develop more specific and effective drugs. It is expected that multiple genes will be responsible for familial atrial fibrillation (as has been the case with hypertrophic and dilated cardiomyopathies and long QT syndromes) and that identification of the

Table 1: Cardiac Diseases with an Identified Genetic Locus or Gene

Cardiomyopathies	Chromosomal Locus
Hypertrophic Cardiomyopathy	1q3, 3p, 7q3, 11q11, 12q, 14q1, 15q2, 19p13
Dilated Cardiomyopathy	1q32, 6q1, 9q12, 10q21-23, 15q1
Dilated Cardiomyopathy with Conduction Defects	1q1, 3p22, 6q23
Arrhythmogenic Right Ventricular Dysplasia	1q12, 2q32, 14q12, 14q23, 3p23
Mitochondrial Cardiomyopathies	Mitochondrial DNA
Conduction Disorders	**Chromosomal Locus**
Long QT Syndrome	3p21-24, 4q24, 7q35, 11p15, 21q22
Familial Heart Block	19q13, 1q32
WPW Syndrome	7q3
Atrial Arrhythmias	**Chromosomal Locus**
Atrial Fibrillation	10q22
Cardiac Septal Defects	**Chromosomal Locus**
Holt-Oram Syndrome	12q2
DiGeorge Syndrome	22q
Noonan Syndrome	12q
Aortic Disorders	**Chromosomal Locus**
Supravalvar Aortic Stenosis	9q
Marfan Syndrome	15q

various defects in these genes will provide a framework of the various currents responsible for generating the atrial action potential. Furthermore, and more importantly, specific molecules will be available as targets for the development for more specific and effective therapy in the prevention and treatment of atrial fibrillation.

THE EPIDEMIOLOGY OF ATRIAL FIBRILLATION

The most common sustained arrhythmia is atrial fibrillation. It is the most common cause of embolic stroke, accounting for approximately 75,000 strokes per year in the US, and leads to more hospital admissions than any other arrhythmia (6). There are over 3 million cases of AF in the US, with an overall prevalence of 0.5% -1%, increasing to about 10 % in people over the age of 70 years. It is claimed that AF accounts for about one third of strokes over the age of 65 years (7). Since there is no known cure for AF, palliative therapy is directed towards heart rate control and the prevention of systemic emboli.

IDENTIFICATION OF FAMILIES WITH ATRIAL FIBRILLATION

The molecular basis for AF is yet to be determined. It is not generally appreciated that atrial fibrillation may be familial. This is evident from a literature search which showed only four publications (8-13) referring to the familial form of the disease. The first report was in 1943 (8), and while it is probably very uncommon, there has been no systematic study to determine the overall prevalence of the disease. We were fortunate to identify a family with familial atrial fibrillation from Spain and subsequently four other related families with atrial fibrillation (Figure 1). The five families consisted of a total of 103 individuals, 42 of whom presented with atrial fibrillation. The age of diagnosis varied from 1 to 45 years. The penetrance of the disease (proportion of patients with the gene who have the disease) is very high and in the last generation, three individuals were diagnosed in their first month of life. The elderly generations were diagnosed at a later age although the age of presentation of the disease is unknown, due mainly to the lack of symptoms and lack of routine examinations until recently.

CLINICAL FEATURES OF FAMILIAL ATRIAL FIBRILLATION

The majority of the individuals in these five families were asymptomatic. The arrhythmia is well tolerated in the young population with some of the individuals being diagnosed in their 20s during family screening. Six patients have recurrent palpitations, but otherwise continue a normal life. The disease is chronic in all but two individuals. In the individuals with paroxysmal atrial fibrillation, some have symptoms of palpitation but are unaware of any triggering factors for the arrhythmia. The echocardiograms were within the normal range when the patients were diagnosed. Some of them have subsequently developed dilatation of the left atrium. Two patients have developed left ventricular dysfunction, one of them probably related to her advanced age and the other possibly due to a cardiomyopathy secondary to a poorly controlled heart rate. Electrical cardioversion was attempted in six patients but none were converted despite structurally normal hearts.

The lack of symptomatology and the apparent benign nature of the arrhythmia does not exclude the possibility of complications. Eight patients have suffered complications from the disease. Seven had a cerebrovascular accident before age 70 and in one it was fatal. One patient suffered sudden death at age 36. This patient had paroxysmal atrial fibrillation and despite anti-arrhythmic therapy continued to have recurrent episodes. The patient had a cardiac arrest which is believed to be due to a pro-arrhythmic effect of the medication. The heart rates in these patients were controlled primarily by digoxin or β-blockers. Patients above 65 years are treated with warfarin to prevent systematic emboli and some of the younger patients are taking aspirin.

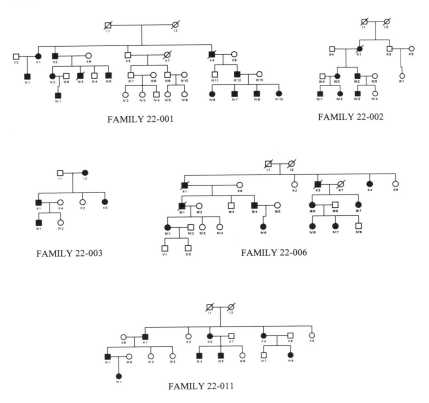

Figure 1: Pedigree of the families collected in Catalonia, Spain with common locus on chromosome 10, segregating with familial atrial fibrillation. Solid blocks represent affected individuals, squares represent males and circles females. The blocks with slash represent deceased individuals.

MAPPING THE CHROMOSOMAL LOCUS FOR ATRIAL FIBRILLATION

The first necessary step in identifying a gene responsible for a disease is to find a family in which several of the members are affected with the disease. The diagnosis is best determined using consistent and objective criteria to stratify into three diagnostic categories: affected, normal and indeterminant. One must also exclude other causes that may simulate the phenotype. For example, in familial atrial fibrillation, it is important to rule out valvular disease, which by itself, could cause atrial fibrillation. The initial diagnostic assessment is a history and physical examination, an electrocardiogram, and an echocardiogram. The genetic studies require a blood sample. DNA is obtained from the white cells and the lymphocytes are cultured in the presence of Epstein-Barr virus to generate immortal cell lines for a renewable source of DNA.

The next step is to map the location of the gene to its precise chromosomal location (chromosomal locus) (14;15). The human genome, which consists of 23 chromosomes, contains three billion bases with between 50,000-100,000 genes. Mendel's laws state that genes are inherited as independent units and therefore the likelihood of a particular gene being inherited is by chance and on the average is about 50%.

The technique used to map the chromosomal locus of a gene is referred to as genetic linkage analysis (16). To map the locus one analyzes the DNA from the whole family (affected and unaffected) for markers of known chromosomal location. These markers are short stretches of DNA whose approximate chromosomal locations are known. For initial screening one chooses a set of 300 markers that span the human genome (all 23 chromosomes) at 10 million bp intervals. The identification of a marker(s) inherited by the affected individuals and not the unaffected, indicate this region contains the gene causing the disease. The marker and the gene are so close together that they are co-inherited more frequently than by chance alone. Thus, it indicates the gene is on that chromosome in close proximity to the marker. This requires a computerized statistical analysis, and to have enough power requires at least 10 affected individuals from a family of two generations.

The next step is to identify the gene (14). There are two overall approaches: 1) the positional candidate gene approach, and 2) positional cloning. The first attempt is always the candidate gene approach which consists of determining whether genes already mapped to the region (region being defined as that between the two flanking markers) are responsible for the disease. The candidate genes are sequenced and if a mutation is present and is co-inherited in affected individuals but not in normal individuals, it is considered causative. Positional cloning refers to cloning a region knowing its position only in relation to marker to identify novel genes and determining whether the gene has mutations which could cause the disease. Ultimate proof is induction of the disease in an animal by a mutated transgene.

Genetic linkage analysis was performed in the families we have recruited (17) using chromosomal markers as outlined. The locus responsible for the disease was shown to be on the long arm of chromosome 10q22-q24 (18). The affected members of the family shared an area of 28 cM (28 million base pairs). With the additional four other families, several genetic crossovers were identified which narrowed the region containing the gene to less than 0.5 cM. We have sequenced several candidate genes including a β-adrenergic receptor, α-adrenergic receptor, G-protein-coupled receptor kinase, and a potassium channel, none of which contained a mutation and thus were excluded. We then proceeded to positional cloning of the region and have cloned the entire region in Bacterial Artificial Chromosomes (BACs). Two novel genes have been identified that are presently being sequenced.

SCREENING FOR ADDITIONAL FAMILIES

Familial atrial fibrillation would appear to be rather uncommon based on clinical experience and the few reports in the literature. To further ascertain the frequency of familial atrial fibrillation, we established a toll-free number through the internet and encouraged individuals, who are below the age of 50 years with a diagnosis of atrial fibrillation, a family history of the disease, and structural heart disease to respond or see their physician. Subsequently, individuals with atrial fibrillation would undergo the regular screening for genetic cardiac disease, namely, history, physical, electrocardiogram, echocardiogram and a blood sample for DNA analysis. The response we received suggests familial atrial fibrillation is much more common than previously anticipated. We identified more than 100 probands with the familial form of the disease in the United States and 15 probands from six other countries (18). Analysis of four of these families has shown that they are not linked to chromosome 10. This means that familial atrial fibrillation is a heterogeneous disease, caused by more than one gene. This fact is not at all surprising given the experience with other cardiac diseases like congenital long QT syndrome or hypertrophic cardiomyopathy in which several disease-causing genes have been identified.

FUTURE IMPLICATIONS

Identification of the gene(s) responsible for familial atrial fibrillation should provide some understanding of the mechanisms responsible for atrial fibrillation. It is most likely that the pathways interrupted by the genetic defect that induces atrial fibrillation is the same pathway involved with normal atrial conduction and the same pathway disrupted by acquired disease to induce atrial fibrillation. Despite the familial form being very uncommon, no study has been performed to evaluate the prevalence. We particularly recommend screening family members of individuals affected with the so called "lone" atrial fibrillation to rule out the familial form. The disease is better tolerated if it develops in early stages of life and it is generally resistant to cardioversion even with normal size atria.

SUMMARY

The molecular basis for atrial fibrillation continues to be largely unknown, and therapy remains unchanged, aimed at controlling the heart rate and preventing systemic emboli with anticoagulation. Familial atrial fibrillation is more common than previously suspected. While atrial fibrillation is commonly associated with acquired heart disease, a significant proportion of individuals have early onset without other forms of heart disease, referred to as "lone" atrial fibrillators. It is also well recognized that atrial fibrillation occurs on a reversible or functional basis, without associated structural heart disease, such as with hyperthyroidism or following surgery. It remains to be determined what percentage of atrial fibrillation in these individuals is familial or due to a genetic predisposition.

Mapping the locus for familial atrial fibrillation is the first step towards the identification of the gene. Isolation of the gene and subsequent identification of the responsible molecular genetic defect should provide a point of entry into the mechanism responsible for the familial form and the common acquired forms of the disease and eventually provide more effective therapy. We know that the ionic currents responsible for the action potential of the atrium is due to multiple channel proteins as is electrical conduction throughout the atria. Analogous to the ongoing genetic studies in patients with familial long QT syndrome, it is highly likely that defects in each of these channel proteins will be manifested in familial atrial fibrillation. Through their identification one can elucidate the molecular basis for the generation of the atrial action potential and its conduction throughout the atria.

ACKNOWLEDGMENTS

This work is supported in part by grants from the National Heart, Lung, and Blood Institute, Specialized Centers of Research (P50-HL42267-01), the NIH Training Center in Molecular Cardiology (T32-HL07706), the American Heart Association, Bugher Foundation Center for Molecular Biology (86-2216), ACC/Merck Fellowship Awards/International Exchange Committee Award (ID#67567), and the Fundacion MAPFRE MEDICINA, Madrid, Spain.

REFERENCES

1. Jarcho JA, McKenna W, Pare JAP, et al. Mapping a gene for familial hypertrophic cardiomyopathy to chromosome 14q1. *N Engl J Med* 1989;321:1372-1378.
2. Geisterfer-Lowrance AA, Kass S, Tanigawa G, et al. A molecular basis for familial hypertrophic cardiomyopathy: A beta-cardiac myosin heavy chain gene missense mutation.*Cell* 1990;62:999-1006.
3. Roberts R. A glimpse of the future from present day molecular genetics. Cardiology at the Limits II 1999;(In Press)
4. Wang Q, Chen Q, Li H, Towbin JA. Molecular genetics of long QT syndrome from genes to patients. *Current Opinion in Cardiology* 1997;12:310-320.

5. Kirsch CQ, Zhang GE, Brugada R, Brugada J, Brugada PPD,Moya A, Borggrefe M, Breithardt G, Ortiz-Lopez R, Wang Z, Antzelevitch C, O'Brien RE,Schulze-Bahr E, Keating MT, Towbin JA, Wang Q. Genetic basis and molecular mechanism for idiopahic ventricular fibrillation. *Nature* 1998;392:293-296.

6. Feinberg WM, Blackshear JL, Laupacis A, Kronmal R, Hart RG. Prevalence, age distribution, and gender of patients with atrial fibrillation. *Arch Intern Med* 1995;155:469-473.

7. Albers GW. Atrial fibrillation and stroke: Three new studies, three remaining questions.*Arch Intern Med* 1994;154:1443-1448.

8. Wolff L. Familial auricular fibrillation. *N Engl J Med* 1943;229:396-397.

9. Gould WL. Auricular fibrillation. *Arch Intern Med* 1957;100:916-926.

10. Girona J, Domingo A, Albert D, Casaldaliga J, Mont L, Brugada J, Brugada R. Fibrilacion auricular familiar. *Rev Esp Cardiol* 1997;50:548-551.

11. Tikanoja T, Kirkinen P, Nikolajev K, Eresmaa L, Haring P. Familial atrial fibrillation with fetal onset. *Heart* 1998;79:195-197.

12. Poret P, Mabo P, Deplace C, Leclercq C, Gras D, Marec BL, Daubert C. Isolated atrial fibrillation genetically determined? Apropos of a familial history. *Arch Mal Coeur Vaiss* 1996;89:1197-1203.

13. Beyer F, Paul T, Luhmer I, Bertram H, Kallfelz HC. Familial idiopathic atrial fibrillation with bradyarrhythmia. *Z Kardiol* 1993;82:674-677.

14. Roberts R. ed. Molecular Basis of Cardiology. 1 Ed. Cambridge, MA: Blackwell Scientific, 1993:1-518.

15. Marian AJ, Roberts R. Recent advances in the molecular genetics of hypertrophic cardiomyopathy. *Circulation* 1995;92:1336-1347.

16. Ott J. Analysis of human genetic linkage. Baltimore: The Johns Hopkins University Press, 1991:

17. Brugada R, Tapscott T, Czernuszewicz GZ, Marian AJ, Iglesias A, Mont L, Brugada J, Girona J, Domingo A, Bachinski LL, Roberts R. Identification of a genetic locus for familial atrial fibrillation. *N Engl J Med* 1997;336:905-911.

18. Brugada R, Bachinski LL, Hill R, Roberts R. Familial atrial fibrillation is a genetically heterogeneous disease.*J Am Coll Cardiol* 1998;31:349A(Abstract)

8

THE MOLECULAR CARDIOLOGY OF HEART BLOCK

Robert M. Hamilton, M.D., FRCP(C)

The Hospital for Sick Children, Toronto, Ontario, CANADA

INTRODUCTION

Heart block in children is most frequently acquired as a result of traumatic injury to the conduction system during repair of structural congenital heart disease. Nevertheless, a significant proportion of pediatric heart block is acquired either *in utero* or during childhood due to molecular causes. The most common of these rare disorders is "congenital" complete heart block associated with the presence of maternal autoantibodies in pregnancies of women with clinical or subclinical connective tissue disease. Other possible autoimmune conduction system disorders include Chagas disease and Lyme disease.

Non-immune molecular mechanisms of complete heart block in childhood may include conduction disorders associated with heterotaxia, ventricular inversion, Kearns-Sayre syndrome and related mitochondrial myopathies. Indeed, it was a patient with heterotaxia and dextrocardia that stimulated Yater's 1929 classic definition of congenital complete heart block. (1) Many of the molecular mechanisms underlying these disorders remain at least partially speculative. This chapter will review the current state of knowledge and major hypotheses of these disorders.

CONGENITAL COMPLETE HEART BLOCK

Congenital heart block was described by Morquio in 1901 and defined as "A syndrome of slow pulse, syncopal attacks, and sudden death, often occurring in families". (2) From such a description, it is easy to understand why this disease was suspected to be a genetically transmitted disorder. Complete heart block is usually present at birth, but lesser degrees of block are occasionally present. Many patients are asymptomatic at birth and not detected until later in childhood. A series of case reports led investigators to suspect a relationship with maternal connective tissue disease. (3, 4) Chameides and colleagues reported a series of 6 infants born to mothers with systemic lupus erythematosus, including an infant whose post-mortem study demonstrated thickening of the annulus fibrosus. (5) McCue et al reported that 14 of 22 children with complete heart block were born to mothers with connective tissue disease. (6) They suggested that trans-placental passage of IgG antinuclear antibodies may be responsible for injury to the fetal conduction system.

Serological studies

Esscher and colleagues studied 67 infants and suggested that one in three mothers of children with complete heart block will have or develop connective tissue disease. (7) However, this connective tissue disease may be significantly delayed. (8, 9) Lee and colleagues described the immunology and genetics of this association in 1983. (10) They assessed six affected families and demonstrated that the mothers almost invariably had anti-SSA/Ro antibodies, but that these antibodies disappeared in the children in mid-infancy. Certain HLA antigens predominated in the six seropositive mothers (DR3 in 5, MB2 in 5, MT2 in 6, and B8 in 6), but no associations were found in the affected infants. They concluded that certain HLA antigens were associated with autoantibody production in the mothers, but not with cardiac tissue injury in the infants. However, some HLA markers are more common in the newborn affected by heart block than the unaffected newborn. It is hypothesised that they may play a role by affecting antigen presentation and targeting for the maternal immune response. (11)

The identification of anti-Ro antibody in mothers of children with congenital complete heart block depends on the time of sampling in relation to the affected pregnancy, and the method of analysis. Anti-Ro (SSA) antibody was present in 34/41 mothers when analysed by immunodiffusion, but the majority of samples were collected more than three months after the birth of the affected child. (12) When assessed by more sensitive techniques and collected at or near the time of pregnancy, the prevalence of anti-Ro antibodies in mothers of children with congenital heart block is 97%.(13) Unfortunately, autoantibodies to soluble cellular ribonucleoproteins are interrelated and closely linked. (14) Clustering of autoantibody specificity is a consistent finding in patients with systemic auto-immune diseases. (15) This is considered to result from intermolecular spreading of the immune response. (16) Such spreading limits the ability of serological studies to identify the actual antibody involved in the pathophysiology of congenital heart block. Conversely, in the presence of maternal antibodies, heart block is found in only a few cases. Ramsay Goldman found congenital heart block in only 6 of 96 pregnancies in women with anti-SS- A (anti-Ro) antibodies and this was associated with high-titre levels. (17) Others have found that titres did not differ between mothers of affected or unaffected children. (18)

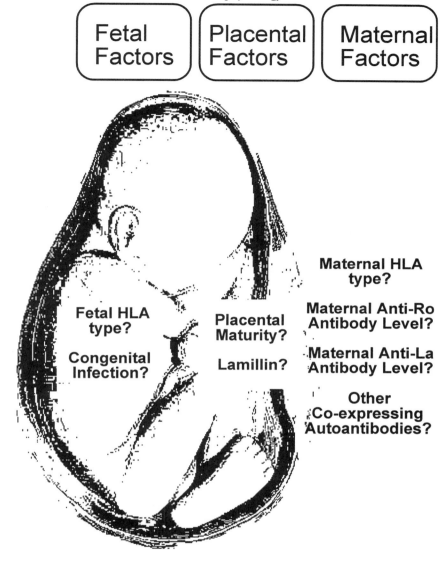

Figure 1. The maternal-fetal dyad in autoimmune congenital heart block

The enigmas of congenital heart block

Anti-Ro antibodies are almost invariably found in mothers of infants with congenital heart block if a sufficiently sensitive assay is performed on sera collected at the time of pregnancy or delivery. However, it remains unclear why the majority of infants born to mothers with anti-Ro antibodies are unaffected. (19, 20) It has been noted that mothers with both anti-Ro/SSA and anti-La/SSB are more likely to have infants with NLE than mothers with anti-Ro/SSA alone.

(21) In subsequent pregnancies to mothers with one affected infant, only 22% of subsequent siblings are affected. In addition, twin pregnancies are usually discordant for heart block, whether fraternal(22) HLA-identical(23-25) or monozygotic(25) . Whatever the true pathophysiology of congenital heart block, it should explain each of the above findings.

Candidate antigens in conduction system disease

Ro proteins are relatively conserved across species; (26) their sub-cellular location is controversial, and their function has been unclear. (27) The intracellular locations of 60 kD Ro and 52 kD Ro are markedly different, at least in keratinocytes. (28) Observations of Pourmand and colleagues indicate a cytoplasmic location of the 52 kD Ro protein. (29)

Calreticulin, a calcium binding protein that resides in the endoplasmic and sarcoplasmic reticulum, is frequently reactive with human Ro/SS- A autoimmune sera. (30) The protein sequence demonstrates significant homology with 60 kD Ro. (31) Anticalreticulin antibodies are frequently present in maternal lupus, but also arise in other diseases, such as onchocerciasis. (32-34) Although calreticulin was considered to be the 60 kD Ro antigen, (35-37) this does not appear to be the case. (38) Although anticalreticulin antibodies are often present in children with congenital heart block or their mothers, this finding is less sensitive than the presence of anti-Ro antibodies, and less specific. (39) Molecular spreading of the immune response from the Ro proteins to calreticulin frequently occurs in experimental models of autoimmunity. (40)

Anti-La antibodies bind preferentially to human fetal hearts, possibly due to binding to cell surface laminin (based on murine studies). (41) Laminin, the major component of the cardiac sarcolemmal membrane, cross-reacts with both anti-La antibodies and human Chagasic Serum. (42, 43) Cross-reaction with placental laminin is postulated to decrease the load of anti-La antibodies to the fetus. (44)

Connexins are an attractive candidate for the antigen involved in congenital heart block. Multiple cardiac connexins exist (Cx40, 43, 45) which have differing cell to cell conduction properties. These cardiac connexins have degrees of expression within the heart which vary with cardiac tissue type and embryologic developmental stage. (45-49) Connexin expression also varies between cell types within a single structure. (50) Connexin 43 begins to be expressed from embryonic day 13 in prenatal rat hearts, but never becomes expressed in the sinus node or atrioventricular node. (48, 51) Connexin 43 is expressed in myocyte-myocyte gap junctions, but not in myocyte-fibroblast gap junctions. (52) Connexin 40 is primarily expressed in the specialised atrioventricular conduction system(53, 54) , particularly in the atrioventricular node. (55) Tissue-specific pattern of connexin expression may contribute to differences in the conduction properties between specialised conduction tissue and the remainder of the myocardium. (56, 57) Developmental reduction in the expression of connexin 40 appears to coincide with developmental changes in the conduction system in the fetal mouse. (58) Connexin 45 is preferentially associated with the ventricular conduction system. (59) Connexin 43 membrane expression, conduction and function are reduced in tissue culture infected with Trypanosoma cruzi. (60, 61) Removal of connexin 40 function in knockout mouse models results in slowed myocardial conduction, resulting in electrocardiographic changes compatible with atrioventricular and His-Purkinje conduction disease. Knockout mouse models for connexin 43 demonstrate reduced conduction velocity in ventricular, but not atrial tissue. (62)

The beta-1 adrenergic receptor is another potential antigen in immune conduction system disorders. IgG from human Chagasic serum binds to this receptor and exerts noncompetitive inhibition. (63, 64) This may be due to molecular mimicry between a ribosomal protein in the spirochete and the structure of the beta-adrenoreceptor. (65-67) Antibodies from Trypanosoma cruzi infected mice also demonstrate this effect. (68) In a rabbit model, these effects can be blocked by introduction of the antigen. (69) A similar mechanism has been suggested in congenital complete heart block. (70) Circulating IgG antibodies can noncompetitively inhibit both beta adrenoreceptors and muscarinic receptors. (71) Circulating antibodies against muscarinic receptors have been identified in Sjogren's syndrome, (72) and are specific to neonatal tissue(73) , probably due to a different muscarinic receptor, the M1 sub-type. (74, 75) They have also been identified in human Chagas' disease, (64, 68, 76-81) and may cause the bradycardia frequently observed in these patients. (82) Antiacetylcholinesterase antibodies have also been identified in human and experimental Chagas' disease. (83)

More recently, the L-type calcium channel has been implicated as the target of injury in the heart block associated with neonatal lupus erythematosus. It has been demonstrated in adult rabbit and human fetal hearts that sera containing anti-SSA/Ro antibodies induce atrioventricular block and inhibit L-type calcium currents. (84-86) However, these studies were performed in ventricular tissue, which is not the primary tissue of injury in congenital heart block.

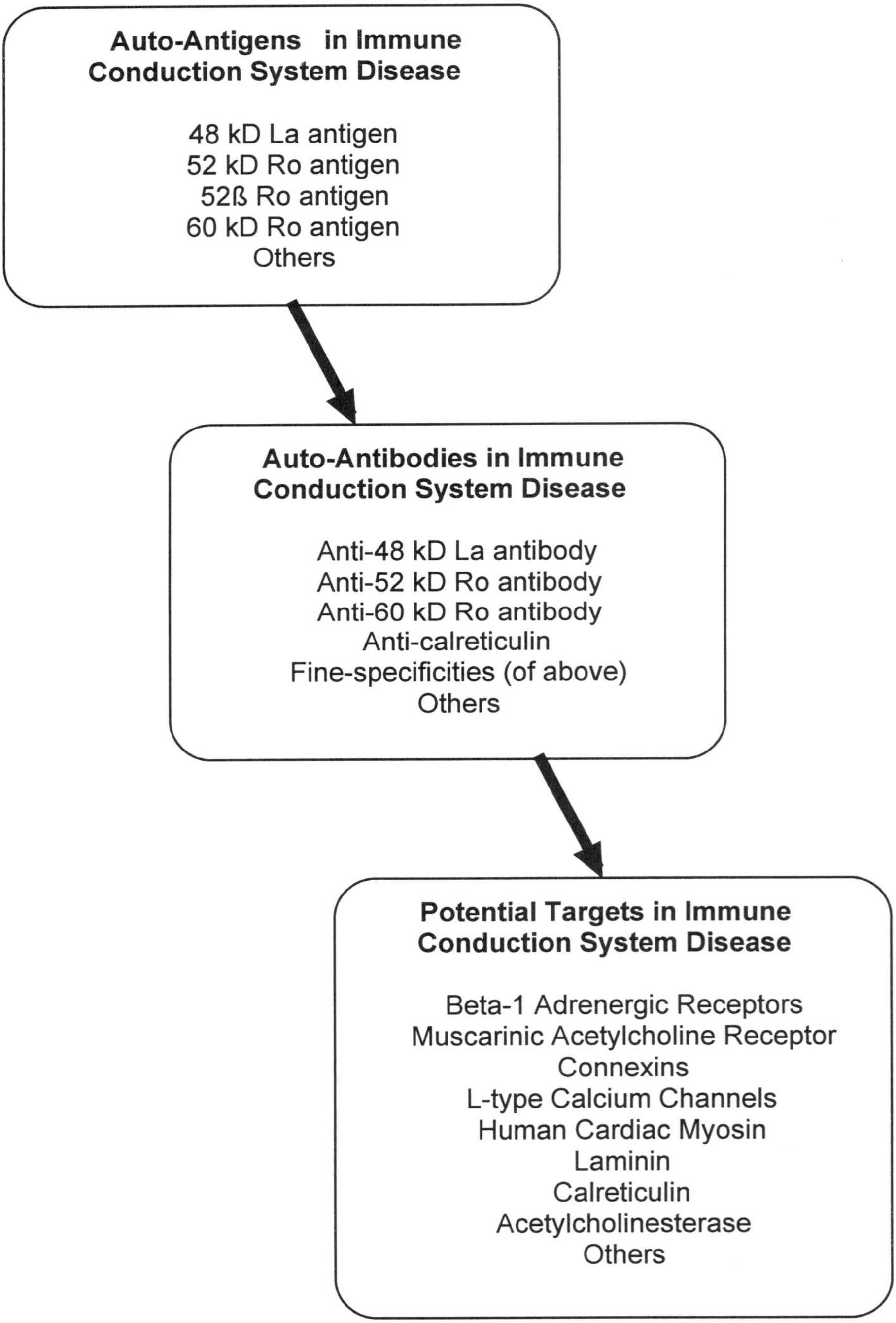

Figure 2. Auto-antigens, auto-antibodies and putative sites of action in immune conduction system diseases

Potential Therapies

Since congenital heart block is actually a fetally acquired disease, potential therapy or prevention should begin in utero. Maternal lupus erythematosus is also associated with significant fetal wastage, (87) possibly related to heart block, (88) and this also should be prevented. An early recommended prevention was plasmapheresis, with the intent of reducing the antibody load to the fetus. (89, 90) The use of this therapy in a pregnancy was reported in 1987 and demonstrated apparent improvement in myocardial dysfunction, but no reversal of heart block. (91) Pregnancies to mothers with systemic lupus erythematosus, a previously affected child, high anti-Ro and anti-La titers and HLA DR3 are considered at highest risk. (92) Although prophylactic plasmapheresis has been suggested, experience demonstrates at best a limited success. (93) Plasmapheresis did appear to reduce fetal wastage in pregnancies complicated by systemic lupus erythematosus with positive antiphospholipid antibodies in a small series of patients. (94)

Maternal therapy with steroids during pregnancy has been reported since 1969. (95) Most reports indicate that steroid therapy is unable to reverse complete heart block once it has been established, (96, 97) although there are rare exceptions in case reports(98) or small series. (99, 100) However, ascites and pericardial effusion may resolve or substantially decrease. (101) It has been suggested that therapy should be initiated by 16 weeks of gestation. (97)

Although preventive therapies of plasmapheresis and steroid administration have been practised by some for more than 10 years, there remains no sensitive method of identifying pregnancies at risk prior to heart block *in utero*. Thus, to avoid unnecessary therapy in the many unaffected pregnancies to mothers with auto-immune disease, a more sensitive method of detecting pregnancies at risk is necessary. An alternative approach would be to identify the affected fetus early in the course of the disease, and interrupt the pathophysiology. Although sequential ultrasound screening might be expected to identify conduction disorders short of complete (3°) AV block, second degree AV block has not been detected in fetal echocardiographic studies and it is difficult to identify subtle changes in PR interval (1°AV block) by this technique. The non-invasive fetal electrocardiogram (ECG) may provide a rapid simple alternative for screening pregnancies at risk.

CHAGAS DISEASE

American trypanosomiasis, or Chagas disease, is a parasitic disease caused by the haemoflagellate protozoa, Trypanosoma cruzi. The human infection occurs only in the Americas, where it is widely distributed in the periurban and rural areas of tropical and subtropical countries, from Mexico to Argentina and Chile. It is transmitted to man and other mammals mainly through insects, the triatomine bugs. As an enzootic disease, it extends from approximately latitude 42.5 degrees N (northern California and Maryland) to latitude 43.5 degrees S (southern Argentina and Chile). The results of several serological surveys indicate an overall prevalence of 16-18 million infected individuals. Up to 30% of those infected will develop the cardiac and/or hollow viscera irreversible lesions that characterise chronic Chagas disease. The endemic countries can be divided into four groups according to several indicators such as the number of confirmed human cases, the prevalence of sero-positive tests in blood donors and population samples, the presence of infected vectors and reservoirs, and the existence or absence of co-ordinated actions towards the control of this disease. The domestic cycle of transmission, involving man and domestic animals such as dogs, cats, and domestic triatomine bugs, is the one that maintains the infections in the rural and peri-urban areas. Although heart block does occur, the poor prognosis in Chagas disease appears to be more related to ventricular arrhythmias than to AV conduction disturbances. (102, 103)

The molecular pathology of Chagas disease has been suspected to be due to a hypersensitivity reaction to antigens present on subcellular fragments of the parasite Trypanosoma Cruzi. Multiple investigators have suggested that the autoimmune mechanisms that underlie Chagas disease are similar to those of a subset of patients with systemic lupus erythematosus. (104, 105)   Such a reaction has been reproduced in a rabbit model demonstrating myocarditis as early as 1975. (106) Autoimmunity against gap junction proteins, resulting in altered cellular distribution of these proteins and modified cellular electrophysiology have been proposed. (61)

LYME DISEASE

Fluctuating degrees of AV block is the most common cardiac manifestation of Lyme disease in young patients, although it was typically brief (three days to six weeks) (107)   and rarely require pacemaker therapy. (108-111)   This manifestation may be related to acute lymphocytic carditis, (112) and respond to systemic steroids. (113) The heart block is usually supra-Hisian, (112, 114) although HV prolongation may also occur. (115, 116) The concept that auto-immunity may play a role in Lyme disease was first proposed in relation to its neurological manifestations. (117, 118) Indeed, triggering of an auto-immune process has been implicated for multiple infectious diseases, including those with cardiac effects of transient heart block such as Lyme disease and acute rheumatic fever. (119)   Thus although Lyme disease starts as an active cardiac infection which does respond to antibiotic therapy, late or persistent manifestations may be due to local inflammatory or systemic immune responses to pathogenic antigens. (120-122)

ANIMAL MODELS OF IMMUNE CONDUCTION DISEASE

Rabbit

The rabbit was first used as a model of autoimmune conduction system injury in experimental Chagas disease. (106, 123) Ouaissi and colleagues suggested that acetylcholinesterase was the cross reacting antigen in Chagas disease. An alternate finding was that ribonucleoproteins were the cross-reacting antigens in both rabbit and mouse models of the disease. (124) De Oleivera and colleagues have demonstrated that sera from chronic chagasic patients depress conduction in isolated Langendorff-perfused rabbit hearts. (125) These abnormalities can be suppressed by introduction of Trypanosoma cruzi antigens, presumably through competition for auto-antibodies. (69)

Mamula and colleagues then demonstrated that human Ro antigen was immunogenic in a rabbit model. (126) Alexander and colleagues demonstrated that sera and IgG- enriched fractions from anti-SS-A/Ro SS-B/La-positive individuals preferentially bind to cardiac cells and inhibit repolarization in neonatal compared to adult rabbits. (127) Mamula also demonstrated that human and rabbit anti-Ro antibodies behaved similarly both in terms of assay and binding. (128) Alexander and colleagues then went on to demonstrate in their rabbit model that anti-Ro antibodies selectively bind to neonatal cardiac cells and alter membrane repolarization. They concluded that anti-Ro/SS-A antibodies may play a pathophysiologic role in the development of congenital heart block in neonatal lupus. (129)

Garcia and colleagues were the first to demonstrate the production of heart block in Langendorff perfused isolated hearts from adolescent rabbits using IgG-rich sera from mothers with systemic lupus erythematosus (albeit whose children did not have heart block). (130) We were unable to reproduce this finding in similar adolescent rabbit hearts using unconcentrated sera from mothers of children with complete heart block, but were able to demonstrate AV block when neonatal rabbit hearts were used. (131) Supporting their original findings, Viani, Garcia and colleagues were able to demonstrate that affinity purified anti-52 kD Ro/SSA antibodies from mothers with healthy infants are capable of causing in vitro cardiac conduction disturbance. (132)

The Mouse
Circulating antibodies from human and murine chagasic sera bind noncompetitively to both beta-adrenergic receptors and muscarinic cholinergic receptors, leading to increased intracellular levels of cyclic AMP and cyclic GMP respectively. (64, 79) Connexins have been studied in mouse models, including genetic "knockouts".(133) They demonstrate unique patterns of distribution to conduction tissue and developmental changes in isoform concentration and distribution as well. (58, 59) When the conduction system is stressed by esophageal pacing, AV conduction disturbances can be demonstrated in connexin "knockout" mice. (134) Little work has been done to investigate these gap junction proteins as potential targets of autoantibodies.

Anti-La antibodies have been demonstrated to bind to mouse laminin at the myocardial cell surface. (135) Alternately, binding of autoantibodies to laminin in the placenta may modulate neonatal exposure to these potential pathogens. (44) Electrocardiograms of neonatal mice from mothers with experimental SLE demonstrate a high percentage with defects in their conduction system including first, second, and third degree heart block; significant bradycardia; and wide QRS complex. (136, 137) This finding was also demonstrated by Miranda Carus and colleagues who used human recombinant 48 kD La and 60 kD Ro and two transcripts of human recombinant 52 kD Ro antigens to generate their murine SLE model. The found conduction system defects, albeit infrequently, only in the offspring of mothers immunized with 52ß Ro antigen. However, the offspring were not assessed in utero. (138) Mazel and colleagues attempted to generate heart block in a murine model with passive infusion of human autoantibodies, but were able to generate only bradycardia or first degree AV block. (139)

Future Directions
Current animal and tissue culture models, combined with a molecular approach, may allow for more expeditious testing of proposed hypotheses related to the pathogenesis of congenital heart block. (131) The development of human fetal cardiac myocyte cultures demonstrating expression of SSA/Ro and SSB/La may contribute to our ability to investigate this disease. (140) Alternately, it may be that the pathophysiology would be better explored in the isolated AV node. It has been suggested that a second factor may be required for the production of congenital heart block. Such a mechanism has been proposed and evaluated in a tissue culture model relating to skin manifestations of congenital heart block. Ro antigen is usually located in the intracellular cytoplasm. (141) In fibroblast culture, surface expression of Ro antigen is stimulated by the combination of UVB radiation and CMV infection.

A higher occurrence of antibodies to CMV has been found in mothers of affected infants, compared to controls. (142) CMV is a frequently occurring infection, with a high rate of sero-conversion in the general population. Nevertheless, it is known that congenital CMV infection can preferentially affect only one of twins.

MITOCHONDRIAL DISORDERS

The most typical mitochondrial diseases are due to specific mutations of mitochondrial DNA and are usually transmitted through the maternal line via the cytoplasm. These include mitochondrial encephalopathy with lactic acidosis and stroke-like episodes (MELAS), myoclonic epilepsy with ragged red fibers (MERRF) or neuropathy, ataxia and retinitis pigmentosum/maternally inherited Leigh's disease (NARP/MILS). Leber's hereditary optic neuropathy (LHON) is observed more frequently in males than females. Mitochondrial DNA demonstrates significant pleomorphism, and is also more susceptible to mutations than nuclear DNA, and these give rise to myopathies, with or without ophthalmoplegia. The combination of myopathy, opthalmoplegia and fascicular block defines the Kearns-Sayre syndrome (KSS), which usually has large-scale deletions of mitochondrial DNA. Related disorders include Leigh's syndrome, Alpers polydystrophies, myoneurogastrointestinal syndromes such as mitochondrial neurogastrointestinal encephalopathy (MNGIE), Barth's syndrome and Freidrich's disease. A more severe disorder resulting from mitochondrial DNA rearrangement is the lethal childhood disorder , Pearson's Marrow/Pancreas Syndrome. Defects in communication between the mitochondrial genome and nuclear gene defects on chromosomes 3 and 10 give rise to an autosomal dominant chronic progressive external opthalmoplegia. All of these disorders involve, at some level, mitochondrial respiratory chain dysfunction. Some cases of Alzheimers Disease and Parkinson's Disease are also related to mitochondrial base substitutions.

Mitochondrial DNA Disorders

MELAS   Mitichondrial Encephalopathy with Lactic Acidosis and Stroke-like Episodes
MERRF   Myoclonic Epilepsy with Ragged Red Fibers
NARP   Neuropathy, Ataxia and Retinitis Pigmentosum
MILS   Maternally Inherited Leigh's Disease
LHON   Leber's Hereditary Optic Neuropathy
MNGIE   Mitochondrial Neurogastrointestinal Encephalopathy
KSS   Kearns-Sayre Syndrome
Pearson's Marrow/Pancreas Syndrome
Leigh's syndrome
Alpers polydystrophies

Figure 3. Mitochondrial Disorders

The deletions, duplications and rearrangements constituting the Kearns-Sayre syndrome may be broad and varied and may result in multisystem involvement, which may include short stature, gonadal failure, thyroid disease, hyperaldosteronism, hypoparathyroidism, hypomagnesemia, deafness, encephalomyopathy, cerebellar ataxia, diabetes mellitus. Typical Kearns-Sayre syndrome is characterized by an onset before age 20, progressive external opthalmoplegia, pigmentary retinopathy and bifascicular block progressing to complete heart block at the infra-Hisian level. The prognosis in Kearns-Sayre syndrome can be significantly improved by pacemaker intervention at the appropriate time. Similar diseases with manifestations of heart block such as MNGIE syndrome are also associated with a poor prognosis and pacemaker therapy should be considered if symptoms, bifascicular block or heart block are noted. (143) A mouse model of Kearns-Sayre syndrome has been produced by disrupting the function of mitochondrial transcription factor A (TFam), which regulates transcription and regulation of mitochondrial DNA. (144)

HETEROTAXIA

The presence of heart block in some cases of the left atrial isomerism form of heterotaxia has been recognised for approximately thirty years. Garcia and colleagues described six children, aged 12 days to 13 years, with left isomerism and complete atrioventricular block, 5 of whom also had atrio-ventricular septal defects. (145) Roguin and colleagues described an additional three cases and suggested that the overall incidence of AV block is 20% of patients with left atrial isomerism. (146) Shenker suggested that left atrial isomerism and atrioventricular canal is the most likely cause of fetal heart block when there is no evidence for maternal auto-immune disease, and that the prognosis is extremely poor. (147) Wren and colleagues reviewed 67 patients with left atrial isomerism and found complete AV block in ten. This was associated with an atrioventricular septal defect in five of the ten. (148) When patients detected prenatally with AV septal defect also have left atrial isomerism, complete heart block is almost invariably present (11/12). (149-151) Prenatal death is common, and frequently due to congestive heart failure, but these fetal deaths are not usually included in paediatric statistics. The histological mechanism of heart block in these cases was discontinuity between the AV node and ventricular conduction system, rather than between the atria and AV node as in the presence of right atrial isomerism or maternal connective tissue disease. (152) Two separate molecular mechanisms implicate the gap junction in the production of AV conduction disturbances. First, the dorsoventral distribution and function of gap junction connexins in the embryo influence left-right asymmetry in the developing vertebrate embryo. (153) Mutations in the connexin-43 gap-junction gene are associated with visceroatrial heterotaxia. (154) This is thought to be due to abnormal regulation of intercellular communication. (155)

Gap junctions are also necessary for the rapid spread of conduction through the His-Purkinje system. Mice lacking Connexin-40 have first degree AV block and bundle branch conduction disturbances. (156) Connexin type and tissue distribution vary with development, tissue and species. (102, 103)

SUMMARY

Multiple molecular mechanisms, both genetic and autoimmune, should be considered in the assessment conduction system disease presenting in the fetus, infant or child. Our understanding of the physiology and pathophysiology of the specialized cardiac conduction system remains markedly incomplete, partially due to the relative infrequency of these disorders. The use of molecular investigational techniques, particularly in animal and tissue culture models, has great potential to broaden our understanding of these areas.

REFERENCES

1. Yater WM. Congenital heart block: Review of the literature - Report of a case with incomplete heterotaxy: The electrocardiogram in dextrocardia. Am J Dis Child 1929;38:112.
2. Morquio L. Sur une Maladie Infantile et Familiale Caracterisee et la Aort Subite. Arch Med Enfants 1901;4:467.
3. Winkler RB, Nora AH, Nora JJ. Familial congenital complete heart block and maternal systemic lupus erythematosis. Circulation 1977;56:1103-7.
4. Hull D, Binns BA, Joyce D. Congenital heart block and widespread fibrosis due to maternal lupus erythematosus. Arch Dis Child 1966;41:688-90.
5. Chameides L, Truex RC, Vetter V, Rashkind WJ, Galioto FMJ, Noonan JA. Association of maternal systemic lupus erythematosus with congenital complete heart block. N Engl J Med 1977;297:1204-7.
6. McCue CM, Mantakas ME, Tingelstad JB, Ruddy S. Congenital heart block in newborns of mothers with connective tissue disease. Circulation 1977;56:82-90.
7. Esscher E, Scott JS. Congenital heart block and maternal systemic lupus erythematosus. Am J Roentgenol 1979;133:1235-8.
8. Kasinath BS, Katz AI. Delayed maternal lupus after delivery of offspring with congenital heart block. Arch Intern Med 1982;142:2317.
9. Reid RL, Pancham SR, Kean WF, Ford PM. Maternal and neonatal implications of congenital complete heart block in the fetus. Obstet Gynecol 1979;54:470-4.
10. Lee LA, Bias WB, Arnett FCJ, et al. Immunogenetics of the neonatal lupus syndrome. Ann Intern Med 1983;99:592-6.
11. Siren MK, Julkunen H, Kaaja R, Ekblad H, Koskimies S. Role of HLA in congenital heart block: susceptibility alleles in children. Lupus 1999;8:60-7.
12. Scott JS, Maddison PJ, Taylor PV, Esscher E, Scott O, Skinner RP. Connective-tissue disease, antibodies to ribonucleoprotein, and congenital heart block. N Engl J Med 1983;309:209-12.

13. Julkunen H, Kurki P, Kaaja R, et al. Isolated congenital heart block. Long-term outcome of mothers and characterization of the immune response to SS-A/Ro and to SS-B/La. Arthritis Rheum 1993;36:1588-98.

14. Maddison PJ, Skinner RP, Vlachoyiannopoulos P, Brennand DM, Hough D. Antibodies to nRNP, Sm, Ro(SSA) and La(SSB) detected by ELISA: their specificity and inter-relations in connective tissue disease sera. Clin Exp Immunol 1985;62:337-45.

15. Keech CL, Gordon TP, McCluskey J. The immune response to 52-kDa Ro and 60-kDa Ro is linked in experimental autoimmunity. J Immunol 1996;157:3694-9.

16. Tseng CE, Chan EK, Miranda E, Gross M, Di Donato F, Buyon JP. The 52-kd protein as a target of intermolecular spreading of the immune response to components of the SS-A/Ro-SS-B/La complex. Arthritis Rheum 1997;40:936-44.

17. Ramsey Goldman R, Hom D, Deng JS, et al. Anti-SS-A antibodies and fetal outcome in maternal systemic lupus erythematosus. Arthritis Rheum 1986;29:1269-73.

18. Gross KR, Petty RE, Lum VL, Allen RC. Maternal autoantibodies and fetal disease. Clin Exp Rheumatol 1989;7:651-7.

19. McHugh NJ, Reilly PA, McHugh LA. Pregnancy outcome and autoantibodies in connective tissue disease. J Rheumatol 1989;16:42-6.

20. Lockshin MD, Bonfa E, Elkon K, Druzin ML. Neonatal lupus risk to newborns of mothers with systemic lupus erythematosus. Arthritis Rheum 1988;31:697-701.

21. Miyagawa S, Shinohara K, Kidoguchi K, et al. Neonatal lupus erythematosus: studies on HLA class II genes and autoantibody profiles in Japanese mothers. Autoimmunity 1997;26:95-101.

22. Callen JP, Fowler JF, Kulick KB, Stelzer G, Smith SZ. Neonatal lupus erythematosus occurring in one fraternal twin. Serologic and immunogenetic studies. Arthritis Rheum 1985;28:271-5.

23. Kaaja R, Julkunen H, Ammala P, Kurki P, Koskimies S. Congenital heart block in one of the HLA identical twins. Eur J Obstet Gynecol Reprod Biol 1993;51:78-80.

24. Watson RM, Scheel JN, Petri M, et al. Neonatal lupus erythematosus. Report of serological and immunogenetic studies in twins discordant for congenital heart block. Br J Dermat 1994;130:342-8.

25. Cooley HM, Keech CL, Melny BJ, Menahem S, Morahan G, Kay TW. Monozygotic twins discordant for congenital complete heart block. Arthritis Rheum 1997;40:381-4.

26. Wang D, Buyon JP, Chan EK. Cloning and expression of mouse 60kDa ribonucleoprotein SS-A/Ro. Mol Biol Rep 1996;23:205-10.

27. O'Brien CA, Margelot K, Wolin SL. Xenopus Ro ribonucleoproteins: members of an evolutionarily conserved class of cytoplasmic ribonucleoproteins. Proc Natl Acad Sci USA 1993;90:7250-4.

28. Yell JA, Wang L, Yin H, McCauliffe DP. Disparate locations of the 52- and 60-kDa Ro/SS-A antigens in cultured human keratinocytes. J Invest Dermatol 1996;107:622-6.

29. Pourmand N, Blange I, Ringertz N, Pettersson I. Intracellular localisation of the Ro 52kD auto-antigen in HeLa cells visualised with green fluorescent protein chimeras. Autoimmunity 998;28:225-33.

30. McCauliffe DP, Yang YS, Wilson J, Sontheimer RD, Capra JD. The 5'-flanking region of the human calreticulin gene shares homology with the human GRP78, GRP94, and proteindisulfide isomerase promoters. J Biol Chem 1992;267:2557-62.

31. McCauliffe DP, Zappi E, Lieu TS, Michalak M, Sontheimer RD, Capra JD. A human Ro/SS-A autoantigen is the homologue of calreticulin and is highly homologous withonchocercal RAL-1 antigen and an aplysia "memory molecule". J Clin Invest 1990;86:332-5.

32. Meilof JF, Van der Lelij A, Rokeach LA, Hoch SO, Smeenk RJ. Autoimmunity and filariasis. Autoantibodies against cytoplasmic cellular proteins in sera of patients with onchocerciasis. J Immunol 1993;151:5800-9.

33. Lux FA, McCauliffe DP, Buttner DW, et al. Serological cross-reactivity between a human Ro/SS-A autoantigen (calreticulin) and the lambda Ral-1 antigen ofOnchocerca volvulus. J Clin Invest 1992;89:1945-51.

34. Rokeach LA, Haselby JA, Meilof JF, et al. Characterization of the autoantigen calreticulin. J Immunol 1991;147:3031-9.

35. McCauliffe DP, Sontheimer RD. Molecular characterization of the Ro/SS-A autoantigens. J Invest Dermatol 1993;100:73S-79S.

36. Lu J, Willis AC, Sim RB. A calreticulin-like protein co-purifies with a '60 kD' component of Ro/SSA, but is not recognized by antibodies in Sjogren's syndrome sera. Clin Exp Immunol 1993;94:429-34

37. Ben Chetrit E. The molecular basis of the SSA/Ro antigens and the clinical significance of their autoantibodies. Br J Rheumatol 1993;32:396-402.

38. Boehm J, Orth T, Van Nguyen P, Soling HD. Systemic lupus erythematosus is associated with increased auto-antibody titers against calreticulin and grp94, but calreticulin is not the Ro/SS-A antigen. Eur J Clin Invest 1994;24:248-57.

39. Orth T, Dorner T, Meyer Zum Buschenfelde KH, Mayet WJ. Complete congenital heart block is associated with increased autoantibody titers against calreticulin.Eur J Clin Invest 1996;26:205-15.

40. Kinoshita G, Keech CL, Sontheimer RD, Purcell A, McCluskey J, Gordon TP. Spreading of the immune response from 52 kDaRo and 60 kDaRo to calreticulin in experimental autoimmunity. Lupus 1998;7:7-11.

41. Li JM, Horsfall AC, Maini RN. Anti-La (SS-B) but not anti-Ro52 (SS-A) antibodies cross-react with laminin--a role in the pathogenesis of congenital heart block? ClinExp Immunol 1995;99:316-24.

42. Umezawa ES, Shikanai Yasuda MA, Stolf AM. Changes in isotype composition and antigen recognition of anti- Trypanosoma cruzi antibodies from acute to chronic Chagas disease. J Clin Lab Anal 1996;10:407-13.

43. Horsfall AC, Neu E, Forrest G, Venables PJ, Field M. Maternal autoantibodies and congenital heart block: clues from two consecutive pregnancies, one in which there was congenital complete heart block and one in which the fetus was healthy. Arthritis Rheum 1998;41:2079-80

44. Horsfall AC, Li JM, Maini RN. Placental and fetal cardiac laminin are targets for cross-reacting autoantibodies from mothers of children with congenital heart block. J Autoimmun 1996;9:561-8.

45. Gourdie RG, Green CR, Severs NJ, Thompson RP. Immunolabelling patterns of gap junction connexins in the developing and mature rat heart. Anat Embryol (Berl) 1992;185:363-78.

46. Oosthoek PW, Viragh S, Lamers WH, Moorman AF. Immunohistochemical delineation of the conduction system. II: The atrioventricular node and Purkinje fibers. Circ Res 1993;73(3):482-91.

47. De Maziere A, Analbers L, Jongsma HJ, Gros D. Immunoelectron microscopic visualization of the gap junction protein connexin 40 in the mammalian heart. Eur J Morphol 1993;31:51-4.

48. van Kempen MJ, Fromaget C, Gros D, Moorman AF, Lamers WH. Spatial distribution of connexin43, the major cardiac gap junction protein, in the developing and adult rat heart. CircRes 1991;68:1638-51.

49. Davis LM, Rodefeld ME, Green K, Beyer EC, Saffitz JE. Gap junction protein phenotypes of the human heart and conduction system. J Cardiovasc Electrophysiol 1995:813-22.

50. Kwong KF, Schuessler RB, Green KG, et al. Differential expression of gap junction proteins in the canine sinus node. Circ Res 1998;82:604-12.

51. Oosthoek PW, Viragh S, Mayen AE, van K M. J., Lamers WH, Moorman AF. Immunohistochemical delineation of the conduction system. I: The sinoatrial node. CircRes 1993;73:473-81.

52. Rook MB, van Ginneken AC, de JB, el AA, Gros D, Jongsma HJ. Differences in gap junction channels between cardiac myocytes, fibroblasts, andheterologous pairs. Am J Physiol 1992:C959-77.

53. Gourdie RG, Severs NJ, Green CR, Rothery S, Germroth P, Thompson RP. The spatial distribution and relative abundance of gap-junctional connexin40 and connexin43 correlate to functional properties of components of the cardiac atrioventricular conduction system.J Cell Sci 1993:985-91.

54. Bastide B, Neyses L, Ganten D, Paul M, Willecke K, Traub O. Gap junction protein connexin40 is preferentially expressed in vascular endothelium and conductive bundles of rat myocardium and is increased under hypertensive conditions. Circ Res 1993;73:1138-49.

55. Gros D, Jarry Guichard T, Ten Velde I, et al. Restricted distribution of connexin40, a gap junctional protein, in mammalian heart. Circ Res 1994;74:839-51.

56. Kanter HL, Laing JG, Beau SL, Beyer EC, Saffitz JE. Distinct patterns of connexin expression in canine Purkinje fibers and ventricular muscle. Circ Res 1993;72:1124-31.

57. Davis LM, Kanter HL, Beyer EC, Saffitz JE. Distinct gap junction protein phenotypes in cardiac tissues with disparate conduction properties. J Am Coll Cardiol 1994;24:1124-32.

58. Delorme B, Dahl E, Jarry Guichard T, et al. Developmental regulation of connexin 40 gene expression in mouse heart correlates with the differentiation of the conduction system.Dev Dyn 1995;204:358-71.

59. Coppen SR, Dupont E, Rothery S, Severs NJ. Connexin45 expression is preferentially associated with the ventricular conduction system in mouse and rat heart. Circ Res 1998;82:232-43.

60. de Carvalho AC, Tanowitz HB, Wittner M, et al. Gap junction distribution is altered between cardiac myocytes infected with Trypanosoma cruzi. Circ Res 1992;70:733-42.

61. de Carvalho AC, Masuda MO, Tanowitz HB, Wittner M, Goldenberg RC, Spray DC. Conduction defects and arrhythmias in Chagas' disease: possible role of gap junctions and humoral mechanisms. J Cardiovasc Electrophysiol 1994;5:686-98.

62. Thomas SA, Schuessler RB, Berul CI, et al. Disparate effects of deficient expression of connexin43 on atrial and ventricular conduction: evidence for chamber-specific molecular determinants of conduction. Circulation 1998;97:686-91.

63. Sterin Borda L, Cantore M, Pascual J, et al. Chagasic IgG binds and interacts with cardiac beta adrenoceptor-coupled adenylate cyclase system. Int J Immunopharmacol 1986;8:581-8.

64. Cremaschi G, Zwirner NW, Gorelik G, et al. Modulation of cardiac physiology by an anti-Trypanosoma cruzi monoclonal antibody after interaction with myocardium.Faseb J 1995;9:1482-8.

65. Elies R, Ferrari I, Wallukat G, et al. Structural and functional analysis of the B cell epitopes recognized by anti-receptor autoantibodies in patients with Chagas' disease. J Immunol 1996;157:4203-11.

66. Ferrari I, Levin MJ, Wallukat G, et al. Molecular mimicry between the immunodominant ribosomal protein P0 of Trypanosoma cruzi and a functional epitope on the human beta 1-adrenergic receptor. J Exp Med 1995;182:59-65.

67. Kaplan D, Ferrari I, Bergami PL, et al. Antibodies to ribosomal P proteins of Trypanosoma cruzi in Chagas disease possess functional autoreactivity with heart tissue and differ from anti-P autoantibodies in lupus. Proc Natl Acad Sci U S A 1997;94:10301-6.

68. Mijares A, Verdot L, Peineau N, Vray B, Hoebeke J, Argibay J. Antibodies from Trypanosoma cruzi infected mice recognize the second extracellular loop of the beta 1-adrenergic and M2-muscarinic receptors and regulate calcium channels in isolated cardiomyocytes. Mol CellBiochem 1996;164:107-12.

69. Masuda MO, Levin M, De Oliveira SF, et al. Functionally active cardiac antibodies in chronic Chagas' disease are specifically blocked by Trypanosoma cruzi antigens. Faseb J 1998;12:1551-8.

70. Camusso JJ, Borda ES, Bacman S, et al. Antibodies against beta adrenoceptors in mothers of children with congenital heart block. Acta Physiol Pharmacol Ther Latinoam 1994;44:94-9.

71. Bacman S, Sterin BL, Camusso JJ, Hubscher O, Arana R, Borda ES. Circulating antibodies against neurotransmitter receptor activities in children with congenital heart block and their mothers. Faseb J 1994;8:1170-6.

72. Bacman S, Sterin BL, Camusso JJ, Arana R, Hubscher O, Borda E. Circulating antibodies against rat parotid gland M3 muscarinic receptors in primary Sjogren's syndrome. Clin Exp Immunol 1996;104:454-9

73. Borda E, Camusso JJ, Perez Leiros C, et al. Circulating antibodies against neonatal cardiac muscarinic acetylcholine receptor in patients with Sjogren's syndrome. Mol Cell Biochem 1996;164:335-41.

74. Borda ES, Perez LC, Camusso JJ, Bacman S, Sterin Borda L. Differential cholinoceptor subtype-dependent activation of signal transduction pathways in neonatal versus adult rat atria. Biochem Pharmacol 1997;53:959-67.

75. Borda E, Leiros CP, Bacman S, Berra A, Sterin Borda L. Sjogren autoantibodies modify neonatal cardiac function via M1 muscarinic acetylcholine receptor activation. Int J Cardiol 1999;70:23-32.

76. Goin JC, Perez Leiros C, Borda E, Sterin Borda L. Modification of cholinergic-mediated cellular transmembrane signals by the interaction of human chagasic IgG with cardiac muscarinic receptors. Neuroimmunomodulation 1994;1:284-91.

77. Goin JC, Borda E, Leiros CP, Storino R, Sterin Borda L. Identification of antibodies with muscarinic cholinergic activity in human Chagas' disease: pathological implications. JAuton Nerv Syst 1994;47:45-52.

78. Goin JC, Perez Leiros C, Borda E, Sterin Borda L. [Interaction of chagasic autoantibodies with the third extracellular domain of the human heart muscarinic receptor.Functional and pathological implications]. Medicina (B Aires) 1996;56:699-704.

79. Goin JC, Leiros CP, Borda E, Sterin Borda L. Interaction of human chagasic IgG with the second extracellular loop of the human heart muscarinic acetylcholine receptor. Faseb J 1997;11:77-83.

80. Leiros CP, Sterin Borda L, Borda ES, Goin JC, Hosey MM. Desensitization and sequestration of human m2 muscarinic acetylcholine receptors by autoantibodies from patients with Chagas' disease. J Biol Chem 1997;272:12989-93.

81. Sterin Borda L, Leiros CP, Goin JC, et al. Participation of nitric oxide signaling system in the cardiac muscarinic cholinergic effect of human chagasic IgG. J Mol Cell Cardiol 1997;29:1851-65.

82. Goin JC, Borda ES, Auger S, Storino R, Sterin Borda L. CardiacM(2) muscarinic cholinoceptor activation by human chagasic autoantibodies: association with bradycardia. Heart 1999;82:273-278.

83. Ouaissi A, Cornette J, Velge P, Capron A. Identification of anti-acetylcholinesterase and anti-idiotype antibodies in human and experimental Chagas' disease. Eur J Immunol 1988;18:1889-94.

84. Buyon JP. Neonatal lupus: bedside to bench and back [editorial]. Scand J Rheumatol 1996;25:271-6.
85. Boutjdir M, Chen L, Zhang ZH, et al. Arrhythmogenicity of IgG and anti-52-kD SSA/Ro affinity-purified antibodies from mothers of children with congenital heart block. Circ Res 1997;80:354-62.
86. Boutjdir M, Chen L, Zhang ZH, Tseng CE, El SN, Buyon JP. Serum and immunoglobulin G from the mother of a child with congenital heart block induce conduction abnormalities and inhibit L-type calcium channels in a rat heart model. Pediatr Res 1998;44:11-9.
87. Zurier RB, Argyros TG, Urman JD, Warren J, Rothfield NF. Systemic lupus erythematosus. Management during pregnancy. Obstet Gynecol 1978;51:178-80.
88. Julkunen H, Kaaja R, Siren MK. Recurrent miscarriage, congenital heart block and systemic lupus erythematosus. Aust N Z J Obstet Gynaecol 1999;39:26-7.
89. Buyon J, Szer I. Passively acquired autoimmunity and the maternal fetal dyad in systemic lupus erythematosus. Springer Semin Immunopathol 1986;9:283-304.
90. Hubbard HC, Portnoy B. Systemic lupus erythematosus in pregnancy treated with plasmapheresis. Br J Dermatol 1979;101:87-9.
91. Buyon JP, Swersky SH, Fox HE, Bierman FZ, Winchester RJ. Intrauterine therapy for presumptive fetal myocarditis with acquired heart block due to systemic lupus erythematosus. Experience in a mother with a predominance of SS-B (La) antibodies. Arthritis Rheum 1987;30:44-9.
92. Muller Ladner U, Benning K, Rother E, Lang B. [Neonatal lupus erythematosus as an example of passively acquired autoimmunity]. Immun Infekt 1992;20:117-21.
93. Olah KS, Gee H. Antibody mediated complete congenital heart block in the fetus. Pacing Clin Electrophysiol 1993;16:1872-9.
94. Nakamura Y, Yoshida K, Itoh S, et al. Immunoadsorption plasmapheresis as a treatment for pregnancy complicated by systemic lupus erythematosus with positive antiphospholipid antibodies. Am J Reprod Immunol 1999;41:307-11.
95. Verztman L, Lima EF, Rubinstein J, Lederman R, Leite N. [Systemic lupus erythematosus and pregnancy]. Hospital (Rio J) 1969;75:1595-609.
96. Herreman G, Betous F, Batisse P, Bessis R, Lesavre P, Ferme I. [Intra-uterine detection of atrio-ventricular block in two children whose mother had Sjogren's syndrome].Nouv Presse Med 1982;11:657-60.
97. Shinohara K, Miyagawa S, Fujita T, Aono T, Kidoguchi K. Neonatal lupus erythematosus: results of maternal corticosteroid therapy. Obstet Gynecol 1999;93:952-7.
98. Ishimaru S, Izaki S, Kitamura K, Morita Y. Neonatal lupus erythematosus: dissolution of atrioventricular block after administration of corticosteroid to the pregnant mother. Dermatology 1994;1:92-4.
99. Copel JA, Buyon JP, Kleinman CS. Successful *in utero* therapy of fetal heart block. Am J Obstet Gynecol 1995;173:1384-90.
100.   Buyon JP, Waltuck J, Kleinman C, Copel J.*In utero* identification and therapy of congenital heart block. Lupus 1995;4:116-21.
101.   Watson WJ, Katz VL. Steroid therapy for hydrops associated with antibody-mediated congenital heart block. Am J Obstet Gynecol 1991;165:553-4.
102.   Coppen SR, Severs NJ, Gourdie RG. Connexin45 (alpha 6) expression delineates an extended conduction system in the embryonic and mature rodent heart. Dev Genet 1999;24:82-90
103.   van Kempen MJ, ten Velde I, Wessels A, et al. Differential connexin distribution accommodates cardiac function in different species. Microsc Res Tech 1995;31:420-36.
104.   Skeiky YA, Benson DR, Parsons M, Elkon KB, Reed SG. Cloning and expression of Trypanosoma cruzi ribosomal protein P0 andepitope analysis of anti-P0 autoantibodies in Chagas' disease patients. J Exp Med 1992;176:201-11.
105.   Bonfa E, Viana VS, Barreto AC, Yoshinari NH, Cossermelli W. Autoantibodies in Chagas' disease. An antibody cross-reactive with human and Trypanosoma cruzi ribosomal proteins. J Immunol 1993;150:3917-23.
106.   Teixeira AR, Teixeira ML, Santos Buch CA. The immunology of experimental Chagas' disease. IV. Production of lesions in rabbits similar to those of chronic Chagas' disease in man. Am J Pathol 1975;80:163-80.
107.   Steere AC, Batsford WP, Weinberg M, et al. Lyme carditis: cardiac abnormalities of Lyme disease. Ann Intern Med 1980;93:8-16.
108.   Kishaba RG, Weinhouse E, Chusid MJ, Nudel DB. Lyme disease presenting as heart block. Clin Pediatr 1988;27:291-3.
109.   Kuiper H, de Jongh BM, Senden PJ. [Pacemaker implantation for complete atrioventricular block due to Lyme borreliosis]. Ned Tijdschr Geneeskd 1988;132:2109-11.

110. Nagi KS, Thakur RK. Lyme carditis: indications for cardiac pacing. Can J Cardiol 1995;11:335-8.

111. van der Linde MR, Crijns HJ, de Koning J, et al. Range of atrioventricular conduction disturbances in Lyme borreliosis: a report of four cases and review of other published reports. Br Heart J 1990;63:162-8.

112. Reznick JW, Braunstein DB, Walsh RL, et al. Lyme carditis. Electrophysiologic and histopathologic study. Am J Med 1986;81:923-7.

113. Bedell SE, Pastor BM, Cohen SI. Symptomatic high grade heart block in Lyme disease. Chest 1981;79:236-7.

114. Kapusta P, Fauchier JP, Cosnay P, Huguet R, Grezard O, Rouesnel P. [Sinoatrial and atrioventricular conduction disorders in Lyme disease.Apropos of 2 case reports]. Arch Mal Coeur Vaiss 1986;79:1361-6.

115. Rey MJ, Zimmermann M, Adamec R, Fleisch M, Viquerat C, de Freudenreich J. Intra-hisian 2:1 atrioventricular block secondary to Lyme disease. Eur Heart J 1991;12:1048-51.

116. Rubin DA, Sorbera C, Baum S, McAllister A, Nadelman R. Acute reversible diffuse conduction system disease due to Lyme disease. Pacing Clin Electrophysiol 1990:1367-70.

117. Doutlik S, Kucera V, Vacek Z, Hancil J, Jirous J, Picha D. An immunological study of Lyme disease. Czech Med 1990;13:71-8.

118. Doutlik S, Kucera V, Vacek Z, Hancil J, Jirous J, Picha D. [Immunologic study of Lyme borreliosis]. Cas Lek Cesk 1989;128:392-5.

119. Ehrenstein M, Isenberg D. Autoimmunity associated with infection: leprosy, acute rheumatic fever and Lyme disease. Curr Opin Immunol 1991;3:930-5.

120. Hu LT, Klempner MS. Host-pathogen interactions in the immunopathogenesis of Lyme disease. J Clin Immunol 1997;17:354-65.

121. Sigal LH. Immunologic mechanisms in Lyme neuroborreliosis: the potential role of autoimmunity and molecular mimicry. Semin Neurol 1997;17:63-8.

122. Sigal LH. Lyme disease: a review of aspects of its immunology and immunopathogenesis. Annu Rev Immunol 1997;15:63-92.

123. Teixeira AR, Santos Buch CA. The immunology of experimental Chagas' disease. II. Delayed hypersensitivity to Trypanosoma cruzi antigens. Immunology 1975;28:401-10.

124. Sosa Miatello C, Fiorotto ER. Ribosomal antibody response in rabbits and mice infected with Trypanosoma cruzi [erratum in Rev Argent Microbiol 1990;22:30]. Rev Argent Microbiol 1989;21:141-5.

125. de Oliveira SF, Pedrosa RC, Nascimento JH, Campos de Carvalho AC, Masuda MO. Sera from chronic chagasic patients with complex cardiac arrhythmias depress electrogenesis and conduction in isolated rabbit hearts. Circulation 1997;96:2031-7.

126. Mamula MJ, Fox OF, Yamagata H, Harley JB. The Ro/SSA autoantigen as an immunogen. Some anti-Ro/SSA antibody binds IgG. J Exp Med 1986;164:1889-901.

127. Alexander EL, Buyon JP, Lane J, Lafond WA, Provost TT, Guarnieri T. Anti-SS-A/Ro SS-B/La antibodies bind to neonatal rabbit cardiac cells and preferentially inhibit in vitro cardiac repolarization. J Autoimmun 1989;2:463-9.

128. Mamula MJ, O'Brien CA, Harley JB, Hardin JA. The Ro ribonucleoprotein particle: induction of autoantibodies and the detection of Ro RNAs among species. Clin Immunol Immunopathol 1989;52:435-46.

129. Alexander E, Buyon JP, Provost TT, Guarnieri T. Anti-Ro/SS-A antibodies in the pathophysiology of congenital heart block in neonatal lupus syndrome, an experimental modelIn vitro electrophysiologic and immunocytochemical studies. Arthritis Rheum 1992;35:176-89.

130. Garcia S, Nascimento JH, Bonfa E, et al. Cellular mechanism of the conduction abnormalities induced by serum from anti-Ro/SSA-positive patients in rabbit hearts. J Clin Invest 1994;93:718-24.

131. Hamilton RM, Lee Poy M, Kruger K, Silverman ED. Investigative methods of congenital complete heart block. J Electrocardiol 1998:69-74.

132. Viana VS, Garcia S, Nascimento JH, et al. Induction of in vitro heart block is not restricted to affinity purified anti-52 kDa Ro/SSA antibody from mothers of children with neonatal lupus. Lupus 1998;7:141-7.

133. Kirchhoff S, Nelles E, Hagendorff A, Kruger O, Traub O, Willecke K. Reduced cardiac conduction velocity and predisposition to arrhythmias in connexin40-deficient mice.Curr Biol 1998;8:299-302.

134. Hagendorff A, Schumacher B, Kirchhoff S, Luderitz B, Willecke K. Conduction disturbances and increased atrial vulnerability in Connexin40-deficient mice analyzed by transesophageal stimulation. Circulation 1999;99:1508-15.

135.   Horsfall AC, Rose LM. Cross-reactive maternal autoantibodies and congenital heart block. J Autoimmun 1992;5:479-93.

136.   Kalush F, Rimon E, Mozes E. Neonatal lupus erythematosus in offspring of mothers with experimental systemic lupus erythematosus. Am J Reprod Immunol 1992;28:264-8.

137.   Kalush F, Rimon E, Keller A, Mozes E. Neonatal lupus erythematosus with cardiac involvement in offspring of mothers with experimental systemic lupus erythematosus. J Clin Immunol 1994;14:314-22.

138.   Miranda Carus ME, Boutjdir M, Tseng CE, DiDonato F, Chan EK, Buyon JP. Induction of antibodies reactive with SSA/Ro-SSB/La and development of congenital heart block in a murine model. J Immunol 1998;161:5886-92.

139.   Mazel JA, El SN, Buyon J, Boutjdir M. Electrocardiographic abnormalities in a murine model injected with IgG from mothers of children with congenital heart block. Circulation 1999;99:1914-8.

140.   Tseng CE, Miranda E, Di Donato F. mRNA and protein expression of SSA/Ro and SSB/La in human fetal cardiac myocytes cultured using a novel application of the Langendorff procedure. Pediatr Res 1999;45:260-9.

141.   Buyon JP, Ben Chetrit E, Karp S, et al. Acquired congenital heart block. Pattern of maternal antibody response to biochemically defined antigens of the SSA/Ro-SSB/La system in neonatal lupus. J Clin Invest 1989;84:627-34.

142.   Taylor PV, Scott JS, Gerlis LM, Esscher E, Scott O. Maternal antibodies against fetal cardiac antigens in congenital complete heart block. N Engl J Med 1986;315:667-72.

143.   Debouverie M, Wagner M, Ducrocq X, Grignon Y, Mousson B, Weber M. [MNGIE syndrome in 2 siblings]. Rev Neurol (Paris) 1997;153:547-53.

144.   Wang J, Wilhelmsson H, Graff C, et al. Dilated cardiomyopathy and atrioventricular conduction blocks induced by heart-specific inactivation of mitochondrial DNA gene expression. Nat Genet 1999;21:133-7.

145.   Garcia OL, Metha AV, Pickoff AS, et al. Left isomerism and complete atrioventricular block: a report of six cases. Am J Cardiol 1981;48:1103-7.

146.   Roguin N, Pelled B, Freundlich E, Yahalom M, Riss E. Atrioventricular block in situs ambiguus and left isomerism (polysplenia syndrome). Pacing Clin Electrophysiol 1984;7:18-22.

147.   Shenker L, Reed KL, Anderson CF, Marx GR, Sobonya RE, Graham AR. Congenital heart block and cardiac anomalies in the absence of maternal connective tissue disease. Am J Obstet Gynecol 1987;157:248-53.

148.   Wren C, Macartney FJ, Deanfield JE. Cardiac rhythm in atrial isomerism. Am J Cardiol 1987;59:1156-8.

149.   Lopes LM, Cha SC, Sadek L, Iwahashi ER, Aiello VD, Zugaib M. [Fetal atrioventricular block]. Arq Bras Cardiol 1992;59:261-4.

150.   Gembruch U, Hansmann M, Redel DA, Bald R, Knopfle G. Fetal complete heart block: antenatal diagnosis, significance and management. Eur J Obst Gynecol Reprod Biol 1989;31:9-22.

151.   Schmidt KG, Ulmer HE, Silverman NH, Kleinman CS, Copel JA. Perinatal outcome of fetal complete atrioventricular block: a multicenter experience. J Am Coll Cardiol 1991;17:1360-6.

152.   Ho SY, Fagg N, Anderson RH, Cook A, Allan L. Disposition of the atrioventricular conduction tissues in the heart with isomerism of the atrial appendages: its relation to congenital complete heart block. J Am Coll Cardiol 1992;20:904-10.

153.   Levin M, Mercola M. Gap junctions are involved in the early generation of left-right asymmetry. Dev Biol 1998;203:90-105.

154.   Britz-Cunningham SH, Shah MM, Zuppan CW, Fletcher WH. Mutations of the Connexin43 gap-junction gene in patients with heart malformations and defects of laterality. N Engl J Med 1995;332:1323-9.

155.   Paul DL. New functions for gap junctions. Curr Opin Cell Biol 1995;7:665-72.

156.   Simon AM, Goodenough DA, Paul DL. Mice lacking connexin40 have cardiac conduction abnormalities characteristic of atrioventricular block and bundle branch block. Curr Biol 1998;8:295-8.

9

CONGENITAL LONG QT SYNDROMES

G. Michael Vincent, M.D. and Katherine Timothy, B.S.

LDS Hospital, Salt Lake City, UT 84103 USA

INTRODUCTION

Many important advances have been made in the last several years regarding the molecular genetics and physiology of the congenital long QT syndrome. These findings have significantly changed our perceptions of the clinical manifestations of this disorder, and added new diagnostic and therapeutic strategies. Further, the findings have fundamental importance for understanding the molecular mechanisms of arrhythmogenesis in general and, therefore, have broad applicability to clinical cardiology. This chapter reviews the current status of the genetic basis of the congenital long QT syndrome, and provides an overview of the physiologic and phenotypic consequences of the genetic alterations.

Background

Congenital long QT syndrome was defined as a specific entity in publications between 1957 and 1964 (1-3). Commonly referred to as LQTS, it is an inherited disorder of cardiac repolarization caused by abnormalities of ion channel electrophysiology. It is estimated that the frequency of LQTS in the USA is about 1:7000 persons, and that the disease accounts for approximately 3000-4000 sudden deaths in children and young persons each year. The principal symptoms are syncope and sudden death, usually occurring in children and young adults, due to the ventricular tachyarrhythmia torsade de pointes (TdP). Most often, the TdP is self-terminating, producing a syncopal episode. The characteristic signs of LQTS are QT interval prolongation and T wave abnormalities on the electrocardiogram, (Figure 1).

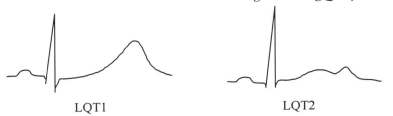

LQT1   LQT2

Figure 1. Computer generated schematics of the two most common T wave patterns in LQTS. In the left panel is the broad based, large area T wave characteristic of LQT1, and in the right panel the bifid T wave, variations of which are quite characteristic of LQT2.

Historically, two forms have been identified, the Jervell and Lange-Nielsen syndrome (J,L-N) associated with congenital deafness and autosomal recessive inheritance (1) and the autosomal dominant Romano-Ward syndrome (R-W) with normal hearing (2,3). The molecular genetics findings have clarified the commonality of these entities, to be discussed in detail later in the chapter. LQTS can also be acquired, usually from administration of drugs which block the I_{Kr} potassium channel, one of the ion channels affected in congenital long QT syndrome (4,5). Drug induced LQTS is an idiosyncratic response, but the mechanism rendering one person vulnerable to TdP upon administration of the drug but not most others is unknown. The acquired form of LQTS is discussed by Dr. Roden in the following chapter. The recognition that both drug-induced and the LQT2 form of congenital LQTS affect the I_{Kr} channel has suggested that patients who have drug induced LQTS have an underlying forme fruste of congenital LQTS. With their underlying defect, they become susceptible to TdP when repolarization is further impaired by administration of drugs which decrease potassium channel function (6,7). Acquired LQTS also occurs as a consequence of a number of acute and chronic neurologic disorders, such as subarachnoid hemorrhage and diabetic autonomic neuropathy (8-10), presumably due to effects of these diseases on the autonomic nervous system center (11,12). An association between Long QT syndrome and sudden infant death syndrome (SIDS) has also been suggested (13). As is well known, electrolyte disturbances such as hypokalemia and hypomagnesemia also cause QT prolongation, T wave abnormalities, and arrhythmias.

Jervell, Lange-Nielsen Syndrome

Long QT syndrome was first clearly defined by Jervell and Lange-Nielsen (1) in a Norwegian family in which 4 of 6 children showed congenital deaf-mutism, markedly prolonged QT intervals, "fainting spells" beginning at ages 3-5 years, and sudden death in 3 of the 4 children at ages 4, 5 and 9 years of age. The transmission of the disorder in this and subsequent publications appeared to be consistent with an autosomal recessive trait. It is quite rare, making up less than 1% of congenital LQTS patients. It is associated with more marked QT prolongation and T wave abnormality, and earlier and more severe symptoms, than the Romano-Ward form.

Cardiac events are precipitated by emotion, particularly startle, fright and anger, and by physical activity. The molecular genetics of J, L-N have provided a new genetic paradigm, to be described later in the chapter.

Romano-Ward Syndrome

Romano-Ward syndrome (2,3) is the common form of LQTS. It is inherited as an autosomal dominant condition and patients have normal hearing. Each child of an affected parent has a 50% chance of inheriting the disease. Most gene carriers live normal life spans and bear children, so transmission of the gene is frequent. The QT interval averages 0.49 seconds, with a range from 0.41 to over 0.60 seconds. There is significant overlap of QTc intervals with those of normals, (Figure 2). Approximately 12% of gene carriers have a normal QTc, defined as ≤ 0.44 seconds, with an additional 30% demonstrating a QTc between 0.45-0.47 seconds, values which overlap with normals.

There is reduced penetrance and expressivity of the prolonged QT phenotype, as about 12% of gene carriers have a normal QTc of ≤ 0.44 seconds, and another 30% have a borderline QTc of 0.45 - 0.47 seconds, values which overlap with that of normal individuals. Thus, the diagnosis cannot be excluded by a normal QTc, and diagnosis by ECG criteria may be difficult. The presence of typical T wave patterns (14), as shown in Figure 1 can assist in the correct diagnosis of LQTS in the

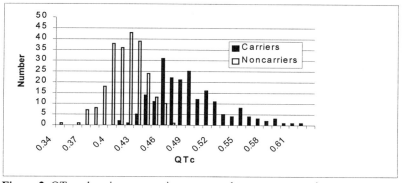

Figure 2. QTc values in gene carriers compared to non-gene carriers.

presence of a borderline QTc interval. Recently, other T wave patterns have been described which may be relatively genotype specific (15). Aside from the ECG changes, no structural or physiological abnormalities have been identified, although possible relationships with asthma, diabetes mellitus and depression have been suggested, primarily because of the physical proximity of genes for these conditions to the LQTS genes. Syncope, due to self-terminating TdP is the most common symptom. It most often occurs during exercise and emotion, but may occur during sleep, or while awake and without apparent provocation. The triggering events are related to the specific genetic defect (16). Patients with mutations affecting the I_{Ks}

channel (LQT1, LQT5, Jervell, Lange-Nielsen) have events almost exclusively during exercise or emotion, for example startle, fright and anger. Those with mutations of the SCN5A gene, the LQT3 patients, have the majority of their events during sleep. The HERG gene carriers, or LQT2, have events about equally divided between exercise/emotion and sleep/rest. There is some physiologic rationale for these differences, which will be discussed in the section on pathophysiology. Patients may have one to more than one hundred syncopal episodes. The symptoms can begin anytime from birth to the fourth or fifth decade of life, rarely thereafter, with the peak age of onset and of sudden death being in the preteen to early teenage years in LQT1 and in the late teenage years to twenties in the LQT2 patients. There are relatively few LQT3 patients for analysis, but they may have later events. It is not entirely clear how often sudden death occurs. Previous reports have included primarily highly symptomatic patients and small family groups. When complete family groups are studied, including asymptomatic and briefly symptomatic patients, and normal QTc carriers, sudden death appears to occur in about 15-20% of untreated patients, about 4% per year over the at risk years, and perhaps 5% of all gene carriers. Importantly, sudden death may be the first manifestation of the disease, and thus, our recommendation is that asymptomatic patients should be treated prophylactically with beta-blockers, as one cannot accurately predict the risk in a given patient and a "second chance" may not be available. At least one-third of gene carriers never experience syncope or other evidence of arrhythmia. Why some gene carriers are asymptomatic throughout life, others have one to a few syncopal episodes during childhood and then none thereafter, and others have multiple episodes and/or sudden death, is unknown and one of the critical questions in LQTS. The clinical features, such as ECG changes, do not discriminate between these groups, nor does the genotype or specific mutation.

MOLECULAR GENETICS

LQTS is caused by mutations of genes which encode for cardiac ion channels. Five genes have thus far been discovered, and one other locus mapped to chromosome 4, (Table 1). The genes have been numbered in the order of discovery as LQT1, LQT2, etc. Different designations have been given over time, and the names in parentheses represent other designations for the gene.

Table 1. Genes associated with Congenital Long QT Syndrome

LQT No.	Gene	Chromosome	Encoded protein	Ion Channel
LQT1	KvLQT1 (KCNQ1)	11p15.5	$I_{Ks}\alpha$ subunit	I_{Ks}
LQT2	HERG	7q35-36	$I_{Kr}\alpha$ subunit	I_{Kr}
LQT3	SCN5A	3p21-24	Na^+ channel unit	I_{Na}
LQT4	Unknown	4q25-27	Unknown	Unknown
LQT5	MinK (IsK, KCNE1)	21q22.1-2	$I_{Ks\beta}$ subunit	I_{Ks}
LQT6	MiRP1 (KCNE2)	21q22.1	$I_{Kr\beta}$ subunit	I_{Kr}

Over 175 different mutations of these five genes have so far been described, and additional mutations are being described regularly. Thus, LQTS demonstrates considerable genetic heterogeneity. A few families share the same mutation, for example the KPQ deletion of SCN5A, or have different substitutions for alanine at the 212 position on KvLQT1, but for the most part, each family has it's own mutation, and no real "hot spots" are evident. This makes screening for mutations very time consuming, as the entire gene(s) needs to be screened in each case.

KvLQT1 and MinK
The KvLQT1 and MinK genes coassemble to form the delayed rectifier potassium channel I_{Ks}, so they are discussed together for clarity.

The first genetic locus for LQTS was mapped to chromosome 11p15.5 in 1991 in a large family of Danish origin with exercise and emotion precipitation of syncope and sudden death (17). We had followed this family for 18 years, and had expanded the pedigree to about 900 members with over 100 clinically affected individuals (18). Subsequently, the gene was identified by positional cloning (19) and named KvLQT1 as it appeared to encode a novel voltage gated potassium channel with a predicted shaker-like potassium channel topology, with six transmembrane spanning domains, a voltage sensor in the S4 domain, and the signature pore sequence between the S5 and S6 domains, (Figure 3).

Congenital Long QT Syndromes

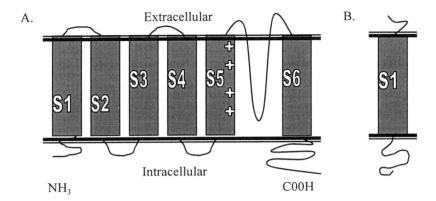

Figure 3. A. The predicted Shaker-like structure of the KvLQT1 and HERG genes. B. The predicted structure of the MinK and MiRP1 genes.

Further studies revealed KvLQT1 to coassemble with MinK (LQT5) (20,21) forming the I_{Ks} delayed rectifier potassium channel. KvLQT1 encodes for the larger α subunit and MinK the small β subunit of the I_{Ks} protein. KvLQT1 consists of 16 exons, spans 400kb, has relatively small amino and carboxy termini, and encodes a protein of 676 amino acids (22). At least 78, mostly missense, mutations have been reported in KvLQT1, primarily occurring in the membrane spanning domains and the pore region. Because of the large number of known mutations and the frequent recognition of new mutations, no attempt is made to show the position of all the mutations in any of the genes. Approximately 45% of the currently known LQTS mutations are in the KvLQT1 gene.

MinK (KCNE1, IsK)
MinK is a small protein of just 3 exons, spanning approximately 40kb and encoding a protein of 129 amino acids. It is predicted to have a single transmembrane spanning domain with small intra-and extracellular components, (Figure 3). Only a few mutations of this gene have been identified, accounting for about 2% of known LQTS mutations (22).

As noted above, MinK coassembles with KvLQT1 to form the I_{Ks} delayed rectifier potassium channel (20,21). The stochiometry of the α-β subunit complexes is not clear. While it is thought that four α subunits assemble as a tetramer to make the functional channel, (Figure 4) the number of β subunits which are involved in the assembly of the channel protein is not known.

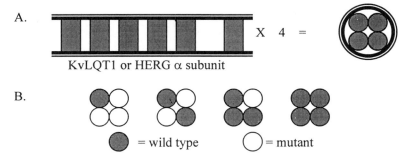

Figure 4. A. Schematic of the tetrameric assembly of KvLQT1 or HERG proteins. B. The potential combinations of wild type and mutant α units.

It has been reported than MinK coassembles with HERG (23), as well as KvLQT1. This report antedated the identification of the MiRP1 gene and it is possible that the protein identified was really MiRP1 rather than MinK, as the two are very similar. However, it also seems possible that both MinK and MiRP1 can coassemble with both KvLQT1 and HERG, producing a variety of heterotetramers. It appears that there may be a large family of small, MinK like genes which modify other proteins. Thus, there may be many β subunits which assemble with the LQTS genes and a variety of assembly stoichiometric relationships, and the possible combinations of protein assembly and presumably function could be numerous. This may explain the remarkable heterogeneity of certain phenotype features, such as the QT interval as shown in Figure 2, which exists within genotypes, mutation types, and even single families.

The mutations of KvLQT1 decrease channel function. The degree of reduction of the repolarizing current is dependent upon the specific mutation. Most mutations alter channel function by a dominant-negative mechanism in which the combination of mutant and wild type units (Figure 4) produces a severe reduction in channel current. This is due to a "poison pill" effect, in which the mutant units adversely affect the wild type units, causing more dysfunction than would be expected just from the ratio of wild type to mutant units. In other mutations, the degree of channel dysfunction is modest, suggesting no dominant-negative effect. Thus, there is physiologic heterogeneity of channel function dependent upon the specific mutation. Added to this cause of heterogeneity of channel dysfunction is the probability that the channels are not uniformly distributed in the myocardium.

The reduction of I_{Ks} current prolongs the action potential duration, particularly in the mid myocardial (M cell) myocytes (24), predisposing the cells to development of early afterdepolarizations (EADs) which appear to be the triggering mechanism for the TdP.

The Genetics of Jervell, Lange-Nielsen Syndrome

A mutation of one KvLQT1 or MinK allele, the heterozygous condition, causes the chromosome 11 or LQT1 form of the Romano-Ward syndrome. Being autosomal genes, boys and girls are equally affected. Each offspring of an affected parent has a 50% chance of inheriting the mutant allele, as the affected parent has a 50-50 chance of contributing the mutant allele to each child. Jervell, Lange-Nielsen syndrome occurs when a child inherits two mutant alleles, one from each parent, either two mutant KvLQT1 or MinK alleles (the homozygous condition) or one mutant allele of KvLQT1 and one of MinK (the compound heterozygous condition). This inheritance usually occurs in a cosanguinous marriage, such as between second cousins, in which both have a mutant KvLQT1 or MinK gene (25-29). The affected homozygote or compound heterozygote has a "double dose" of dysfunctional ion channels, thereby producing the more severe form of LQTS, with longer QT intervals, earlier and more severe symptoms, and a higher rate of sudden death than in heterozygotes with Romano-Ward syndrome. The deafness is related to the absence of the KvLQT1 gene. KvLQT1 is expressed in the inner ear, as well as lung and kidney, in addition to the heart (30). At least one normal KvLQT1 allele is necessary for production of the potassium rich endolymph. In the homozygote or compound heterozygote Jervell, Lange-Nielsen syndrome patient, there is no endolymph or organ of Corti formation, and the patient has severe congenital deafness along with Long QT syndrome. The homozygous condition would be expected in 25% of the offspring of two affected parents, 50% would be heterozygous, and 25% would be expected to be normal. Now for the new genetic paradigm. The heterozygotes in the Jervell, Lange-Nielsen families have autosomal dominant Romano-Ward Long QT syndrome. The mutations causing Jervell, Lange-Nielsen syndrome produce a less severe physiologic defect than those causing the more typical, and obvious, Romano-Ward syndrome. The heterozygotes have lesser degrees of QT prolongation, averaging about 0.46 seconds or less, and fewer symptoms than the typical Romano-Ward patients. However, the heterozygotes are not without risk of cardiac events (31), and all potentially affected family members need to be carefully screened by ECG for heterozygous LQTS. The new paradigm is the combination of a recessive trait, the deafness, and a dominant trait, the Long QT syndrome, both existing in members of the same family, caused by the same genetic defect.

The LQT1 genotype is the form of LQTS most often described in the literature, with exercise and emotion induced cardiac arrhythmias. The I_{Ks} channel is responsive to adrenergic stimulation and is the principal current responsible for altering action potential duration in response to changes in cycle length. In LQT1 patients, the QT interval does not shorten appropriately with increments in heart rate, a finding which can be of diagnostic importance (32). Thus, there is a physiologic rationale for the adrenergic precipitation of cardiac events in LQT1 in that the mutant channels respond differently to adrenergic stimulation than do the wild type channels, producing marked heterogeneity of recovery and the substrate for the TdP arrhythmia. This physiologic defect also explains the abnormal cycle length-QT interval relationship so commonly described in LQTS in which the QT fails to shorten appropriately with exercise induced increases in heart rate

HERG and MiRP1

HERG, the "human ether-a-go-go related" gene, is the LQT2 gene, mutations of which cause chromosome 7 linked LQTS (33). MiRP1, the recently described LQT6 gene, is a small protein similar in size and function to MinK and sitting adjacent to MinK on chromosome 21. HERG and MiRP1 coassemble to form the channel conducting the rapidly activating delayed rectifier current I_{Kr} (4,34). HERG encodes for the α subunit, and MiRP1 the β subunit, in a fashion similar to KvLQT1 and MinK, (Figure 1). Mutations of HERG produce a loss of function abnormality, usually but not always by a dominant-negative mechanism. The degree of channel impairment is variable, depending upon the specific mutation (34). The loss of function causes prolongation of APD, particularly of the M cells, rendering the cells vulnerable to EADs and the patient to torsade de pointes. Experimental studies suggest more heterogeneity of transmural APD in the baseline state than with KvLQT1 and MinK mutations, perhaps explaining the higher incidence of cardiac events during sleep or at rest in the LQT2 patients. HERG has a putative Shaker-like structure (Figure 3) similar to KvLQT1, but has more extensive amino and carboxyl termini than does KvLQT1. HERG consists of 16 exons, spans 55kb, and encodes a protein of 1159 amino acids. More than 81 mutations of the gene have been thus far identified, representing approximately 46% of the known LQTS gene mutations (35). Most mutations are in the spanning domains and the pore region, but unlike KvLQT1 there are also many mutations in the amino and carboxyl termini. As in KvLQT1, there are no real "hot spots".

Prior to the report that HERG coassembles with MiRP1 to form the I_{Kr} channel (36), it was reported that HERG coassembles with MinK (23). Whether HERG coassembles with both is uncertain, as discussed above. I_{Kr} is the current affected by the majority of QT prolonging drugs (37,38) providing a rational relationship between congenital LQTS and drug induced LQTS.

During the initial studies on HERG channel function, it was discovered that the current is inversely proportional to the extracellular potassium ion concentration (4). This paradoxical effect suggested that increased serum potassium might have therapeutic benefit in patients with the HERG genotype. Acute trials of potassium loading in a small number of patients with chromosome 7 LQTS showed impressive shortening of the QT interval and normalization of T wave morphology (39). Longer term trials to determine the therapeutic effectiveness of this regimen are underway, but one report indicates the difficulty of maintaining elevated serum potassium over time (40), and it may be difficult to achieve effective therapy over the many years required for protection from syncope and sudden death.

MiRP1

MiRP1, or the "MinK related peptide 1", is the LQT6 gene, the most recent to be recognized. It has properties similar to MinK and appears to encode the β subunit for I_{Kr}, complexing with HERG in a fashion similar to the KvLQT1/MinK complex (36). The mutant channels open slowly and close rapidly, thereby diminishing potassium current as compared to the wild type. The predicted topology is similar to that of MinK, with one spanning domain, with small intra and extracellular components, and it encodes a protein of 127 amino acids, (Figure 3). Three missense mutations have been identified. Two were associated with only modest QT prolongation. The third was associated with a borderline QT interval, and the disorder was only recognized during clarithromycin administration, giving rise to an apparent drug induced LQTS. This observation and others (6) provides additional evidence for the concept that drug induced LQTS may occur in the setting of an underlying abnormal I_{Kr} (or other) channel.

SCN5A

The cardiac Na^+ channel gene SCN5A is the LQT3 gene (41-43), and mutations cause chromosome 3 linked LQTS. The gene consists of 28 exons spanning 80kb. SCN5A appears to encode a complete ion channel (without complexing with a β subunit) with 2016 amino acids. SCN5A consists of four homologous domains, DI-DIV, each of which consists of a protein with six transmembrane spanning domains, a voltage sensor in the S4 domain, and a pore region between the S5 and S6 domains, (Figure 5).

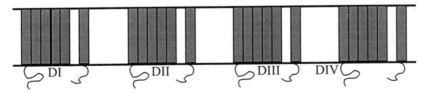

Figure 5. Schematic of the cardiac Na+ channel structure

At least thirteen mutations of this gene have been described, making up approximately 6% of known LQTS mutations. Different from the effect of mutations on the K^+ genes, the Na^+ gene mutations cause an unusual abnormality, a gain of function abnormality. The normal Na^+ channel opens briefly to allow a large influx of Na^+ ions into the cell which depolarizes the cell. The channel quickly inactivates leaving just a small persistent inward current. The mutations of SCN5A interfere with inactivation of the channel, allowing short or longer burst repetitive re-openings throughout the action potential. This persistent inward current causes prolongation of the APD, with marked prolongation in M cells, as opposed to epi- and endocardial cells, seen in experimental models of LQT3 (44-46). Thus, while the K^+ channel mutations produce a loss of channel function abnormality, and the Na^+ channel mutations a gain of function abnormality, the end result is the same, namely prolongation of the APD, delayed repolarization, and vulnerability to EADs and TdP. Expression studies of several mutations of the SCN5A gene have been reported, including missense mutations and a 9 base pair deletion involving 3 amino acids, the dKPQ mutation. The KPQ deletion was found to cause both brief and longer lasting reopenings, whereas the substitutions resulted in only brief reopenings. As a consequence, the gain of function was greater with the KPQ deletion (46). However, as noted with the K^+ channel mutations, it is not obvious that the phenotype in the patients with the dKPQ genotype is more severe than in those with missense mutations.

The identification of the molecular genetics and the physiology of SCN5A mutations suggested therapeutic strategies in LQT3. Once the channel reopenings were identified, it was postulated that drugs like Mexiletine might prevent the repetitive, inappropriate openings and restore channel function to a more normal state. Both molecular and clinical experiments support this hypothesis (47-49). However, it is unknown if sodium channel blocker treatment will prevent TdP, syncope and sudden death, and clinical trials are underway in LQT3 patients.

LQT4
This locus was identified by linkage analysis in one French family (50), but even several years later the gene has not yet been reported. It is probable that this is a very rare genotype, and may be unique to this single family. The phenotype in LQT4 is unusual among the LQTS genotypes, with a high incidence of atrial fibrillation and unusual T wave morphology.

Relative Frequency of the LQTS Genotypes
The relative frequency of the known genotypes is not yet entirely certain. Among genotyped patients, the KvLQT1 gene is the most common, being found in about 50% of patients. HERG accounts for about 40-45% of cases. Thus, mutations of the potassium genes KvLQT1 and HERG together cause about 90-95% of cases. The SCN5A gene accounts for about 3-5% of the cases. The LQT4 genotype is very rare. The MinK and MiRP1 genes are found in about 1% each. In approximately 50% of subjects who appear to have LQTS by clinical criteria, genetic analysis fails to identify a specific genetic locus. They may have mutations of other, at present unidentified, genes or the lack of result may be due to limitations of current genotyping tools. Perhaps supporting this hypothesis, the symptom and ECG phenotypes in those without a genotype result suggest that most have the LQT1 or LQT2 genotypes. Perhaps mutations of other β subunits which coassemble with KvLQT1 or HERG, as discussed above, are responsible for these cases. As these families are genotyped, the frequency distribution of genotypes may be somewhat different than the figures mentioned above.

PATHOPHYSIOLOGY

The feature common to these diverse genetic defects is heterogeneous prolongation of the action potential duration, manifest by QT interval prolongation and T wave abnormalities on the ECG. In the potassium channel mutations this occurs by a reduction in the outward, repolarizing, potassium current. In the sodium channel mutations it is caused by the sustained inward current. In each case the prolongation renders cells susceptible to the development of early afterdepolarizations (EADs), perhaps by activation of L-type Ca 2^+ channels (51). Several clinical studies using monophasic action potential recordings have demonstrated EAD like potentials in patients (52-54) which may increase with adrenergic stimulation and which appear to initiate TdP. TdP is often initiated by a long-short cycle sequence, (55) but the relationship of this physiologic perturbation to specific genotypes is not fully understood.

Several experimental models have provided additional insights into the pathophysiology of the syndrome. In one series of important studies, models of the LQT1, LQT2 and LQT3 genotypes were created using the I_{Ks} blocker chromanol 293B, the I_{Kr} blocker d-sotalol and ATX-II, which increases late inward sodium current, respectively, to mimic the genetic cellular defect. A transmural ECG and transmembrane action potentials from epicardial, endocardial and M cells were simultaneously recorded in an arterially perfused wedge from the canine left ventricle (24,56,57) In the LQT1 model Chromanol 293B prolonged the APD_{90} of all three cell types without increasing transmural dispersion of recovery or inducing TdP. The administration of isoproterenol abbreviated the epicardial and endocardial, but not the M cell, action potentials, producing an increase in transmural dispersion of recovery and EAD induced TdP. This model simulates clinical LQT1 in which TdP is usually precipitated by exercise and emotion, times of increased adrenergic activity. Propranolol and Mexiletine prevented the increase in transmural dispersion and the TdP. The T wave morphology in this model simulated the broad and large area T wave characteristic of LQT1. In the LQT2 model, induced by administration of d-sotalol, the drug preferentially increased the M cell APD, increasing transmural dispersion and inducing EADs in the baseline preparation. The markedly disparate APDs produced a bifid T wave in the transmural ECG, similar to that seen in LQT2. Mexiletine reduced the M cell APD and reduced transmural dispersion and TdP. In the LQT3 model, ATX-II markedly prolonged the M cell APD and transmural dispersion of recovery, with spontaneous TdP. T morphology and the long WT segment were similar to that seen in LQT3 patients. Mexiletine shortened the M cell APD and prevented the TdP. These models place considerable importance on the differential response of the M cell versus endocardial and epicardial cells. In addition to the transmural dispersion measured in these studies, there is likely to be additional heterogeneity of recovery from the non-uniform distribution of channels within the myocardium and the variable reduction of channel current based on the coassembly of α and β subunits as discussed earlier in the chapter. Plus, the patients have more complex biochemical interactions and the autonomic nervous system. Thus, the heterogeneity in patients may be greater, and more complex, than seen in these models.

Other studies have also aided our understanding of the mechanisms of initiation and maintenance of the TdP arrhythmia. Both animal and clinical studies have demonstrated early afterdepolarizations to be the initiating beats for TdP, as noted above. With respect to maintenance, recent animal model studies have indicated that TdP is due to a complex, rotating scroll-like, re-entry mechanism (58,59) and that the characteristic QRS morphology is a consequence of the rotating scrolls and functional block. TdP ends when the reentrant excitation is terminated by functional conduction block.

The syncopal episodes in patients are due to spontaneously terminating TdP, as seen in these animal models. In some patients, however, the TdP does not terminate and sudden death ensues. The patients are in ventricular fibrillation (VF) when seen by the medical personnel, so presumably the TdP degenerates into VF at some point and the patient has sudden death. Why TdP degenerates to ventricular fibrillation in some (the minority) cases, but not in others is unknown, and the risk of such an event in a given patient is unpredictable. It is a particularly important question, as once the underlying substrate is known, it may be possible to detect this substrate and treat those patients with the particular substrate in a more appropriate and successful manner. It seems reasonable to suspect that the degree of dispersion of recovery at the time of the TdP plays an important role. Unfortunately, the clinical findings, i.e., the QT interval, T wave morphology, and presence or frequency of symptoms do not accurately distinguish the patient at risk for sudden death from those with non-fatal syncope nor from those who remain asymptomatic.

TREATMENT

The gold standard for treatment is the administration of beta-blocker medications. There have been no controlled trials of the efficacy of this approach. However, many years of empiric observations have suggested a significant degree of efficacy, with a variety of publications proposing that 80-90% of patients are effectively treated by beta-blockers. Our current belief is that beta-blockers are highly effective in the LQT1 genotype, with adrenergic mediation of their events. Dose is critical, and particularly in young children the dose must be increased in response to growth. Some measure of efficacy other than cessation of symptoms is important, as symptoms are often infrequent and sporadic. In the LQT1 patients, the abnormal cycle-length/QT interval relationship can be a useful measure (60). Beta-blockers normalize this relationship, and prevent the development of a terminal component of the T wave, which appears to be responsible for the absolute or relative QT lengthening. PVC's are not common in most LQTS subjects, and are not generally induced during exercise. Equally important in preventing death in LQTS patients is assuring compliance with the medication. Most physicians know that about half their patients either do not take a prescribed medication or don't take it as prescribed. In LQTS, this can be a fatal mistake. Careful and thoughtful discussion with patient, and with parents in the case of children, with education as to the importance of daily usage, can markedly diminish the rate of non-compliance and the resultant disasters.

LQT2 patients usually respond well to beta-blockers, but the response may not be as consistent as in LQT1. Episodes are triggered by exercise or emotion in about 60% of LQT2 patients (16) and our own experience is that these patients respond well to beta-blockers. Whether those who are more prone to the sleep/rest events respond better or less well to beta-blockers is unknown. At present it seems prudent to treat all LQT2 patients with beta-blockers, and to be prepared to intervene with other measures if symptoms develop or return.

The side effects of beta-blockers are troublesome to an important percentage of patients, particularly the fatigue. Some patients tolerate one beta-blocker when they don't tolerate others, and it is worth experimenting. We have found that starting with a low dose, allowing the patient to adjust for several weeks or longer, and then increasing the dose in increments until the desired dose is obtained, has been quite successful in avoiding this side effect. The best approach for patients with asthma or other relative contraindications to beta-blockers is not clear. We have had very good success in treating patients with infrequent to mild asthma. In those with exacerbation of asthma, Mexiletine or interventional therapy should be considered.

LQT3 presents even more complexities. LQT3 is uncommon, as noted above, thus, there is relatively little clinical experience from which to draw conclusions. Some experts believe LQT3 patients respond less well to beta-blockers and evidence from experimental models suggests the possibility that beta-blockers may aggravate the pathophysiology in that genotype (56). While no definitive conclusions appear warranted at the present time, it seems advisable to consider alternative forms of therapy for the LQT3 patients. Since most have events during sleep (16), and bradycardia may be more prominent in this genotype than the others, consideration should be given to pacemaker intervention if unusual nocturnal bradycardia is demonstrated.

The role of interventional therapy for LQTS patients is not well defined. Pacemaker therapy is appropriate for those with symptomatic bradycardia. It's role in other situations is less clear. Beta-blockers should be continued whenever possible. ICD insertion is commonly employed in those who have had a cardiac arrest or continued symptoms on pharmacologic therapy. It does not seem desirable to implant ICD's in patients who have syncope but who have not been treated with medications, as most will do very well on beta-blocker therapy. We have had success in a few LQT1 and LQT2 patients with Mexiletine when beta-blockers were not completely effective, or produced significant side effects, and the benefit has been present over a number of years. Interestingly, the experimental models of LQTS suggest that Mexiletine may be beneficial in all three genotypes (24,56).

Molecular genotype based therapeutic strategies are now being investigated, and have been mentioned earlier in the chapter. There are no data yet to determine if these strategies are effective in preventing sudden death and syncope. Clinical trials are underway with potassium loading and Mexiletine administration but it will be several years before a definitive answer as to their effectiveness is known. In the interim, clinicians must use judgement and the circumstances surrounding each patient to make the best therapeutic decisions for each LQTS patient.

Finally, it is appropriate to ask families with highly symptomatic members to learn CPR. It is wise to have a "buddy" system for younger patients, in which a responsible and knowledgeable "buddy" is present during sports, swimming, etc. This person can summon help, indicate to bystanders and medical personnel the possible nature of the syncope/arrest, and even perform CPR. It is reasonable to consider recommending to families of high risk persons that an automatic external defibrillator be purchased, the family members well trained in it's use, and that it be available in those sites and circumstances during which events might be more likely to occur, i.e. sports, swimming, etc.

REFERENCES

1. Jervell A, Lange-Nielsen F. Congenital deaf-mutism, functional heart disease with prolongation of the QT interval, and sudden death. Am Heart J 1957;54:59-68.
2. Romano C, Genrme G, Pongiglione R. Aritmie cardiache rare dell'eta pediatrica. Clin Pediatr 1963;45:656-683.
3. Ward OC. A new familial cardiac syndrome in children. J Ir Med Assoc 1964;54:103-106.
4. Sanguinetti MC, Jiang C, Curran ME, Keating MT. A mechanistic link between an inherited and an acquired cardiac arrhythmia: HERG encodes the IKr potassium channel. Cell 1995;81:299-307.
5. Roden DM, Lazzara R, Rosen M, Schwartz PJ, Towbin JA, Vincent GM. Multiple mechanisms in the long-QT syndrome: current knowledge, gaps, and future directions. For the SADS Foundation Task Force on LQTS. Circulation 1996;94:1996-2012.
6. Priori SG, Napolitano C, Schwartz PJ, Ballabio A, Paganini V, Cantu F, Pinnavaia A, Aquaro G, Casari G. KvLQT1 mutation in drug induced torsade de pointes. Eur Heart J 1997;18:324(Abstract).
7. Donger C, Denjoy I, Berthet M, et al. KVLQT1 C-terminal missense mutation causes a forme fruste long-QT syndrome. Circulation 1997;96:2778-2781.
8. Grossman MA. Cardiac arrhythmias in acute central nervous system disease. Arch Intern Med 1976;136:203-207.
9. Ewing DJ. Diabetic autonomic neuropathy and the heart. [Review]. Diabetes Res Clin Pract 1996;30 Suppl:31-36.
10. Kahn JK, Sisson J, Vinik A. QT interval prolongation and sudden cardiac death in diabetic autonomic neuropathy. J Clin Endocrinol Metab 1987;64:751-754.
11. Yanowitz F, Preston JB, Abildskov JA. Functional distribution of right and left stellate innervation to the ventricles. Production of neurogenic electrocardiographic changes by unilateral alterations of sympathetic tone. Circ Res 1966;18:416
12. Abildskov, J. A., Vincent, G. M. "The autonomic nervous system in reltaion to electrocardiographic waveform and cardiac rhythm." In *Neural Regulation of the Heart,* W. C. Randall. ed. Boston: Oxford University Press, 1977.
13. Schwartz PJ, Stramba-Badiale M, Segantini A, et al. Prolongation of the QT interval and the sudden infant death syndrome. N Engl J Med 1998;338:1709-1714.

14. Moss AJ, Zareba W, Benhorin J, et al. ECG T-wave patterns in genetically distinct forms of the hereditary long QT syndrome. Circulation 1995;92:2929-2934.

15. Guili LC, Zhang L, Timothy KW, Handrahan AJ, Moss AJ, Zareba W, Schwartz PJ, Lehmann MH, Keating MT, Towbin JA, Vincent GM. Long QT genotype can be identified by ECG phenotype. J Am Coll Cardiol 1998;31:192A(Abstract).

16. Schwartz PJ, Moss AJ, Priori SG, Wang Q, Lehmann MH, Timothy KW, Denjoy I, Haverkamp W, Guicheney P, Paganini V, Scheinman MM, Karnes PS. Gene-specific influence on the triggers for cardiac arrest in the long QT syndrome. Circulation 1997;96 (suppl I):I-204(Abstract).

17. Keating MT, Atkinson D, Dunn C, Timothy KW, Vincent GM, Leppert M. Linkage of a cardiac arrhythmia, the long QT syndrome, and the Harvey ras-1 gene. Science 1991;252:704-706.

18. Vincent, G. M. "Long-term follow-up of a family with Romano-Ward prolonged QT interval syndrome." In *Clinical Aspects of Ventricular Repolarization.*, G. S. Butrous, P. J. Schwartz. eds. London: Farrand Press, 1989.

19. Wang Q, Curran ME, Splawski I, et al. Positional cloning of a novel potassium channel gene: KVLQT1 mutations cause cardiac arrhythmias. Nat Genet 1996;12:17-23.

20. Barhanin J, Lesage F, Guillemare E, Fink M, Lazdunski M, Romey G. KvLQT1 and IsK (minK) proteins associate to form the IKs cardiac potassium current. Nature 1996;384:78-80.

21. Sanguinetti MC, Curran ME, Zou A, et al. Co-assembly of KvLQT1 and minK (IsK) proteins to form cardiac Iks potassium channel. Nature 1996;384:80-83.

22. Splawski I, Shen J, Timothy KW, Vincent GM, Lehmann MH, Keating MT. Genomic structure of three long QT syndrome genes: KVLQT1, HERG, and KCNE1. Genomics 1998;51:86-97.

23. McDonald T.V., Yu Z., Ming Z, et al. A minK-HERG complex regulates the cardiac potassium current I(Kr). Nature 1997;388:289-292.

24. Shimizu W, Antzelevitch C. Cellular basis for the ECG features of the LQT1 form of the long-QT syndrome: effects of beta-adrenergic agonists and antagonists and sodium channel blockers on transmural dispersion of repolarization and torsade de pointes. Circulation 1998;98:2314-2322.

25. Splawski I, Timothy KW, Vincent GM, Atkinson DL, Keating MT. Molecular basis of the long-QT syndrome associated with deafness. Proc Assoc Am Physicians 1997;109:504-511.

26. Neyroud N, Tesson F, Denjoy I, et al. A novel mutation in the potassium channel gene KVLQT1 causes the Jervell and Lange-Nielsen cardioauditory syndrome. Nat Genet 1997;15:186-189.

27. Duggal P, Vesely MR, Wattanasirichaigoon D, Villafane J, Kaushik V, Beggs AH. Mutation of the gene for IsK associated with both Jervell and Lange-Nielsen and Romano-Ward forms of Long-QT syndrome. Circulation 1998;97:142-146.

28. Schulze-Bahr E, Haverkamp W, Wedekind H, et al. Autosomal recessive long-QT syndrome (Jervell Lange-Nielsen syndrome) is genetically heterogeneous. Hum Genet 1997;100:573-576.

29. Schulze-Bahr E, Wang Q, Wedekind H, et al. KCNE1 mutations cause Jervell and Lange-Nielsen syndrome. Nat Genet 1997;17:267-268.

30. Vetter DE, Mann JR, Wangemann P, et al. Inner ear defects induced by null mutation of the isk gene. Neuron 1996;17:1251-1264.

31. Splawski I, Timothy KW, Vincent GM, Atkinson DL, Keating MT. Molecular basis of the long-QT syndrome associated with deafness. N Engl J Med 1997;336:1562-1567.

32. Vincent GM. The heart rate of Romano-Ward long QT syndrome patients. Circulation 1985;72:III-44(Abstract).

33. Curran ME, Splawski I, Timothy KW, Vincent GM, Green ED, Keating MT. A molecular basis for cardiac arrhythmia: HERG mutations cause long QT syndrome. Cell 1995;80:795-803.

34. Sanguinetti MC, Curran ME, Spector PS, Keating MT. Spectrum of HERG K+-channel dysfunction in an inherited cardiac arrhythmia. Proc Natl Acad Sci U S A 1996;93:2208-2212.

35. Splawski I, Shen J, Timothy KW, Vincent GM, Lehmann MH, Keating MT. Genomic structure of three long QT genes: KVLQT1, HERG and KCNE1. Circulation 1998;98:(Abstract).

36. Abbott GW, Sesti F, Splawski I, et al. MiRP1 forms IKr potassium channels with HERG and is associated with cardiac arrhythmias. Cell 1999;97:175-187.

37. Spector PS, Curran ME, Keating MT, Sanguinetti MC. Class III antiarrhythmic drugs block HERG, a human cardiac delayed rectifier K+ channel. Open channel block by methanesulfonanilides. Circ Res 1996;78:499-503.

38. Roden DM. Current status of class III antiarrhythmic drug therapy. [Review]. Am J Cardiol 1993;72:44B-49B.

39. Compton SJ, Lux RL, Ramsey MR, et al. Genetically defined therapy of inherited long-QT syndrome. Correction of abnormal repolarization by potassium. Circulation 1996;94:1018-1022.

40. Tan HL, Alings M, VanOlden RW, Wilde AAM. Long-term (subacute) potassium treatment in congenital HERG-related long QT syndrome (LQTS2). J Cardiovasc Electrophysiol 1999;10:229-233.

41. Wang Q, Shen J, Splawski I, et al. SCN5A mutations associated with an inherited cardiac arrhythmia, long QT syndrome. Cell 1995;80:805-811.

42. Wang Q, Shen J, Li Z, et al. Cardiac sodium channel mutations in patients with long QT syndrome, an inherited cardiac arrhythmia. Hum Mol Genet 1995;4:1603-1607.

43. Wang Q, Li Z, Shen J, Keating MT. Genomic organization of the human SCN5A gene encoding the cardiac sodium channel. Genomics 1996;34:9-16.

44. Bennett PB, Yazawa K, Makita N, George AL, Jr. Molecular mechanism for an inherited cardiac arrhythmia. Nature 1995;376:683-685.

45. Chandra R, Starmer CF, Grant AO. Multiple effects of KPQ deletion mutation on gating of human cardiac Na+ channels expressed in mammalian cells. Am J Physiol 1998;274 (5 Pt 2):H1643-H1654

46. Dumaine R, Wang Q, Keating MT, et al. Multiple mechanisms of Na+ channel-linked long QT syndrome. Circ Res 1996;78:916-924.

47. Priori SG, Napolitano C, Cantu F, Brown AM, Schwartz PJ. Differential response to Na+ channel blockade, beta-adrenergic stimulation, and rapid pacing in a cellular model mimicking the SCN5A and HERG defects present in the long QT syndrome. Circ Res 1996;78:1009-1015.

48. Schwartz PJ, Priori SG, Locati EH. QTc responses to mexiletine and to heart rate changes differentiate LQT1 from LQT3 but not from LQT2 patients. Circulation 1996;94:I204(Abstract).

49. Schwartz PJ, Priori SG, Locati EH, et al. Long QT syndrome patients with mutations of the SCN5A and HERG genes have differential responses to Na+ channel blockade and to increases in heart rate: implications for gene-specific therapy. Circulation 1995;92:3381-3386.

50. Schott JJ, Charpentier F, Peltier S, et al. Mapping of a gene for long QT syndrome to chromosome 4q25-27. Am J Hum Genet 1995;57:1114-1122.

51. January CT, Riddle JM. Early afterdepolarizations: mechanism of induction and block. A role for L-type Ca2+ current. Circ Res 1989;64:977-990.

52. Gavrilescu S, Luca C. Right ventricular monophasic action potentials in patients with long QT syndrome. Br Heart J 1978;40:1014-1018.

53. Shimizu W, Ohe T, Kurita T, et al. Early afterdepolarizations induced by isoproterenol in patients with congenital long QT syndrome. Circulation 1991;84:1915-1923.

54. Shimizu W, Yamada K, Arakaki Y, Kamiya T, Shimomura K. Monophasic action potential recordings during T-wave alternans in congenital long QT syndrome. Am Heart J 1996;132:699-701.

55. Viskin S, Alla SR, Barron HV, et al. Mode of onset of torsade de pointes in congenital long QT syndrome. J Am Coll Cardiol 1996;28:1262-1268.

56. Shimizu W, Antzelevitch C. Sodium channel block with mexiletine is effective in reducing dispersion of repolarization and preventing torsade de pointes in LQT2 and LQT3 models of the long-QT syndrome. Circulation 1997;96:2038-2047.

57. Sicouri S, Antzelevitch D, Heilmann C, Antzelevitch C. Effects of sodium channel block with mexiletine to reverse action potential prolongation in in vitro models of the long term QT syndrome. J Cardiovasc Electrophysiol 1997;8:1280-1290.

58. Asano Y, Davidenko JM, Baxter WT, Gray RA, Jalife J. Optical mapping of drug-induced polymorphic arrhythmias and torsade de pointes in the isolated rabbit heart. J Am Coll Cardiol 1997;29:831-842.

59. El-Sherif N, Chinushi M, Caref EB, Restivo M. Electrophysiological mechanism of the characteristic electrocardiographic morphology of torsade de pointes tachyarrhythmias in the long-QT syndrome: detailed analysis of ventricular tridimensional activation patterns. Circulation 1997;96:4392-4399.

60. Vincent GM, Jaiswal D, Timothy KW. Effects of exercise on heart rate, QT, QTc and QT/QS2 in the Romano-Ward inherited long QT syndrome. Am J Cardiol 1991;68:498-503.

10

MOLECULAR GENETICS OF THE ACQUIRED LONG QT SYNDROME

Dan M. Roden, M.D.

Director, Division of Clinical Pharmacology
Vanderbilt University School of Medicine, Nashville, TN USA 37232

INTRODUCTION

The previous chapter has outlined the clinical conditions under which arrhythmias occur in patients with the congenital long QT syndrome (LQTS). One such condition - identified in only a handful of patients to date - is administration of a QT-prolonging drug; this finding indicates that the congenital form of LQTS and the drug-associated form overlap. Moreover, as the availability of molecular genotyping expands, individuals with mutations in LQTS disease genes with no manifest phenotype are being identified, and anecdotal clinical data also support the contention that drug administration in such individuals may unmask the genotype by provoking Torsades de Pointes (TdP). More generally, it seems increasingly clear that abnormal repolarization is a common feature of acquired heart disease, and may play a role in the development of arrhythmias in diverse settings, such as heart failure (1), hypertrophy (2), or atrial fibrillation (3). It is the goal of this chapter to outline the role genetic factors may play a role in determining cardiac repolarization and arrhythmias in the "acquired" long QT syndrome, i.e. that provoked by administration of drugs or the presence of heart disease.

Clinical features of acquired long QT syndrome

Any mechanism to explain the apparently "idiosyncratic" development of sporadic TdP should take into account clinically-identified risk factors (Table 1). Identification of risk factors for drug-associated TdP should not only allow clinicians to better predict risk but also provide a framework for basic scientists to better understand mechanisms underlying development of the arrhythmia.

Drugs that have been commonly associated with TdP are listed in Table 2. For most antiarrhythmics that cause TdP, the incidence has been estimated at 2-10%. These estimates derive from retrospective series (in the case of quinidine (5) and sotalol (6)) as well as prospective evaluations with some newer agents (ibutilide (7) and dofetilide). Hypokalemia and hypomagnesemia are often reported (8). Women appear to be at 2-3 fold increase risk of TdP on exposure to a QT-prolonging antiarrhythmic (9), highly reminiscent of the situation in the congenital syndromes where post-pubertal females are similarly at increased risk (10). The presence of underlying heart disease is another important risk factor.

This has long been suggested in the literature, and data to support this contention has come from analysis of large databases presented to the FDA. In the sotalol ventricular arrhythmia experience, the risk of TdP was increased by sotalol dose, by female gender and by the presence of heart failure (11). In the dofetilide database presented to the FDA (but not yet published), the incidence of TdP could be limited by appropriate monitoring and patient selection to <1% in patients with structurally near-normal hearts, but was as high as 3.3% in patients with advanced heart failure.

Table 1. Risk Factors for Acquired Torsades de Pointes

female gender
hypokalemia
hypomagnesemia
bradyarrhythmias[1]
ion channel gene mutations
congestive heart failure[2]
recent conversion from atrial fibrillation
excessively rapid intravenous drug administration rate
digoxin therapy[3]

[1]The heart rate may actually rise in the minutes prior to an episode of drug-associated TdP (4); this effect has been attributed to adrenergic activation. However, drug-associated TdP itself most often occurs after a pause or in the setting of bradycardia (e.g. heart block).
[2]TdP probably also occurs more commonly in patients with other forms of structural heart disease, often associated with increased QT intervals (2).
[3]One as yet unpublished case control series suggests digitalis therapy as an additional risk factor (Crijns et al.)

Table 2. Drugs Which May Prolong Repolarization

antiarrhythmics
    quinidine
    disopyramide
    procainamide
    sotalol
    ibutilide
    dofetilide
    amiodarone only rarely

calcium channel blockers
    bepridil

antihistamines
    terfenadine
    astemizole
antibiotics
    erythromycin[2]
    clarithromycin
    ketoconazole

anti-psychotics, antidepressants
    haloperidol
    thioridazine
    some tricyclics

gastric motility agent
    cisapride

[1]This list presents only commonly implicated agents; for patients very prone to long QT-related arrhythmias, such as those with LQTS mutations and manifest QT prolongation, the drugs listed (and potential others) should be avoided or used with great caution. [2]High concentrations of erythromycin, as seen with intravenous therapy, can cause TdP. In addition, erythromycin and other CYP 3A4 inhibitors (such as ketoconazole) may potentiate TdP by causing accumulation of other drugs (e.g. terfenadine) that rely on CYP 3A4 for their clearance.

For most drugs, the incidence of TdP rises as a function of drug dose and plasma concentration; an exception is quinidine, for which a possible explanation is offered below. It is not strictly well-established that pre-drug QT prolongation is a risk factor, since most large contemporary antiarrhythmic drug databases derive from drug development programs, and these generally exclude patients with pre-existing QT prolongation. Nevertheless, retrospective analyses of case control studies of patients developing TdP do support the idea that pre-drug QT prolongation (e.g. QTc > 485 msec) is a risk factor (12). QT dispersion developing during administration of a drug is thought to be a potential marker for impending TdP (13,14). Among patients treated with QT prolonging agents for atrial fibrillation or flutter, the period immediately following restoration of sinus rhythm appears to be one of special risk. In our own study, we found that an infusion of dofetilide that caused only minimal QT prolongation when patients were in atrial fibrillation produced marked QT prolongation (and TdP) in some, but not all, patients when administered within 24 hours of DC cardioversion (15).

Drug interactions and TdP
Although TdP is now well-recognized during therapy with non-cardioactive agents, its actual incidence seems much lower than with antiarrhythmics, likely reflecting use of the drugs in patients with little underlying heart disease, as well as the rarity of specific drug interactions that often underlie the development of the arrhythmia. An underlying mechanism has been best worked out with cisapride and terfenadine. Both of these compounds are cleared almost exclusively by hepatic and intestinal oxidative metabolism by CYP3A. Indeed, in most patients, presystemic clearance in these two sites is so efficient that the parent drugs cannot ordinarily be measured in plasma unless specialized techniques are used. When CYP3A activity is saturated (as in overdose), decreased (as in liver disease), or inhibited by co-administration of drugs such as azole antifungals (e.g. ketoconazole) or macrolide antibiotics (e.g. erythromycin), the drugs accumulate in plasma because there are no alternate pathways for their elimination. Since both terfenadine and cisapride are very potent action potential prolonging compounds *in vitro* (16-18), their accumulation to high plasma concentrations is associated with TdP. CYP3A function varies widely among human subjects, for reasons that are actually not well understood; no polymorphism in the coding region of the gene has yet been identified. It is not known whether CYP3A activity might be sufficiently low in rare individuals that TdP might occur even in the absence of interacting drugs. Despite exposure of millions of subjects, there are only a handful of cases suggesting this possibility; nevertheless, these incidence figures must be taken with a healthy grain of salt, since the important and potentially fatal interactions were not even picked for the fist 6 years terfenadine was on the market. It is assumed (but not established) that factors such as female gender, the presence of organic heart disease, or recent conversion from atrial fibrillation further increase risk among patients receiving these agents.

The finding of TdP during drug interactions with terfenadine, and the commercial availability of the terfenadine metabolite (fexofenadine, or Allegra[R]) whose generation is CYP3A-dependent, led to the withdrawal of terfenadine. Although *in vitro* studies suggest fexofenadine is devoid of I_{Kr} blocking action (16), a single case of apparent fexofenadine-related TdP has now been reported (19). This occurred in a man with baseline QT prolongation, suggesting that other factor(s) played a role.

Arrhythmia mechanisms in TdP
Genes in which mutations have been associated with the long QT syndrome are

described in detail in the previous chapter (20). However, animals have not yet been developed in which LQTS mutations have been introduced and typical TdP has occurred. Thus, studies of mechanisms in TdP have used drugs that modify repolarizing currents. When drugs reduce net repolarizing current (either by reducing outward potassium current or augmenting inward current), action potential prolongation is the predictable result. This effect is exaggerated at slow rates and by low extracellular potassium, and is especially pronounced in some tissues, notably those from the conducting system (Purkinje fibers (21-23)) and from mid-myocardium (M cells) (24,25). Marked action potential prolongation in turn is often associated with interruptions in the smooth trajectory of phase 3 repolarization (Figure 1); these interruptions are termed early afterdepolarizations (EADs). EADs, in turn, may lead to generation of spontaneous secondary upstrokes, or triggered activity. Since the *in vitro* conditions eliciting EAD-related triggering so closely resemble those associated with the development of drug-induced TdP, it has been postulated that these phenomena underlie initiation of the drug-induced arrhythmia. Further, the marked heterogeneity of action potential prolongation produced by the experimental conditions generating EAD-mediated triggered activity (hypokalemia, slow driving rates, action potential prolonging drugs) is thought to play an important role in the maintenance of the arrhythmia. Because action potentials are much longer under these conditions in the M cell region compared to epicardium and endocardium, the initiating triggered beat is thought to encounter islands of refractoriness at some sites (e.g. M cell layer), but not at others, initiating re-entrant excitation. The re-entrant circuit then meanders slowly through the wall of the heart in a "scroll"-fashion, lending TdP its distinctive morphology (25,26). Studies in whole heart preparations support the idea that TdP initiates in the subendocardium (i.e. in the Purkinje system), and is perpetuated by functional reentry of the type described here.

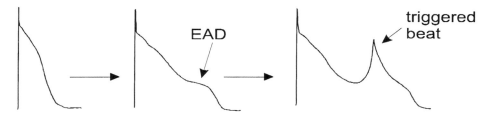

Since, as described below, most drugs that cause TdP are I_{Kr} blockers, it seems likely that this description will also apply to forms congenital LQTS that disrupt I_{Kr} function (i.e. HERG and MiRP1 mutations). Computer modeling suggests different rate dependencies for the genesis of triggered activity in different LQTS variants, and available data support the idea that the clinical provokers of the arrhythmia vary among subtypes (27,28). Thus, it is conceivable that mechanisms different from those outlined above are operative in other forms of congenital LQTS. For example, mutations that disrupt I_{Ks} function would be expected to produce their greatest effect at fast rates, where EADs are usually not provoked. In this situation, intracellular calcium overload and arrhythmias triggered by delayed afterdepolarizations may be an important contributor (29,30). As our understanding of mechanisms in defined subtypes of congenital LQTS expands, it seems likely that new mechanisms to explain arrhythmias in the broader category of "acquired" LQTS -- as in heart failure or hypertrophy for example -- may be identified.

I_{Kr} and TdP

Almost without exception, drugs that have been associated with TdP are potent blockers of I_{Kr}, the current encoded by the human ether à-go-go-related gene (HERG). For some drugs (e.g. dofetilide, sotalol, terfenadine, cisapride) this appears to be the sole, or major, effect on cardiac ion currents. In the case of racemic sotalol, it is possible that ancillary beta blocking properties modify the incidence of TdP. Ibutilide blocks I_{Kr} (31), and also activates an inward sodium current in some animal models (32). Whether the latter effect contributes to TdP with this agent is not known. Interestingly, we have found amiodarone to be a relatively potent I_{Kr} blocker, but it very rarely causes TdP (33). Here, it is likely that other actions, such as inhibition of inward movement through calcium current or other phenomena possibly involved in the development of triggered upstrokes from EADs (34), are sufficiently potent to override any proarrhythmic risk conferred by I_{Kr} block. Similarly, verapamil can be shown to be a relatively potent I_{Kr} blocker, but has never been associated with TdP, and indeed has been proposed as a therapy (35). Again, the drug's calcium channel blocking properties are probably sufficiently potent that any proarrhythmic potential of I_{Kr} block is completely eliminated.

Quinidine and TdP

Quinidine is an instructive case. Quinidine is a potent blocker of I_{Kr} (36), a much less potent blocker of I_{Ks} and other potassium currents (37-39), and also a sodium channel blocker (40). Block of inward current through sodium channels is an action potential shortening effect which can be shown to eliminate triggered activity and EADs *in vitro*. Thus, at very low concentrations, quinidine markedly prolongs action potentials at slow rates *in vitro*, whereas at higher concentrations action potentials actually shorten toward baseline, reflecting the drug's multiple actions. Taken together, these findings suggest that the extent to which quinidine administration confers risk for TdP depends on the extent to which I_{Kr}, I_{Ks}, sodium current, and other currents operative during the plateau contribute to repolarization in an individual subject. In a subject in whom repolarization highly dependent on I_{Kr} block, even a single dose of quinidine might be sufficient to trigger TdP. On the other hand, in a subject with a robust I_{Ks}, quinidine may be much less likely to produce TdP.

Evidence that ion channel gene mutations predispose to TdP

This line of reasoning, and the finding that most drugs associated with TdP block I_{Kr}, raises a more general hypothesis: that patients developing TdP during administration of drugs do so because of dysregulation of other currents controlling repolarization, notably I_{Ks}. There are now three lines of evidence that lend some, albeit indirect, support to this concept. *First,* occasional cases have now been reported of TdP developing on drug exposure in patients with "mild" or "subclinical" mutations in LQTS genes, and in particular, in KvLQT1 (one of the genes whose expression underlies I_{Ks}) (41-43). *Second,* the penetrance of congenital LQTS can be incomplete in some families; i.e. mutation carriers in such families may display normal baseline QT intervals (44). *Third,* the Jervell-Lange-Nielsen (JLN) LQTS variant, associated with congenital deafness and an especially malignant phenotype, is now recognized to arise when a child inherits mutant *KvLQT1* or *minK* alleles from both parents (45,46). Although JLN parents are traditionally viewed as phenotypically normal, these molecular-genetic findings indicate that in fact they should more correctly be viewed as carriers of usually subclinical LQTS mutations. Indeed, sudden presumed arrhythmic death has rarely been reported in JLN parents (47). To date, no systematic analysis of a large database of patients with drug-associated TdP has yet been completed to answer the question of how frequently affected patients actually harbor phenotypically-silent mutations in the coding regions of LQTS genes. Preliminary reports suggest that this mechanism is unusual, perhaps accounting for 5-10% of cases of TdP (48,49).

It is also possible that mutations may confer altered sensitivity to drug block. A MiRP1 mutation identified in a patient with TdP in association with hypertensive heart disease, intravenous erythromycin, oral clarithromycin, and hypokalemia, was found to confer a 3-fold increase in sensitivity to block by clarithromycin of HERG + mutant MiRP1 I_{Kr} channels, compared to block of HERG + wild-type MiRP1 (50). It is also possible that other genetic influences, such as polymorphisms in promoter regions of these or other genes, play a role.

SUMMARY

The unifying hypothesis of reduced repolarization reserve
Normal repolarization is accomplished by multiple ionic currents. We hypothesize that under normal circumstances, mild dysfunction of one of these mechanisms results in either no discernible phenotype or very subtle QT prolongation. Such dysfunction may be on the basis of gender, recent conversion from atrial fibrillation, presence of congestive heart failure, or a subclinical mutation in an ion channel gene. When the further stress of a QT-prolonging agent, in particular an I_{Kr} blocker, is added in such a patient, reserve mechanisms that accomplish normal repolarization may be completely overwhelmed, resulting in catastrophic failure of repolarization, i.e. TdP. In this context, the acquired long QT syndrome then becomes a general manifestation of altered expression or function of any one of the multiple genes whose protein products (ion channels or other proteins) play a role in maintaining normal "repolarization reserve".

REFERENCES

1. Tomaselli GF, Beuckelmann DJ,Calkins HG, et al. Sudden cardiac death in heart failure.The role of abnormal repolarization. *Circulation* 1994;90:2534-2539.

2. Hart G. Cellular electrophysiology in cardiac hypertrophy and failure*Cardiovasc Res* 1994;28:933-946.

3. Wijffels MC, Kirchhof CJ, Dorland R, Allessie MA. Atrial fibrillation begets atrial fibrillation. *Circulation* 1995;92:1954-1968.

4. Locati EH, Maison-Blanche P, Dejode P, Cauchemez B, Coumel P. Spontaneous sequences of onset of torsades de pointes in patients with acquired prolonged repolarization: Quantitative analysis of Holter recordings. *J Am Coll Cardiol* 1995;25:1564-1575.

5. Lown B, Wolf M. Approaches to sudden death from coronary heart disease*Circulation* 1971; 44:130-140.

6. Hohnloser SH, Arendts W, Quart B. Incidence, type, and dose-dependence of proarrhythmic events during sotalol therapy in patients treated for sustained VT/VF. *PACE* 1992;15:551-555.

7. Stambler BS, Wood MA, Ellenbogen KA, Perry KT,Wakefield LK, VanderLugt JT, The Ibutilide Repeat Dose Study Investigators. Efficacy and safety of repeated intravenous doses of ibutilide for rapid conversion of atrial flutter or fibrillation. *Circulation* 1996;94:1613-1621.

8. Roden DM, Woosley RL, Primm RK. Incidence and clinical features of the quinidine-associated long QT syndrome: implications for patient care. *Am Heart J* 1986;111:1088-1093.

9. Makkar RR, Fromm BS, Steinman RT, Meissner MD, Lehmann MH. Female gender as a risk factor for torsades de pointes associated with cardiovascular drugs. *JAMA* 1993;270:2590-2597.

10. Locati EH, Zareba W, Moss AJ, et al. Age- and sex-related differences in clinical manifestations in patients with congenital long-QT syndrome: findings from the International LQTS Registry. *Circulation* 1998;97:2237-2244.

11. Hohnloser SH. Proarrhythmia with class III antiarrhythmic drugs: types, risks, and management. *Am J Cardiol* 1997;80:82G-89G.

12. Houltz B, Darpo B, Edvardsson N, et al. Electrocardiographic and clinical predictors of torsades de pointes induced by almokalant infusion in patients with chronic atrial fibrillation or flutter. *PACE* 1998;21:1044-1057.

13. Day CP, McComb JM, Campbell RWF. QT dispersion: An indication of arrhythmia riskin patients with long QT intervals. *Br Heart J* 1990;63:342-344.

14. Hii JT, Wyse DG, Gillis AM, Duff HJ, Solylo MA, Mitchell, LB. Precordial QT interval dispersion as a marker of torsades de pointes. Disparate effects of class Ia antiarrhythmic drugs and amiodarone. *Circulation* 1992;86:1376-1382.

15. Choy AMJ, Darbar D, Dell'Orto S, Roden DM. Increased sensitivity to QT prolonging drug therapy immediately after cardioversion to sinus rhythm. *J Am Coll Cardiol* 1999 in press

16. Woosley RL, Chen Y, Freiman JP, Gillis RA. Mechanism of the cardiotoxic actions of terfenadine. *JAMA* 1993;269:1532-1536.

17. Carlsson L, Amos GJ, Andersson B, Drews L, Duker G, Wadstedt G. Electrophysiological characterization of the prokinetic agents cisapride andmosapride in vivo and in vitro -- implications for proarrhythmic potential. *J Pharmacol Exp Ther 1997;*282:220-227.

18. Drolet B, Khalifa M, Daleau P, Hamelin BA, Turgeon J. Block of the rapid component of the delayed rectifier potassium current by the prokinetic agent cisapride underlies drug-related lengthening of the QT interval. *Circulation* 1998;97:204-210.

19. Pinto YM, Van Gelder IC, Heeringa M, Crijns HJGM. QT lengthening and life-threatening arrhythmias associated with fexofenadine. *Lancet* 1999;353:980-5

20. Roden DM, Lazzara R, Rosen MR, Schwartz PJ, Towbin JA,Vincent GM, The SADS Foundation Task Force on LQTS. Multiple mechanisms in the long QT syndrome: Current knowledge, gaps, and future directions. *Circulation* 1996;94:1996-2012.

21. Strauss HC, Bigger JT, Hoffman BF. Electrophysiological and beta-receptor blocking effects of MJ1999 on dog and rabbit cardiac tissue. *Circ Res* 1970;26:661-678.

22. Dangman KH, Hoffman BF. In vivo and in vitro antiarrhythmic and arrhythmogenic effects of N-acetyl procainamide. *J Pharmacol Exp Ther* 1981;217:851-862.

23. Roden DM, Hoffman BF. Action potential prolongation and induction of abnormal automaticity by low quinidine concentrations in canine Purkinje fibers. *Circ Res* 1985;56:857-867.

24. Antzelevitch C, Sicouri S, Litovsky SH, et al. Heterogeneity within the ventricular wall: Electrophysiology and pharmacology of epicardial, endocardial, and M cells*Circ Res* 1991;69:1427-1449.

25. Antzelevitch C, Sun ZQ, Zhang ZQ, Yan GX. Cellular and ionic mechanisms underlying erythromycin-induced long QT intervals and torsades de pointes. *J Am Coll Cardiol*1996;28:1836-48.

26. El-Sherif N, Chinushi M, Caref EB, Restivo M. Electrophysiological mechanism of the characteristic electrocardiographic morphology of torsades de pointes tachyarrhythmias in the long-QT syndrome: detailed analysis of ventricular tridimensional activation patterns. *Circulation* 1997;96:4392-4399.

27. Hondeghem LM, Snyders, DJ. Class III antiarrhythmic agents have a lot of potential, but a long way to go:Reduced effectiveness and dangers of reverse use- dependence*Circulation* 1990;81:686-90.

28. Viswanathan P, Rudy Y. Rate dependencies of arrhythmias in different forms of the congenital long QT syndrome. *Cardiovasc Res* 1999 In press

29. Burashnikov A, Antzelevitch C. Acceleration-induced action potential prolongation and early afterdepolarizations. *J Cardiovasc Electrophysiol* 1998;9:934-948.

30. Wu Y, Roden DM, Anderson ME. CaM kinase inhibition prevents development of the arrhythmogenic transient inward current. *Circ Res* 1999 In press

31. Yang T, Snyders DJ, Roden DM. Ibutilide, a methanesulfonanilide antiarrhythmic, is a potent blocker of the rapidly-activating delayed rectifier K+ current (I_{Kr}) in AT-1 cells: Concentration-, time-, voltage-, and use-dependent effects. *Circulation* 1995;91:1799-1806.

32. Lee KS. Ibutilide, a new compound with potent class III antiarrhythmic activity, activates a slow inward Na+ current in guinea pig ventricular cells. *J Pharmacol Exp Ther 1992;*262:99-108.

33. Lazzara R. Amiodarone and torsades de pointes. *Ann Int Med* 1989;111:549-551.

34. Mason JW, Hondeghem, LM, Katzung, BG. Block of inactivated sodium channels and of depolarization- induced automaticity in guinea pig papillary muscle by amiodarone*Circ Res* 1984;55:277-285.

35. Shimizu W, Ohe T, Kurita T, et al. Effects of verapamil and propranolol on early afterdepolarizations and ventricular arrhythmias induced by epinephrine in congenital long QT syndrome. *J Am Coll Cardiol* 1995;26:1299-1309.

36. Yang T, Roden DM. Extracellular potassium modulation of drug block of I_{Kr}: Implications for torsades de pointes and reverse use-dependence. *Circulation* 1996;93:407-411.

37. Balser JR, Bennett PB, Hondeghem LM, Roden DM. Suppression of time-dependent outward current in guinea pig ventricular myocytes. Actions of quinidine and amiodarone. *Circ Res* 1991;69:519-529.

38. Balser JR, Roden DM, Bennett PB. Single inward rectifier potassium channels in guinea pig ventricular myocytes. Effects of quinidine. *Biophys J* 1991;59:150-161.

39. Imaizumi Y, Giles WR. Quinidine-induced inhibition of transient outward current in cardiac muscle. *Am J Physiol* 1987;253:H704-H708.

40. Johnson EA, McKinnon MG. The differential effect of quinidine andpyrilamine on the myocardial

action potential at various rates of stimulation. *J Pharmacol Exp Ther* 1957;120:460-468.

41. Donger C, Denjoy I, Berthet M, et al. KVLQT1 C-terminal missense mutation causes aforme fruste long-QT syndrome. *Circulation* 1997;96:2778-2781.

42. Napolitano C, Priori SG, Schwartz PJ, et al. Identification of a long QT syndrome molecular defect in drug-induced torsades de pointes. *Circulation* 1997;96:I-211

43. Schulze-Bahr E, Haverkamp W, Hordt M, Wedekind H, Borggrefe M,Funke K. Do mutations in cardiac ion channel genes predispose to drug-induced (acquired) long QT syndrome*Circulation* 1997;96:I-211

44. Priori, SG, Napolitano C, Schwartz PJ. Low penetrance in the Long-QT syndrome: clinical impact. *Circulation,* 1999 in press

45. Neyroud N, Tesson F, Denjoy I, et al. A novel mutation in the potassium channel gene KVLQT1 causes the Jervell and Lange-Nielsen cardioauditory syndrome. *Nature Genetics* 1997;15:186-189.

46. Schulze-Bahr E, Wang Q, Wedekind H, et al. KCNE1 mutations cause Jervell and Lange-Nielsen syndrome. *Nature Genetics* 1997;17:267-268.

47. Splawski I, Timothy KW, Vincent GM, Atkinson DL, Keating MT. Molecular basis of the long QT syndrome associated with deafness. *N Engl J Med* 1997;336:1562-1567.

48. Wei J, Abbott GW, Sesti F, et al. Prevalence of *KCNE2* (Mirp1) mutations in acquired long QT syndrome. *Circulation* 1999 submitted

49. Wei J, Yang IC, Tapper AR, et al. *KCNE1* polymorphism confers risk of drug-induced long QT syndrome by altering kinetic properties of IKs potassium channels. *Circulation* 1999 submitted

50. Abbott GW, Sesti F, Splawski I, et al. MiRP1 forms I_{Kr} potassium channels with HERG and is associated with cardiac arrhythmia. *Cell* 1999;97:175-187.

11

BRUGADA SYNDROME GENETICS

[1,2,3]Jeffrey A. Towbin, M.D., [1]Matteo Vatta, Ph.D., [4]Koonalee Nademanee, M.D., [5]Ramon Brugada, M.D., [6]Josep Brugada, M.D., [7]Charles Antzelevitch, Ph.D., [8]Pedro Brugada, M.D.

Departments of Pediatrics (Cardiology),[1] Cardiovascular Sciences,[2] Molecular and Human Genetics,[3] and Medicine,[5] Baylor College of Medicine, Houston, Texas; Department of Medicine,[4] University of Southern California, Los Angeles, California; [6]Cardiovascular Institute Hospital Clinic, University of Barcelona, Barcelona, Spain; [7]Masonic Medical Research Laboratory, Utica, New York; [8]Cardiovascular Center, OLV Hospital, Aalst, Belgium

INTRODUCTION

Sudden cardiac death is a significant problem in the United States, with an incidence reported to be greater than 300,000 persons per year (1). Interest in identifying the underlying cause of the death has been focused on cases of unexpected arrhythmogenic death, which is estimated to represent 5% of all sudden deaths (2). In cases in which no structural heart disease can be identified, the long QT syndrome and ventricular preexcitation are most commonly considered as likely causes. Recently, Brugada syndrome (also known by some investigators as idiopathic ventricular fibrillation, IVF), a disease associated with an electrocardiographic (ECG) abnormality of right bundle branch block with ST-elevation in the right precordial leads (V1-V3), has been added to the list of possible causes of sudden death in otherwise healthy, young individuals. The purpose of this chapter is to describe the clinical disorder and the genetics of this disease.

CLINICAL ASPECTS OF BRUGADA SYNDROME

The first identification of the ECG pattern of right bundle branch block (RBBB) with ST-elevation in leads V1-V3 was reported by Osher and Wolff (3), who noted this finding in three apparently healthy males. Shortly thereafter, Edeiken (4) identified persistent ST-elevation without RBBB in another ten asymptomatic males and Levine et al (5) described ST-elevation in the right chest leads and conduction block in the right ventricle in patients with severe hyperkalemia. Although multiple other reports of patients with variations of this ECG pattern exists (6-10), this ECG abnormality was largely ignored as being associated with sudden death until Martini et al (11) and Aihara et al (12) focused attention on the possible link. This association was further confirmed in 1991 by Pedro and Josep Brugada (13), who described four patients with sudden and aborted sudden death with ECGs demonstrating RBBB and persistent ST-elevation in leads V1-V3. In 1992, these authors characterized what they believed to be a distinct clinical and electrocardiographic syndrome (14).

The finding of ST-elevation in the right chest leads has been observed in a variety of clinical and experimental settings and is not unique or diagnostic of Brugada syndrome by itself. Situations in which these ECG findings occur include electrolyte or metabolic disorders, pulmonary or inflammatory diseases, abnormalities of the central or peripheral nervous system. In the absence of these abnormalities, the term idiopathic ST-elevation is often used and may identify Brugada syndrome patients. The prevalence of idiopathic ST-elevation varies from 2.1% - 2.65% (15), with elevation of the ST-segment limited to the right precordial leads occurring in less than 1% of all cases of ST-elevation (8).

The ECG findings and associated sudden and unexpected death has been reported as a common problem in Japan and Southeast Asia where it most commonly affects men during sleep (16). This disorder, known as sudden and unexpected Death Syndrome (SUDS) Sudden Unexpected Nocturnal Death Syndrome (SUNDS), has many names in Southeast Asia including bangungut (to rise and moan in sleep) in the Philippines, non-laitai (sleep-death) in Laos, lai-tai (died during sleep) in Thailand, and pokkuri (sudden and unexpectedly ceased phenomena) in Japan, General characteristics of SUDS include young, healthy males in whom death occurs suddenly with a groan, usually during sleep late at night. No precipitating factors are identified and autopsy findings are generally negative (17). Life-threatening ventricular tachyarrhythmias as a primary cause of SUDS has been demonstrated, with VF occurring in most cases (18).

The *complete syndrome* is characterized by episodes of rapid polymorphic VT in patients with an ECG pattern of right bundle branch block and ST segment elevation in leads V_1 to V_3 (Figures 1-2).

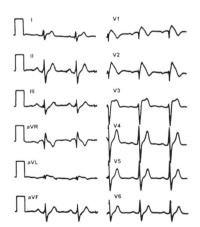

Figure 1. Typical ECG of Brugada syndrome. Note the ST-segment elevation and the pattern resembling a right bundle branch block in leads V_1 to V_3. There is a slight prolongation of the PR interval. Paper speed 25 mm/s.

Panel B 10:12:46P1   Chan. 2

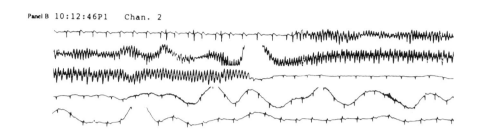

Figure 2. Self-terminating polymorphic ventricular tachycardia (continuous recording) in a patient with the Brugada syndrome. Closely coupled premature ventricular contractions precede the onset of tachyarrhythmias, with disappearance of the repolarization abnormalities following the arrhythmia.

The manifestations of the syndrome are caused by episodes of polymorphic VT/VF (Table 11-1). When the episodes terminate spontaneously, the patient develops syncopal attacks. When the episodes are sustained, full-blown cardiac arrest and eventually sudden death occurs. Thus, these manifestations can range widely: at one end of the spectrum are asymptomatic individuals and at the other end of the spectrum are those who die suddenly (Table 11-1). Other symptoms include seizures and agonal respiration. Those patients who suffer an episode at night during sleep are witnessed as having labored respiration, agitation, loss of urinary bladder control, and not uncommonly, recent memory loss (perhaps due to brain anoxia). Many patients who have the disease can appear to be otherwise healthy and active, vigorously engaging in strenuous activity or exercise. Physical examinations are typically normal. Initial evaluation of these patients commonly is consistent with benign episodes of vasovagal origin. Many patients undergo a tilt-table test, and in many are positive. However, despite appropriate therapy for vasovagal syncope, the patient may subsequently die suddenly. As seen in other clinical-ECG syndromes, there is a wide spectrum of presentations of the disease (i.e., clinical heterogeneity).

There exist *asymptomatic* individuals in whom the characteristic ECG is detected during routine examination. This ECG cannot be distinguished from that seen in symptomatic patients. In other patients, the characteristic ECG is recorded during screening after the sudden death of a family member with the disease. On the other hand, there is the group of *symptomatic* patients who have been diagnosed as suffering syncopal episodes of unknown cause, or of vasovagal origin, or have a diagnosis of idiopathic VF. Some of these patients are diagnosed at follow-up, when the ECG changes spontaneously from normal to the typical pattern of the Brugada syndrome (Figure 3). This is also the case for those individuals in whom the disease is unmasked by the administration of an antiarrhythmic drug given for other arrhythmias, such as atrial fibrillation.

Recent studies indicate that patients displaying the ECG characteristics of the syndrome have an incidence of arrhythmia and sudden death similar to that of patients in whom the ECG manifestation must be unmasked with a sodium channel-blocking agent. Up to 40% of individuals develop a new or a first episode of polymorphic VT or sudden death during a 2- to 3-year follow-up period. Hence, it does not appear to matter whether this ECG pattern occurs with or without symptoms, appearing spontaneously or after the administration of medications; in either circumstance, it is a marker of sudden death.

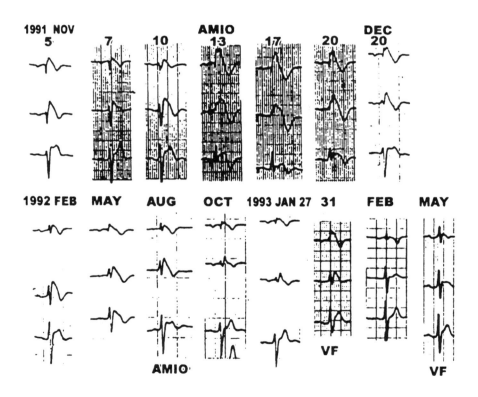

Figure 3. ECG leads V_1, V_2, and V_3 are shown from a single patient to illustrate the variability of the ECG pattern during follow-up. Note that the ECG can be extremely abnormal (top tracings) but sometimes completely normal (bottom).

Table 11-1.
Brugada Syndrome: Clinical Manifestations

a. Complete syndrome (symptomatic individuals)
    • Typical ECG with symptoms consisting of recurrent syncope or sudden
      death (aborted or not) caused by polymorphic ventricular tachycardia
b. Clinical variants
    • Typical ECG in symptomatic individual without family history of
      sudden death or Brugada syndrome
    • Typical ECG in asymptomatic individual, family member of a
      symptomatic individual with the syndrome
    • Typical ECG after administration of a drug in an asymptomatic
      individual without family history of sudden death or Brugada syndrome
    • Typical ECG after administration of a drug in an asymptomatic
      individual with the syndrome
    • Typical ECG after administration of a drug in patient with recurrent
      syncope or resuscitated sudden death (ventricular fibrillation diagnosed
      as idiopathic)
c. Electrocardiographic variants
    • Typical ECG with clear right bundle branch block, ST elevation and P-R
      prolongation
    • Typical ECG with ST elevation but no right bundle branch block, nor P-
      R prolongation
    • Incomplete right bundle branch block with saddle-type ST elevation
    • Incomplete right bundle branch block without ST segment elevation
    • Isolated P-R interval prolongation

INCIDENCE AND DISTRIBUTION

Because the syndrome has been identified only recently, it is difficult to ascertain its incidence and distribution in the world. Analysis of the data from the different published studies, suggests the disease is responsible for 4% to 12% of unexpected sudden deaths, and for up to 50% of all sudden deaths in patients with apparently normal hearts. The incidence may even be greater in the younger population. Indeed, this syndrome is the most common cause of sudden death in individuals younger than 50 years of age in Southeast Asia with no underlying cardiac disease (13). Based on a database of 48 individuals who died suddenly without evidence of structural heart disease, 57% had the right bundle branch block (RBBB) pattern with ST-elevation in leads V1 through V3. It is striking that all patients who had this pattern were male.

Several reasons exist which suggest that the disease is under-reported. One of the difficulties in estimating the incidence and prevalence of the disease is the peculiar characteristics of Brugada syndrome. It is a syndrome that in some cases presents with a typical ECG pattern, but in other cases the pattern is concealed or intermittent (i.e., the ECG is normal at certain times). Several studies have provided important clues for identifying these concealed forms; firstly, medical provocation is useful. Ajmaline continues to be the best medication to unmask the characteristics (see later). Procainamide and flecainide are useful but less sensitive. Unfortunately, these tests at present are not utilized routinely, leading to under-diagnosis.

This syndrome had already been recognized in virtually all parts of the world. In Europe there are cases in Spain, Italy, Belgium, the Netherlands, Greece, Germany, Austria, Switzerland, Poland, Ukraine, and France. In the Americas cases have been described in the United States, Canada, Uruguay, Brazil, and Argentina; and in Asia in Japan, Thailand, China, India, Laos, Vietnam, Singapore, and Cambodia. It is likely that the lack of cases in other countries is probably due more to the lack of recognition than to the absence of the disease. Hence, the disease is likely to be found worldwide, not a surprising finding given the high mobility of the population and the genetic basis of the disease. In the future, a sizeable increase in the number of identified cases is expected as the recognition of the disease grows.

A prospective study of an adult Japanese population (22,027 subjects) showed an incidence of 0.05% of ECGs compatible with the syndrome (19). A second study (20) of adults in Awa, Japan showed an incidence of 0.6% (66 cases out of 10,420). However, a third study (21) in children from Japan showed an incidence of ECGs compatible with the syndrome of only 0.0006 % (1 case in 163,110). These results suggest that the syndrome manifests primarily during adulthood, which is in concordance with the mean age of sudden death. As noted, the ECG pattern is variable over time, with periods in which it is clearly normal.

CLINICAL GENETICS OF BRUGADA SYNDROME

Most of the families thus far identified with Brugada syndrome have apparent autosomal dominant inheritance (22-28). In these families, approximately 50% of offspring of affected patients develop the disease. Although the number of families reported has been small, it is likely that this is due to under-recognition as well as premature and unexpected death (20,23-26).

DIAGNOSIS OF BRUGADA SYNDROME

The diagnosis of the syndrome is usually made by electrocardiography when the patient presents the typical ECG pattern and there is a history of aborted sudden death or syncope caused by a polymorphic VT or VF. The ST-segment elevation in leads V1 to V3 with or without a right bundle branch block pattern is characteristic. The ST-segment changes are different from the ones observed in acute septal ischemia, pericarditis, ventricular aneurysm, and in some normal variants such as early repolarization (29). Some patients, however, have ECGs that are not characteristic, and these patients are recognized only by a physician who is aware of the syndrome. There are also patients with a normal ECG in whom the syndrome can be recognized only when the typical pattern appears on follow-up ECG, or after administration of ajmaline, procainamide, or flecainide (Figure 4).

It is possible that the ECG patterns differ depending on the genetic abnormality, as is the case in other genetic diseases such as the long QT syndrome (30,31). Although mutations have been discovered in the Brugada syndrome (see section on Molecular Genetics), it will be necessary to identify more mutations and make genotype-phenotype correlations to establish clinical links (25).

Additional diagnostic problems are caused by changes in the ECG induced by the autonomic nervous system and by antiarrhythmic drugs (Figure 5). Miyazaki et al (32) were the first to identify variability of the ECG pattern in the syndrome. Despite the fact that the syndrome was initially described as a persistent ECG pattern, it was later recognized that it is variable over time, depending on modifying influences such as the autonomic interaction and the administration of antiarrhythmic drugs (33-35). Adrenergic stimulation decreases the ST-segment elevation while vagal stimulation accentuates it. The administration of class Ia, Ic and III drugs increase the ST-segment elevation, while exercise decreases ST-segment elevation in some patients but increase it in others (32-35). The changes in heart rate induced by atrial pacing are accompanied by changes in the degree of ST-segment elevation as well. When the heat rate decreases, the ST-segment elevation increases; on the other hand, when heart rate increases, ST-segment elevation decreases (35). However, the contrary can also be observed. Based on this information, patients with syncope of unknown cause should be challenged with antiarrhythmic drugs in order to exclude the possibility of this syndrome as a cause of ventricular arrhythmias and syncope.

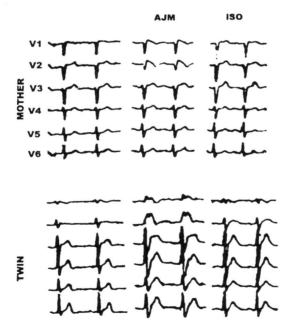

Figure 4. Effects of the intravenous administration of ajmaline on the ECG of the mother and a twin brother of a patient with Brugada syndrome. The ST-segment elevation becomes evident in both cases and indicates that both have the genetic defect underlying this syndrome.

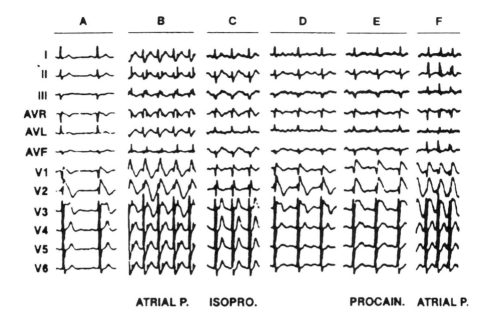

ATRIAL P.   ISOPRO.   PROCAIN.   ATRIAL P.

Figure 5. The different panels illustrate the modulation of ST-segment elevation with atrial pacing (ATRIAL P.), isoproterenol infusion (ISOPRO.), and intravenous procainamide (PROCAIN.) in a patient with the syndrome. Atrial stimulation worsens the RBBB in panel B and results in T wave alternans. Acceleration of heart rate by isoproterenol, on the contrary, results in normalization of the ST-segment, although an incomplete RBBB is still seen. Panel D shows return to baseline. In panel E, procainamide increases ST-elevation, and atrial pacing in F after procainamide results again in bizarre ECG changes and T wave alternans.

ELECTROPHYSIOLOGICAL SUBSTRATE

Patients with this ECG pattern clearly have a proclivity to develop rapid polymorphic VT/VF (26,36). Before the episode, the patients present with a regular sinus rhythm, with no changes in the QT interval. In some rare cases it seems that the ST-segment elevation increases just prior to the onset of polymorphic VT. Rarely, the triggering of the arrhythmia occurs after a short-long-short cycle. It is clear that these patients have an electrophysiological substrate for VT/VF as evidenced by the fact that the majority of patients who have the syndrome have inducible polymorphic VT/VF and an abnormal signal averaged ECG. This is despite normal cardiac function and lack of gross structural cardiac abnormalities. When comparing patients with abnormal ECG patterns to those with normal ECGs in the SUDS (Sudden Unexpected Death Syndrome) study (16), VF was induced in 93% of patients with the Brugada syndrome pattern, but in only 11% of those patients with a normal ECG. Patients with the syndrome have also been shown to have prolonged His-Purkinje conduction (H-V interval). Whether this abnormality contributes to VF occurrence is unclear.

ELECTROPHYSIOLOGICAL AND HEMODYNAMIC FINDINGS

During invasive electrophysiological investigation, sinus node function is normal in the large majority of patients. However, isolated patients have manifest sinus node disease and are pacemaker-dependent. Approximately, about 10% of patients have paroxysmal atrial fibrillation. No detailed studies exist on the ability to induce this arrhythmia by programmed electrical stimulation, however.

All published studies agree on the inducibility of polymorphic VT by programmed electrical stimulation in symptomatic patients (13,14,16,23) (Figure 6). Approximately 80% are inducible by providing one or two ventricular premature beats during ventricular pacing. In some patients three premature stimuli are required. In practically all cases, the induced arrhythmia is sustained and results in hemodynamic collapse, which must be terminated by an external DC shock. Polymorphic VT or VF induced by programmed stimulation is a nonspecific finding, however, since these arrhythmias can sometimes be induced in patients with a normal heart (37). There exist, however, major differences between the two situations: 1) the clinical context, with symptomatic patients with the Brugada syndrome having suffered from spontaneous ventricular arrhythmias; 2) the percentage of patients inducible to a sustained polymorphic ventricular arrhythmia in the Brugada syndrome (80%) as compared to individuals without the syndrome where a sustained polymorphic VT or VF is only rarely induced.

Electrophysiologic studies frequently identify conduction disturbances in patients with Brugada syndrome. The H-V interval is prolonged in about half the patients. The prolongation is not marked—it rarely exceeds 70 ms—but it is clearly abnormal in this population with an average age of 40 years. The H-V prolongation explains the slight prolongation of the P-R interval during sinus rhythm.

Hemodynamic studies are usually found to be normal. SUDS patients with or without the typical ECG also have normal findings. The coronary arteries are normal, as are the right and left ventricular function and contractility in patients with Brugada syndrome and SUDS.

PATHOLOGICAL FINDINGS

At present no patients have had any structural abnormality identified consistently in the heart (36). Despite the suggestion of some authors (38,39), there is no indication that the disease is a form of arrhythmogenic right ventricular dysplasia (ARVD). Noninvasive studies, including nuclear magnetic resonance and echocardiography (available in the majority of the patients) are typically normal. As noted above, there have been some arguments as to whether the syndrome is a variant of ARVD. Burke et al (40) has shown that 15% of normal hearts contain transmural fatty infiltration of the right ventricle. This fact raises an important doubt as to our ability to diagnose ARVD by histology alone. As there is no gold standard for the diagnosis, and no controlled, double-blind studies evaluating endomyocardial biopsies of patients with ARVD, this correlation must await future analyses.

CELLULAR AND IONIC MECHANISMS

The polymorphic VT can often be induced in these patients by programmed electrical stimulation of the heart, suggesting a reentrant mechanism. As will be discussed below, two mechanisms are thought to underlie this syndrome: phase 2 reentry and circus movement reentry.

ST-SEGMENT ELEVATION

The mechanisms responsible for the ST segment elevation and the genesis of VT/VF in the Brugada syndrome are slowly coming into better focus. The available data suggest that a downsloping ST-segment elevation observed in the right precordial leads of patients with Brugada syndrome is the result of depression or loss of the action potential dome in *right* ventricular epicardium (31,35,41-45).

ST-segment elevation is a normal characteristic of the ECG of some rodents (46). This electrocardiographic feature is the result of a much earlier repolarization of the epicardial action potential due to a more intense transient outward current (I_{to}) in epicardium. I_{to} block with 4-aminopyridine (4-AP) eliminates the differences in atrial premature depolarization of rat/mouse epicardium and endocardium, yielding an isoelectric ST-segment (47-49). In larger mammals, an isoelectric ST-segment is the norm, due to the absence of voltage differences in the action potential plateau throughout the ventricular myocardium. As in rodents, I_{to} is differentially distributed across the ventricular wall, but instead of contributing to final repolarization of the action potential, in larger mammals including humans, the current gives rise to an early repolarization phase (phase 1), responsible for notched or "spike and dome" appearance of the epicardial action potential (Figure 7).

It is now well established that a transient outward current (I_{to})-mediated phase 1 is much more prominent in epicardium than in endocardium in canine (50,51), feline (52), rabbit (53), rat (54), and human (55,56) ventricular cells. The spike and dome morphology of the epicardial action potential is absent in neonates and gradually appears over the first few months of life, reaching a plateau between 10 and 20 weeks of age in the dog (59-62). The progressive development of the notch parallels the appearance of I_{to}. Age-related changes in the manifestation of the spike and dome have been described in human atrial (63) and canine Purkinje (64) tissues and rat ventricular (65) cells. The extent to which I_{to2}, a Ca-activated component of transient outward current, differs among the 3 ventricular myocardial cell types is unknown (66).

Initially ascribed to a K^+ current, I_{to2} is believed to be largely due to a calcium-activated chloride current ($I_{cl(Ca)}$) (35). Recent studies also indicate the presence of larger I_{to}-mediated notch in right vs. left canine ventricular epicardium (35,61) (Figure 8).

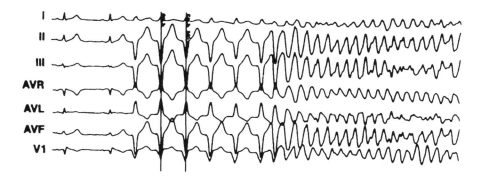

Figure 6. Initiation of ventricular fibrillation in the electrophysiology laboratory by means of programmed ventricular stimulation.

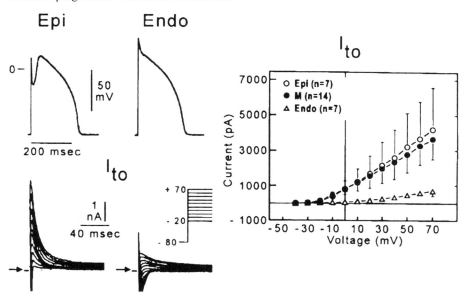

Figure 7. Transmembrane action potentials recorded from canine right ventricular epicardial and endocardial cells and accompanying transient outward current (I_{to}) (bottom). Epicardial cells typically display a much more prominent I_{to}-mediated action potential notch.

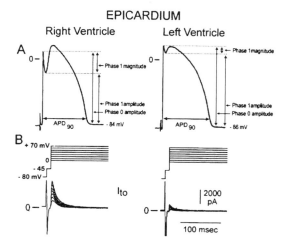

Figure 8. Transmembrane action potentials recorded from isolated right (A) and left (B) canine ventricular epicardial tissues (BCL 5 800 msec) and associated I_{to} current. Right ventricular cells commonly display a more prominent I_{to}-mediated action potential notch than do cells from left ventricular epicardium.

A prominent action potential notch in right ventricular epicardium but not in endocardium gives rise to a transmural voltage gradient during ventricular activation that is responsible for the inscription of the J wave or J point elevation in the ECG[41] (Figure 9). A prominent I_{to}-mediated notch also predisposes canine right ventricular epicardium to all-or-none repolarization under a variety of conditions (22,43,47,48,67). Under normal conditions, developing inward current (principally calcium current I_{ca}) overcomes the outward current (principally I_{to}) active at the end of phase 1, thus producing a secondary depolarization that gives rise to the dome of the epicardial action potential. Under pathophysiological conditions, the balance of current at the end of phase 1 of the epicardial response can change, thus leading to important alterations in action potential morphology and the cycling of cellular calcium. The balance of current active at the end of phase 1 can easily shift outward, causing a loss of the action potential dome. Much of the characterization of this phenomenon has involved studies of canine ventricular epicardium (41-51,58,59,67-78). Under ischemic conditions and in response to a variety of drugs, including sodium and calcium channel blockers, canine ventricular epicardium exhibits an "all-or-none" repolarization as a result of the rebalancing of currents flowing at the end of phase 1 of the action potential. The dome fails to develop when the outward currents (principally I_{to}) overwhelm the inward currents (chiefly I_{Ca}), resulting in a marked (40-70%) abbreviation of the action potential. The dome can be restored by inhibition of I_{to} with 4-AP, supporting the hypothesis that a prominent I_{to} facilitates loss of the action potential dome. In addition to I_{to} block, agents capable of reducing other outward currents (e.g. $I_{K\text{-}ATP}$) or augmenting inward current (I_{Ca}) are also capable of restoring the dome.

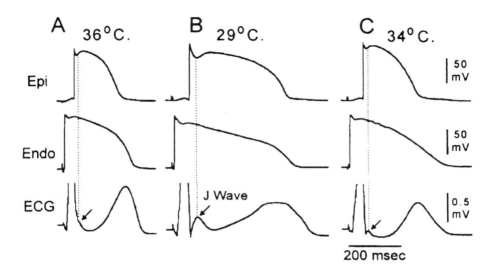

Figure 9. Cellular basis for the J wave. Each panel shows transmembrane recordings obtained from the epicardial (Epi) and endocardial (Endo) regions of an isolated arterially perfused canine left ventricular wedge and a transmural ECG simultaneously recorded. A: A small but distinct action potential notch in epicardium, but not in endocardium, is associated with an elevated J point at the R-ST junction (arrow) under normothermic conditions (36°C). B: A decrease in the temperature of the perfusate and bath to 29°C results in an increase in the amplitude and width of action potential notch in epicardium but not in endocardium, leading to a prominent J wave on the transmural ECG (arrow). C: Rewarming to a temperature of 34°C is attended by a parallel reduction in the amplitude and width of the J wave and epicardial action potential notch.

Loss of the dome in right ventricular epicardium but not endocardium has been demonstrated in variety of studies using tissues isolated from the canine right ventricle, myocytes enzymatically dissociated from the respective regions of the wall, and most recently in studies involving arterially perfused wedges of the canine right ventricle. Studies involving the wedge preparation have provided direct evidence in support of the hypothesis that loss of depression or the action potential dome in epicardium but not endocardium underlies the development of a prominent ST segment elevation (Figure 10). As in tissue and cells, loss of the dome in the wedge preparations can be affected either by augmenting outward current or reducing inward current active at the end of phase 1 or the action potential.

"All-or-none" repolarization of the right ventricular epicardial action potential is caused by an outward shift in the balance of currents active at the end of phase 1 of the action potential. As a consequence, autonomic neurotransmitters (i.e., acetylcholine) facilitate loss of the dome (68) by suppressing I_{Ca} and/or augmenting potassium current, whereas β-adrenergic agents such as isoproterenol and dobutamine restore the dome by augmenting I_{Ca}. Sodium channel blockers also facilitates loss of the canine right ventricular epicardial action potential dome (67,69). Accentuation of the ST-segment elevation in patients with the Brugada syndrome following vagal maneuvers or Class Ia and Ic antiarrhythmic agents (sodium blockers) and reduction of ST-segment elevation following β-adrenergic agents are consistent with these findings in isolated tissue preparations (32).

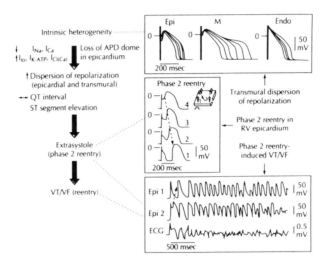

Figure 10. Intrinsic heterogeneity in the form of transmural dispersion of repolarization (*top inset*: action potentials recorded from epicardial (Epi), endocardial (Endo), and M cell (M) regions of canine ventricular wall at rates between 300 - 5000 ms) is amplified as a result of the loss of the epicardial action potential dome, due to a decrease in sodium current (I_{Na}) or calcium current (I_{Ca}) or an increase in transient outward current (I_{to}), ATP-sensitive potassium current (I_{K-ATP}), or calcium-activated chloride current ($I_{Cl\ (Ca)}$). Loss of the dome augments both epicardial and transmural dispersion of repolarization, thus creating a vulnerable window for the development of reentry. Heterogeneous loss of the action potential dome in ventricular epicardium generates a strong voltage gradient that causes the dome of the action potential in regions where it is maintained to propagate to regions where it is lost, and thus to generate a closely coupled premature extrasystole (*middle inset*: phase 2 reentry observed using four simultaneous right ventricular epicardial transmembrane recordings; modified from Antzelevitch (31) with permission). The QT interval may undergo little changes, but the ST-segment is elevated as a consequence of the transmural gradients flowing during the plateau of the action potential. The extrasystole captures the vulnerable window and precipitates ventricular tachycardia/ventricular fibrillation (VT/VF) in an arterially perfused canine right ventricular wedge preparation. Note the downsloping ST- segment elevation in the electrocardiogram (ECG) recorded across the wedge).

THE BRUGADA SYNDROME AND THE J WAVE

In the wedge preparation, loss of the action potential dome is often preceded by accentuation of the epicardial action potential notch, giving rise to abnormally large J waves (Figure 9), as sometimes observe patients with Brugada syndrome just before and after VF (35,79). The electrocardiographic J wave, because it provides an index of the magnitude of the epicardial action potential notch, may be useful to identify individuals at risk for developing idiopathic VF or the Brugada syndrome. Here too, I_{to} block may be of therapeutic value.

RIGHT BUNDLE BRANCH BLOCK

It is unclear whether the right bundle branch block in this syndrome is real or whether it represents early repolarization of the right ventricular epicardium. Clinical and electrophysiological data suggest that both possibilities exist. Some ECGs clearly show a right bundle branch block pattern after normalization of the ST-segment. There is frequently a prolongation of the H-V interval in these patients, which supports an abnormality of the conduction system. On the other hand, ECGs without a right bundle branch block are common when the ST-segment elevation is corrected. Moreover, not all patients have a prolongation of the H-V interval. It is possible that the different ECG patterns result from different ion channel defects, as seen in the long QT syndrome (80). The dispersion of repolarization that forms the substrate for VT/VF can develop with a defect in any one of a number of ion channels, as well as other pathologic influences, as discussed later.

TRIGGERING MECHANISMS

Kasanuki et al have suggested that in some cases of Brugada syndrome the beginning of the arrhythmia is bradycardia-dependent (81). This fact could explain the higher incidence of sudden death at night in individuals with the syndrome. In addition, Proclemer et al reported a patient in whom the episodes of ventricular arrhythmias could be controlled only during fast ventricular pacing (82). Notably, however, not all patients die at night and not all patients are controlled with fast ventricular pacing. For instance, patients from Southeast Asia who have the ECG pattern usually develop VT/VF during sleep. Evaluation of cardioverter-defibrillators in these patients show no evidence of bradycardia-dependence and in many cases the rate preceding the VF episode is relatively fast. Therefore, although some of the triggers are known, others clearly exist.

CHANGES IN HEART RATE AND EXERCISE ON THE ECG

As already discussed in part, this syndrome is characterized by great variability in the ECG pattern. The ECG may be completely abnormal at times, but completely normal at others. This variability has many causes and several explanations, such as autonomic changes influence the ECG pattern (32). An artificial increase in heart rate (by atrial pacing) decreases ST-segment elevation, while a decrease in heart rate increases it. These data are consistent with loss of the action potential dome at the epicardial level as the cause of ST-segment elevation. I_{to} becomes more prominent at slow rates, increasing heterogeneity and ST-segment elevation. These data are also in agreement with the clinical observations in the Asian population documenting a bradycardia dependency and a higher incidence of sudden death during sleep in patients with this syndrome (16).

Normalization of the ST-segment has been identified during exercise in the majority of patients with this syndrome (26). These findings are in line with the mechanisms described, because both an increase in heart rate and adrenergic stimulation decrease ST-segment elevation.

ROLE OF THE AUTONOMIC NERVOUS SYSTEM

The role of the autonomic nervous system in this syndrome is still not fully understood. Vagal stimulation is believed to trigger the arrhythmia in some patients because many episodes occur at night and sympathetic stimulation normalizes the abnormal ECG pattern. In one report from Japan (81), VT/VF induction was facilitated by vagal stimulation or sympathetic blockade. On the other hand, there are patients who suffer the arrhythmia during adrenergic stimulation, while others present with no apparent correlation with changes in the autonomic balance.

One of the observations in patients with the Brugada syndrome that may compel physicians to think that sympathetic blockade and vagal stimulation can enhance the induction or spontaneous occurrence of VT/VF is that the abnormal ECG pattern normalizes with sympathetic stimulation, while vagal stimulation enhances the abnormal pattern. However, at present there is not sufficient data to support the concept that normalization of the ECG correlates with a decreased occurrence of VT/VF. Nor do we know whether it results in an increase of the VF threshold. Future work will need to address this issue.

Kobayashi et al provided information regarding possible alterations in the cardiac innervation in this syndrome (83). Using I-123 MIBG and SPECT, they found a higher washout in patients with the syndrome than in patients with VT due to other etiologies. Previously, however, Miyazaki et al (32) were unable to identify an alteration in the cardiac innervation in a similar group of patients. At present, there is no compelling data to conclude that there is a correlation between this syndrome and abnormalities of the autonomic system or innervation abnormalities. As in other diseases like long QT syndrome, there may be a role for the autonomic nervous system as a modifying factor, but it is unlikely to be a primary cause.

PHASE 2 REENTRY IN ISOLATED SHEETS OF CANINE RIGHT VENTRICULAR EPICARDIUM

Under all of the conditions listed above, loss of the action potential dome is usually inhomogeneous (31,35,61). Loss of the dome at some epicardial sites but not others leads to the development of a marked dispersion of repolarization. Propagation of the action potential dome from sites at which it is maintained to sites at which it is abolished can cause local reexcitation of the impulse within the preparation. This mechanism, termed phase 2 reentry, produces closely coupled extrasystolic beats which can initiate one or more cycles or circus movement reentry (43) (Figure 10).

Under ischemic conditions the contribution of I_{Ca} is reduced, thus shifting the balance of current at the end of phase 1 to net outward in epicardium (43). Similar electrical heterogeneity leading to phase 2 reentry occurs in canine epicardium exposed to: a) K^+ channel openers such a pinacidil (48); b) sodium channel blockers such as flecainide (67); c) increased $(Ca^{2+})_o$; and d) metabolic inhibition (22) (Figure 11). Because the level of I_{to} is pivotal, I_{to} block restores electrical homogeneity and abolishes reentrant activity in all cases.

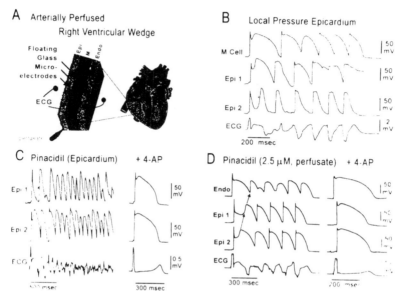

Figure 11. ECG and arrhythmias with typical features of the Brugada syndrome recorded from canine right ventricular wedge preparations. A: Schematic of the arterially perfused right ventricular wedge preparation. B: Local pressure-inducedphase 2 reentry and VT. Shown are transmembrane action potentials simultaneously recorded from 2 epicardial (Epi 1 andEpi 2) and one M region (M) sites, together with a transmural potential dome at that site but not atEpi 1 or M sites, together with a transmural ECG. Local application of pressure nearEpi 2 results in loss of the action then reexcites Epi 2 giving rise to a phase 2 reentrant extrasystole which then triggers a short run of VT. Note the ST segment elevation due to loss of the action potential dome in a segment of epicardium. C: Polymorphic VT/VF induced by local application of the potassium channel opener pinacidil (10 μM) to the pericardial surface of the wedge. Action potentials from 2 epicardial sites (Epi 1 andEpi 2) and a transmural ECG were simultaneously recorded. Loss of the dome atEpi 1 but not Epi2 creates a marked dispersion of repolarization, giving rise to a phase 2 reentrantextrasystole. The extrasystolic beat then triggers a long episode of VF (22 sec). Right panel: Addition of 4-AP (2mM), a specific I_{to} blocker, to the perfusate restored the action potential dome at Epi 1, thus reducing dispersion of repolarization and suppressing all arrhythmic activity. BCL=2000 msec. D: Phase 2renetry gives rise to VT following addition of pinacidil (2.5 μM) to the coronary perfusate. Transmembrane action potentials form 2 epicardial sites (Epi 1 andEpi 2) and one endocardial site (Endo) as well as a transmural ECG were simultaneously recorded. Right panel: 4-AP (lmM) markedly reduces the magnitude of the action potential notch in epicardium, thus restoring the action potential dome throughout the preparation and abolishing all arrhythmic activity.

PHASE 2 REENTRY AS TRIGGER FOR VENTRICULAR TACHYCARDIA AND FIBRILLATION IN THE WALL OF CANINE RIGHT VENTRICLE

These observations point to a depressed right ventricular epicardial action potential dome as the basis for the ST-segment elevation and to phase 2 reentry as a trigger for episodes of VT and VF in patients with the Brugada syndrome (35,61). The available data also indicate that autonomic neurotransmitters like acetylcholine facilitate loss of the action potential dome by suppressing calcium current and augmenting potassium current, and that β-adrenergic agonists such as isoproterenol and dobutamine restore the dome by augmenting I_{Ca}, Sodium channel blockers also facilitate loss of the canine right ventricular action potential dome as a result of a negative shift in the voltage at which phase 1 begins (67,69).

Exaggeration of the ST-segment elevation in patients with the Brugada syndrome following vagal maneuvers or sodium channel blockers, as well as normalization of the ST-elevation following β-adrenergic agents are concordant with these findings in isolated tissue preparations (32,35,41,48,68,69). The appearance of ST-segment elevation only in right precordial leads in patients with the Brugada syndrome is also consistent with the observation that loss of the action potential dome is more easily induced in right vs. left canine ventricular epicardium (5,22), because of the higher density of I_{to} in right vs. left ventricular epicardium (70). It was on the basis of these similarities in electrophysiology, pharmacology, and ECG manifestations, that Antzelevitch and coworkers hypothesized that loss of depression of right ventricular epicardial action potential dome underlies the ST-segment elevation and that phase 2 reentry may provide the trigger for episodes of VF in patients with the Brugada syndrome (26,32,33,35,41,84).

Further tests of these hypotheses have been reported in studies involving arterially perfused canine right ventricular wedge preparations (57-66,70). These preparations provide a direct correlation of transmembrane activity across the right ventricular wall (recorded from the transmural surface using floating glass microelectrodes) with electrocardiographic activity recorded along the same vector and are capable of developing VT and VF. The results obtained using this approach support the hypothesis that ST-segment elevation in patients with the Brugada syndrome may be the result of loss of the action potential dome in right ventricular epicardium, where I_{to} is most prominent, but not in endocardium, where I_{to} is weak. Initiation of VT/VF under these conditions is likely to be via phase 2 reentry secondary to heterogeneous loss of the epicardial action potential dome (41). Extrasystolic beats generated via phase 2 reentry in the wedge preparation are generally very short-coupled, falling on the T wave (Figure 12). This malignant R-on-T phenomenon is always observed in patients with idiopathic VF (16,85).

It is noteworthy that the VT and VF episodes generated in the wedge preparations are often polymorphic, resembling a very rapid form of *torsades de pointes*. Both the Brugada syndrome and long QT syndrome display a large dispersion of repolarization, especially along the transmural axis. In the case of long QT syndrome, dispersion is secondary to a disproportionate prolongation of the M cell action potential in the mid-wall yielding a long QT interval, whereas in the Brugada syndrome, dispersion is secondary to disproportionate abbreviations of the epicardial action potential (QT interval may remain unchanged or abbreviate). In both syndromes, dispersion of repolarization creates a vulnerable period during which a premature beat can succeed in generating a reentrant arrhythmia. In long QT syndrome, the premature beat is thought to be an early after-depolarization-induced triggered beat, whereas in the Brugada syndrome the premature beat appears to be due to phase 2 reentry (31,33,35). In the latter, the substrate that permits the establishment of reentrant activity (dispersion of repolarization) is also responsible for generating the premature beat precipitating the arrhythmia. This syndrome is unique in that the same substrate provides the trigger as well as the means by which circus movement reentry can be sustained. The shorter wavelength (due to a briefer refractory period) in the case of the Brugada syndrome may explain the appearance of a rapid form of *torsades de pointes* in some cases. This activity may be mechanistically related to the migrating spiral wave shown to generate a pattern resembling *torsades de pointes* associated with a normal or long QT interval (86,87).

In both the perfused wedge and in isolated tissues, agents that inhibit I_{to}, including 4-AP, quinidine, and disopyramide (88-90) are effective in restoring the action potential dome, thus restoring electrical homogeneity and aborting all arrhythmic activity (Figures 11-12). Thus, Class Ia antiarrhythmic agents that block I_{Na} but not I_{to} (procainamide and ajmaline) appear to exacerbate or indeed to unmask the Brugada syndrome, whereas those with actions to block both I_{Na} and I_{to} (quinidine and disopyramide) can exert an ameliorative effect (35). The results of Yan et al, demonstrating a therapeutic effect of quinidine may help explain the success of Belhassen and coworkers in treating patients with idiopathic VF (91).

The applicability of these phenomena observed in the canine heart to the human heart must be approached with caution. Extrapolation to the clinic requires that action potentials in human epicardium exhibit a pronounced I_{to}-mediated spike and dome morphology. However, there are indications that this is the case (55,56,92). I_{to} reactivation is much faster in human epicardium than in canine, suggesting that electrical heterogeneity and phase 2 reentry might occur over a much wider range of heart rates and be less influenced by heart rate in the human ventricle. Although ST-segment elevation in some Brugada syndrome patients shows little or no dependence on rate, Matsuo et al (79) reported a direct relationship between the degree of ST-segment elevation and the preceding RR interval, consistent with a relatively slower rate of reactivation of I_{to}.

Further evidence in support of the hypothesis that the Brugada syndrome is a primary electrical disease derives from the recent demonstration (25) that this syndrome is linked to a mutation in an ion channel gene (sodium channel α subunit SCN5A) located on chromosome 3. This finding is consistent with the demonstration that inhibition of the sodium channel is amongst the easiest means to induce ST-segment elevation and phase 2 reentry in isolated tissue preparation (67,69). Sodium channel blockers facilitate loss of the canine right ventricular action potential dome. This action is due to a negative shift in the voltage at which phase 1 begins, thus causing phase 1 to proceed to more negative potentials at which I_{to} can overwhelm I_{Ca}.

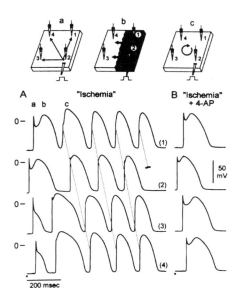

Figure 12. Phase 2 reentry-initiated circus movement tachycardia abolished with transient outward current inhibition. (A) Exposure of canine right ventricular epicardial sheet to simulated ischemia results in loss of the dome at sites 3 and 4 but not at sites 1 and 2 (cycle length=1100 ms). Conduction of the basic beat proceeds normally from the stimulation site (site 2; see schematic a). Propagation of the action potential dome from the right half of the preparation causes reexcitation of the left half via a phase 2 reentry mechanism (see schematic b). The extrasystolic beat generated by phase 2 reentry then initiates a run of tachycardia that is sustained for 4 additional cycles via a typical (phase 0) circus movement reentry mechanism. The proposed reentrant path is shown in schematic c. Note that phase 2 reentry provides an activation front roughly perpendicular to that of the basic beat. (B) Recorded 5 min after addition of 1 mmol/l. 4-aminopyridine (4-AP), an inhibitor of the transient outward current. In the continued presence of ischemia, 4-AP restores the dome at all epicardial recording sites within 3 min. Thus electrical homogeneity is restored and all reentrant activity abolished. Adapted with permission from Lukas and Antzelevitch (43).

THE ROLE OF PHASE 2 REENTRY IN OTHER SYNDROMES

The similarity between the ECG manifestation of the Brugada syndrome and that of acute myocardial infarction suggests that the mechanism responsible for arrhythmogenesis in patients with Brugada syndrome is similar to that responsible for early ventricular arrhythmias in patients with acute MI. The Brugada syndrome model may therefore represent a stable (ischemia-free) model of the early phases of ischemia. This hypothesis has been tested in isolated epicardial tissues (14,42).

These same mechanisms may contribute to the development of arrhythmias in ARVD (39). It is tempting to speculate that the Brugada syndrome may start out as a primary electrical disease that progresses to develop structural abnormalities.

This hypothesis is suggested (93,94) by the observation that electrical remodeling in atrial fibrillation and ventricular hibernation *precedes* structural remodeling (95).

RELATION OF OTHER DISEASES TO BRUGADA SYNDROME

Other diseases may result in ECG manifestations similar to the Brugada syndrome. For instance, in patients with Chagas' disease, Chaiale et al (96) showed that the intravenous administration of ajmaline was of value not only to uncover latent conduction disturbances, but also what they called "latent disease". In patients with positive serology, severe conduction disturbances occurred in one third of patients after the administration of intravenous ajmaline. In 8% of patients they observed the appearance of ventricular arrhythmias and in 7% of patients, elevation of the ST-segment in the right precordial leads was noted. The question arises as to the relationship of Chagas' disease and the Brugada syndrome. Chiale and coworkers suggested that ajmaline challenge is a specific test capable of detecting myocardial damage. In light of the recent discovery of the genetic defect underlying the Brugada syndrome and the response of these patients to ajmaline, the question also arises about the possible occurrence of damage to the sodium channel in Chagas' disease. Although there exist major differences between Chagas' disease and the Brugada syndrome, the final common pathway leading to sudden death may be the same: damage to the Na^+ channel (infectious in Chagas' disease, genetic in Brugada syndrome) with conduction and repolarization disturbances leading to electrical chaos and VF.

Other conditions have been reported to be associated with ECGs simulating the Brugada syndrome, including myotonic dystrophy, pectus excavatum, and mediastinal tumors. These should be excluded before diagnosing the Brugada syndrome. In addition, ARVD and early repolarization syndrome (ERS) have been considered by some investigators to be forms of Brugada syndrome (26). Description of these two entities follows.

Brugada Syndrome and Arrhythmogenic Right Ventricular Dysplasia

Controversy exists concerning the possible association of Brugada syndrome and ARVD, with some investigators arguing that these are the same disorder or at least one is a forme-fruste of the other (38,39,97-101). However, the classic echocardiographic, angiographic and magnetic resonance imaging findings of ARVD are not seen in Brugada syndrome patients. In addition, Brugada syndrome patients typically are without the histopathologic findings of ARVD. Further, the morphology of VT/VF differs. Similarities and differences of these two disorders are compared in Table 2. Notable is the fact that to date, the genes and genetic loci for these two disorders differ. Once the genes are completely identified and characterized, better understanding of these two diseases will be gained.

TABLE 11-2.
Brugada Syndrome vs. ARVD

	ARVD	Brugada
Age	Any	Any
Sex	M>F	M>F
Inheritance	Autosomal Dominant	Autosomal
Dominant ECG	Inverted T, ST elev	epsilon + RBB,V1-3
	Fixed abnormality	Dynamic changes
VT Type	Monomorphic	Polymorphic
H-V Interval	Normal	1/3 normal
Exercise	No effect	Normal or worsening
Isoproterenol	No effect	Normalization
Class I Drugs	No effect	↑ST elevation
Echo/Angio	RV dilation or aneurysms	Normal
MRI	Fatty infiltration	Normal
Pathology	Fibrosis, fatty infiltration	Normal

EARLY REPOLARIZATION AND THE BRUGADA SYNDROME

Because of the similarities between the Brugada syndrome and early repolarization syndrome (ERS), patients with the Brugada syndrome have been misdiagnosed as having early repolarization. A discussion of the similarities, differences, and electrophysiological mechanisms is in order.

The early repolarization syndrome (ERS), although characterized by an ST-segment elevation, differs from the Brugada syndrome in several important ways. Chief among these is the fact that ERS is not associated with life-threatening arrhythmias. The elevated ST-segment in ERS is usually localized to leads V2-V4-5, displaying an upward concavity with a positive T wave polarity accompanied by a notched J point (9), whereas ST-segment elevation in the Brugada syndrome is limited to the right precordial leads, is mildly downsloping, and is followed by a negative T wave.

Early repolarization syndrome and the Brugada syndrome are similarly modulated by drugs, neurotransmitters and autonomic tone, however. As with the Brugada syndrome, isoproterenol reduces or eliminates ST-segment elevation in individuals with ERS, whereas propranolol increases the magnitude of ST-segment elevation (102). Electrocardiographic traces characteristic of ERS are observed in patients with high spinal cord accidents (C5 to C6) in whom injury of the cervical cord disrupts cardiac sympathetic influence from high centers while parasympathetic control remains intact. These observations suggest that reduced sympathetic tone in the presence of normal or strong parasympathetic tone may play a role in the generation of ST-segment elevation (103-105).

ST-segment elevation in both ERS and the Brugada syndrome may be due to depression of the epicardial action potential plateau, while that of endocardium remains normal, thus creating a transmural voltage gradient. The question then arises: why is one syndrome associated with a high incidence of ventricular arrhythmias and the other is not? The answer may lie in the degree to which dispersion of repolarization and refractoriness develops. Whereas "all-or-none" repolarization at some epicardial sites but not endocardium creates a large epicardial and transmural dispersion of repolarization, in early repolarization, a depression of the epicardial action potential may occur without a change in final repolarization, thus causing an ST-segment elevation with little or no dispersion of repolarization. This hypothesis remains to be tested.

MOLECULAR GENETICS OF BRUGADA SYNDROME

In order in identify the gene(s) responsible for Brugada syndrome, moderate size or large families with excellent clinical surveillance is required for gene mapping studies to proceed with subsequent positional cloning or positional candidate gene cloning. In the latter case, genes previously cloned and mapped to a region of interest (i.e., a linked locus) can be screened for mutations to prove that it is responsible for the disease. In cases where excellent electrophysiologic hypotheses exist, candidate genes can also be screened randomly for mutations in small families or sporadic cases.

In Brugada syndrome, several good candidate genes exist. In animal studies, blockade of the calcium-independent 4-aminopyridine-sensitive transient outward potassium current (I_{to}) results in surface ECG findings of elevated, downsloping ST-segments due to greater prolongation in the epicardial action potential compared to the endocardium (which lacks a plateau phase). Loss of the action potential plateau (or dome) in the epicardium but not endocardium would be expected to cause ST-segment elevation and, because loss of the dome is caused by an outward shift in the balance of currents active at the end of phase 1 of the action potential (principally I_{to} and I_{Ca}), autonomic neurotransmitters like acetylcholine facilitate loss of the action potential dome by suppressing calcium current and augmenting potassium current, whereas β-adrenergic agonists (i.e., isoproterenol, dobutamine) restore the dome by augmenting I_{Ca}. Sodium channel blockers also facilitate loss of the canine right ventricular action potential dome as a result of a negative shift in the voltage at which phase 1 begins (67,69). Hence, I_{to}, I_{Ca}, and I_{Na} would be good candidate genes to study. Since I_{Na} (SCN5A) has been shown to cause VT/VF in humans (in the long QT syndrome) this gene certainly is worthy for study (105-108).

We initially reported the findings on six families and several sporadic cases of Brugada syndrome (25). The families were studied by linkage analysis using markers to the known ARVD loci (109-114) and linkage was excluded. More recently, seven other families have also excluded linkage to these loci, thus suggesting that the families recruited with Brugada syndrome to date may indeed by an entity distinct from ARVD. Candidate gene screening using the mutation analysis approach of single strand conformation polymorphism (SSCP) analysis and DNA sequencing was performed and SCN5A was chosen for study. In three families, mutations in SCN5A were identified including (1) a missense mutation (C-to-T base substitution) causing a substitution of a highly conserved threonine by methionine at codon 1620 (T1620M) in the extracellular loop between transmembrane segments S3 and S4 of domain IV (DIVS3 - DIVS4), an area important for coupling of channel activation to fast inactivation; (2) a two nucleotide insertion (AA) which disrupts the splice-donor sequence of intron 7 of SCN5A; and (3) a single nucleotide deletion (A) at codon 1397 which results in an in-frame stop codon that eliminates DIIIS6, DIVS1 – DIVS6, and the carboxy-terminus of SCN5A (Figure 13). Our findings have been confirmed by the identification of missense mutations in the conserved DIII-DIV cytoplasmic linker (R1512W) and in the C-terminal cytoplasmic domain (A1924T) of SCN5A (23).

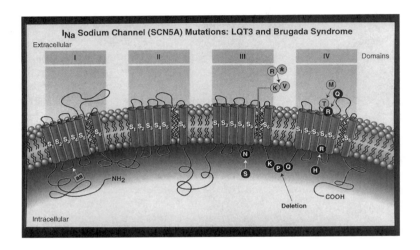

Figure 13. The sodium channel SCN5A and mutations resulting in long QT syndrome (black) and Brugada syndrome (gray). Note that the sodium channel consists of a tetrameric unit of domains I-IV (DI-DIV), each having six transmembrane segments (S1-S6). Pores are seen between S5-S6 of each domain.

Biophysical analysis of the mutants in *Xenopus* oocytes demonstrated a reduction in the number of functional sodium channels in both the splicing mutation and one-nucleotide deletion mutation, which should promote development of reentrant arrhythmias (25). In the T1620M missense mutation, sodium channels recover from inactivation more rapidly than normal. Dumaine et al (115) recently identified temperature-dependence of this mutation. In the setting of reduced functional channels, the presence of both normal and mutant channels in the same tissue would promote heterogeneity of the refractory period, a well-established mechanism of arrhythmogenesis. Inhibition of the sodium channel I_{Na} current causes heterogeneous loss of the action potential dome in the right ventricular epicardium, leading to a marked dispersion of depolarization and refractoriness, an ideal substrate for development of reentrant arrhythmias. Phase 2 reentry produced by the same substrate is believed to provide the premature beat necessary for initiation of the VT and VF responsible for symptoms in these patients. In the case of the other missense mutations, it has been suggested that a negative voltage shift of the steady-state inactivation curve occurs.

Mutations in SCN5A have previously been reported to cause the chromosome 3-linked long QT syndrome, LQT3. It is interesting that the apparent biophysical features of the SCN5A mutations in Brugada syndrome have nearly the opposite features as that seen in LQT3. Further heterogeneity associated with SCN5A mutations has recently been reported by Schott et al (116), who described novel mutations resulting in progressive cardiac conduction disease (PCCD), also known as Lev or Lenegre syndrome. Here, progressive conduction abnormalities with either RBBB or LBBB and wide QRS complex presents initially, with subsequent complete atrioventricular block. Fibrosis is a common feature. The biophysical characteristics of this disorder have not been well characterized to date.

OTHER GENE CANDIDATES FOR THE BRUGADA SYNDROME

Gene mutations that diminish the density or conductance of the sodium channel are therefore prime candidates for the Brugada syndrome. Such mutations may also be consistent with the conduction disturbances that sometimes accompany the Brugada syndrome (14,84). In addition to I_{Na}, other candidates include gene mutations that alter the intensity or kinetics of either I_{to} or I_{Ca} so as to augment the activity of the former and diminish that of the latter during the early phases of the action potential. Genes of autonomic receptors that modulate the activity or expression of these channels as well as those that regulate I_{K-ATP} are also candidates.

FINAL COMMON PATHWAY HYPOTHESIS

As described throughout this chapter, Brugada syndrome is a clinically heterogeneous disease. As noted, the first genetic abnormality causing Brugada syndrome was recently identified by our group as mutations in the ion channel gene SCN5A which encodes the cardiac sodium channel (25). Mutations in this gene result in a loss in function of the channels or rapid recovery from inactivation. SCN5A was previously shown to be the cause of LQT3, a form of Romano-Ward long QT syndrome (106-108,117,118). The differences in the clinical findings between LQT3 and Brugada syndrome occur due to the different biophysical results based on the position of the mutations within this gene. Unlike Brugada syndrome, LQT3 occurs due to a gain of function in SCN5A where persistence of inactivation is seen.

Despite the differences between LQTS and Brugada syndrome, important similarities should be noted. In particular, both of these disorders in which life-threatening ventricular tachyarrhythmias occur are due to mutations in genes encoding ion channels. This similarity is somewhat akin to what has previously been described in familial hypertrophic cardiomyopathy (FHCM) where mutations in genes encoding for sarcomeric proteins have been identified (119-125). Here, eight genes [β-myosin heavy chain (119), α-tropomyosin (120), cardiac troponin T (120), myosin binding protein-C (121,122), myosin essential and regulatory light chain (123), troponin I (124), and actin (125)], all encoding members of the sarcomeric unit have been found mutated in patients with FHCM. The clinical phenotype, including outcome, appears to differ based on the gene mutated and the specific mutation (126,127). Similar findings are emerging in familial dilated cardiomyopathy (FDCM) as well (128) (Figure 14). Thus, it appears that affecting a particular cascade at any point with the "final common pathway" leading to a specific cardiac function (i.e., contractile apparatus resulting in cardiac contractility; ion channels resulting in cardiac rhythm; cytoskeletal proteins resulting in cardiac structural support) results in a spectrum of similar disease (i.e., contractile apparatus mutations cause HCM; ion channel mutations result in LQTS, Brugada syndrome; mutations in cytoskeletal protein genes result in FDCM). This "Final Common Pathway" hypothesis (129-131) is being used in Brugada syndrome to identify the remaining genes responsible for this disorder.

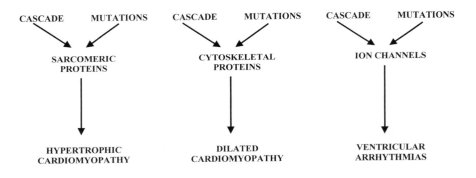

Figure 14. The "final common pathway" hypothesis. The concept that abnormalities of a common group of proteins (i.e., sarcomere, cytoskeletal, ion channel) are responsible for a subgroup of phenotypes (i.e., hypertrophic cardiomyopathy, dilated cardiomyopathy, and ventricular arrhythmias, respectively) is illustrated. Direct single-gene mutations and/or abnormalities in the interacting cascade of pathways are thought to result in the clinical spectrum of these disorders.

PROGNOSIS AND TREATMENT

This syndrome has a very poor prognosis when left untreated. One third of patients who suffer syncopal episodes or are resuscitated from near-sudden death develop a new episode of polymorphic VT within two years (36). Unfortunately, the prognosis of asymptomatic individuals with the typical ECG is also poor. In spite of not having any previous symptoms, one third of these individuals present with the first episode of polymorphic VT or VF within two years of follow-up after diagnosis (Figure 15).

Recurrence or first VF or sudden death

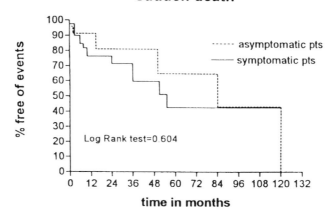

Figure 15. Survival curves in symptomatic and asymptomatic patients with typical Brugada syndrome ECG. About 30% of patients in both categories develop a recurrence or the first episode of polymorphic VT at about 2 years mean follow-up.

Because the heart is structurally normal, and there is no coronary artery disease, these patients do not die from heart failure or complications of ischemic events. Thus, they are ideal candidates for treatment with an implantable cardioverter-defibrillator. It is currently advised that all symptomatic patients should receive this device (Figure 16).

RECURRENCE OR FIRST VF OR SUDDEN DEATH

The observations on prognosis of patients from Europe with the Brugada syndrome are virtually identical to those for SUDS patients in Thailand who show the abnormal ECG pattern. The cumulative proportion of VF or cardiac arrest occurred in approximately 60% of the patients within one year, and 40% were likely to die suddenly if untreated (Figure 17). Furthermore, patients who have recurrent events face the risk of anoxic encephalopathy, from mild to disabling forms. These data are of extreme importance for the delineation of treatment policies of these patients. Because antiarrhythmic drugs (amiodarone or beta blockers) do not protect against sudden cardiac death, the only available treatment currently is the implantable cardioverter-defibrillator. When provided with the implantable defibrillator, total mortality in patients with Brugada syndrome has been 0% with up to 10 years of follow-up. These results are not surprising as these patients are young and usually free of other diseases.

Brugada Syndrome Genetics

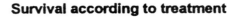
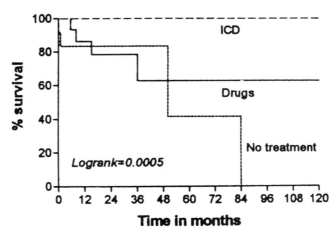

Figure 16. Prognosis of patients depending upon treatment: antiarrhythmic drugs, implantable cardioverter-defibrillator, and no treatment. Only the implantable cardioverter-defibrillator prevents sudden death.

On the other hand, major concerns arise in the treatment of asymptomatic individuals. Of the 6 asymptomatic patients dying suddenly in the study by Brugada et al (36), 4 patients were members of affected families, but 2 were sporadic cases. Data from electrophysiological investigations did not help to predict prognosis, although this may be caused by a type II error (not sufficient number of patients to prove a statistically significant difference). At present, 4 different groups of patients can be distinguished: 1) symptomatic individuals with the disease who require an implantable cardioverter-defibrillator. Patients with transient normalization of the ECG during follow-up have the same prognosis as compared to patients with a permanently abnormal ECG (unpublished observations); 2) asymptomatic patients with a family history of sudden death, a prolonged H-V interval and inducible defibrillator; 3) asymptomatic individuals without a family history of sudden death but with inducible sustained polymorphic ventricular arrhythmias, who also require a defibrillator; and 4) symptomatic individuals without a family history of sudden death and no inducible ventricular arrhythmias who should not be treated but rather followed up carefully for development of symptoms suggesting arrhythmias (particularly syncope). One has to realize, however, that these recommendations may rapidly change depending upon the availability of new data.

SPONTANEOUS TERMINATION OF VF

Bjerregaard et al were the first to report identification of spontaneous termination of VF as detected by ECG monitoring (2). In this report, a typical ECG pattern with right bundle branch block-like QRS and ST-elevation from V1 to V3 was noted.

Since then, many patients implanted with an automatic cardioverter-defibrillator with electrogram storage have been analyzed, with many spontaneous episodes of VT/VF identified. Many of the episodes are self-terminating. This observation helps explain why many patients present with syncope or wake up at night after episodes of agonal respiration or seizures caused by the arrhythmia. It is also possible (since some of these episodes occurred during sleep) that had they not been witnessed, the patients would have been considered asymptomatic, since they were asleep and did not experience the symptoms per se. One also must understand why some episodes self-terminate and why others are sustained and lead to cardiac arrest or even sudden death. Whether certain modulating factors such as drugs, hypokalemia, or sleep-related factors (sleep apnea?) make the episode sustained remains unclear.

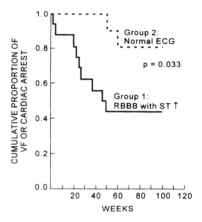

Figure 17. Kaplan-Meier curves showing the high mortality rate due to sudden death occurring in patients with SUDS and the pattern of right bundle branch block and ST elevation from V_1 to V_3 (group 1) as compared to resuscitated victims of almost sudden death with a normal ECG (group 2).

CONCLUSIONS

The syndrome of right bundle block, ST segment elevation from V_1 to V_3 and sudden death is a new entity. This disease is genetically determined and appears to be different from the long QT syndrome and arrhythmogenic right ventricular dysplasia. The genetic cause of this disorder is abnormalities of ion channels (i.e., an ion channelopathy) and is genetically heterogeneous. The incidence of sudden death in this syndrome is very high and, at present, sudden death can only be prevented by implanting a cardioverter-defibrillator. The ECG is a marker of sudden death in symptomatic, but also asymptomatic individuals. As new information on Brugada syndrome is reported, a better understanding of the mechanisms of disease will be gained. This understanding is likely to lead to paradigm shifts in our approach to ventricular arrhythmias and conduction system disease and pave the way for new therapies and reduction in sudden cardiac death.

REFERENCES

1. Myerburg RJ, Kessler KM, Castellanos A. Sudden cardiac death: structure, function and time-dependence of risk. Circulation 1992;85:1-10.
2. Myerburg RJ. Sudden cardiac death in persons with normal (or near normal) heart. Am J Cardiol 1997;79: 3-9.
3. Osher HL, Wolff L. Electrocardiographic pattern simulating acute myocardial injury. Am J Med Sci 1953;226:541-545.
4. Edeiken J. Elevation of RS-T segment, apparent or real in right precordial leads as probable normal variant. Am Heart J 1954;48:331-339.
5. Levine HD, Wanzer SH, Merrill JP. Dialyzable currents of injury in potassium intoxication resembling acute myocardial infarction or pericarditis. Circulation 1956;13:29-36.
6. Roesler H. An electrocardiographic study of high take-off of theR(R')-T segment in right precordial leads. Altered repolarization. Am J Cardiol 1960;6:920-928.
7. Calo AA. The triad secondary R wave, RS-T segment elevation and T waves inversion in right precordial leads: a normal electrocardiographic variant. G Ital Cardiol 1975;5:955-960.
8. Parisi AF, Beckmann CH, Lancaster MC. The spectrum of ST elevation in the electrocardiograms of healthy adult men. J Electrocardiol 1971;4:137-144
9. Wasserburger RH, Alt WJ, Lloyd CJ. The normal RS-T segment elevation variant. Am J Cardiol 1961;8:184-192.
10. Goldman MJ. RS-T segment elevation in mid- and left precordial leads as a normal variant. Am Heart J 1953;46:817-820.
11. Martini B, Nava A, Thiene G, et al. Ventricular fibrillation without apparent heart disease. Description of six cases. Am Heart J 1989;118:1203-1209.
12. Aihara N, Ohe T, Kamakura S, et al. Clinical and electrophysiologic characteristics of idiopathic ventricular fibrillation. Shinzo 1990;22 (Suppl. 2):80-86.
13. Brugada P, Brugada J. A distinct clinical and electrocardiographic syndrome: right bundle-branch block, persistent ST segment elevation with normal QT interval and sudden cardiac death. PACE 1991;14:746.
14. Brugada P, Brugada J. Right bundle-branch block, persistent ST segment elevation and sudden cardiac death: a distinct clinical and ECG syndrome. J Am Coll Cardiol 1992;20:1391-6 (abstr).
15. Sumita S, Yoshida K, Ishikawa T, et al. ST level in healthy subjects with right bundle branch block in relation to Brugada syndrome (abstr). Eur J Cardiac Pacing Electrophysiol 1996;6:270 (1076).
16. Nademanee K, Veerakul G, Nimmannit S, et al. Arrhythmogenic marker for the sudden unexplained death syndrome in Thai men. Circulation 1997;96:2595-2600.
17. Gotoh K. A histopathological study on the conduction system of the so-called Pokkuri disease (sudden unexpected cardiac death of unknown origin in Japan). Jpn Circ J 1976;40:753-768.
18. Hayashi M, Murata M, Satoh M, et al. Sudden nocturnal death in young males from ventricular flutter. Jpn Heart J 1985;26:585-591.
19. Tohyou Y, Nakazawa K, Ozawa A, et al. A survey in the incidence of right bundle branch block with ST segment elevation among normal population. Jpn J Electrocardiol 1995;15:223-226.
20. Namiki T, Ogura T, Kuwabara Y, et al. Five-year mortality and clinical characteristics of adult subjects with right bundle branch block and ST elevation. Circulation 1995;92:I-334(1591). (abstr).
21. Hata Y, Chiba N, Hotta K, et al. Incidence and clinical significance of right bundle branch block and ST segment elevation in V1-V3 in 6-18 year old school children in Japan. Circulation 1997;20:2310.
22. Antzelevitch C, Sicouri S, Lukas A, et al. Clinical implications of electrical heterogeneity in the heart: the electrophysiology and pharmacology of epicardial, M and endocardial cells. In:Podrid P, Kowey P, eds: Cardiac Arrhythmia: Mechanism, Diagnosis and Management. Baltimore: William & Wilkins, 1995:88-107.
23. Alings M, Wilde A. "Brugada" syndrome: clinical data and suggested pathophysiological mechanism. Circulation 1999, 99:666-673.
24. Grace AA. Brugada syndrome. Lancet 1999, 354:445-446.
25. Chen Q, Kirsch GE, Zhang D, et al. Genetic basis and molecular mechanism for idiopathic ventricular fibrillation. Nature 1998;392:293-296.
26. Gussak I, Antzelevitch C, Bjerregaard P, et al. The Brugada syndrome; clinical electrophysiological, and genetic considerations. J Am Coll Cardiol 1999;33:5-15.
27. Brugada J, Brugada P. Further characterization of the syndrome of right bundle branch block, ST segment elevation, and sudden death. J Cardiovasc Electrophysiology 1997;8:325-331.
28. Kobayashi T, Shintani U, Yamamoto T, et al. Familial occurrence of electrocardiographic abnormalities of the Brugada-type. Inter Med 1996;35:637-40.

29. Kambara H, Phillips J. Long-term evaluation of early repolarization syndrome (normal variant RS-T segment elevation). Am J Cardiol 1976;38:157-161

30. Priori SG, Diehl L, Schwartz PJ. Torsades de pointes. In: Podrid PJ, Kowey PR (eds.). Cardiac Arrhythmia. Baltimore, MD, Williams & Wilkins, 1995, 951-963.

31. Antzelevitch C. Ion channels and ventricular arrhythmias: cellular and ionic mechanisms underlying the Brugada syndrome. Curr Opin Cardiol 1999, 14:274-9.

32. Miyazaki T, Mitamura H, Miyoshi S, et al. Autonomic and antiarrhythmic modulation of ST segment elevation in patients with Brugada syndrome. J Am Coll Cardiol 1996;27:1061-1070.

33. Antzelevitch C., The Brugada syndrome. J Cardiovasc Electrophysiol 1998;9:513-6.

34. Fujiki A, Usui M, Anagasawa H, Mizumaki K, et al. ST segment elevation in the right precordial leads induced with class IC antiarrhythmic drugs: insight into the mechanism of Brugada syndrome. J Cardiovasc Electrophysiol 1999, 10:214-218.

35. Yan G-X, Antzelevitch C. Cellular basis for the Brugada syndrome and other mechanisms or arrhythmogenesis associated with ST-segment elevation. Circulation 1999, 100:1660-1666.

36. Brugada J, Brugada R, Brugada P. Right bundle branch block and ST segment elevation in V1-V3: A marker for sudden death in patients with no demonstrable structural heart disease. Circulation 1998;97:457-460.

37. Brugada P, Green M, Abdollah H, et al. Significance of ventricular arrhythmias initiated by programmed ventricular stimulation: Importance of the type of ventricular arrhythmia induced and the number of premature stimuli required. Circulation 1984;69:87-92.

38. Corrado D, Basso C, Nava A, et al. Pathological substrates of right bundle branch block, persistent precordial ST segment elevation and sudden death in young people. Circulation 1996;94:I-627.

39. Corrado D, Nava A, Buja G, et al. Familial cardiomyopathy underlies syndrome of right bundle branch block, ST segment elevation and sudden death. J Am Coll Cardiol 1996;27:443-8.

40. Burke AP, Farb A, Tashko G, Virmani R. Arrhythmogenic right ventricular cardiomyopathy and fatty replacement of the right ventricular myocardium: are they different diseases? Circulation 1998; 97:1571-1580.

41. Yan GX, Antzelevitch C. Cellular basis for the electrocardiographic J wave. Circulation 1996;93: 372-379.

42. Lukas A, Antzelevitch C. Differences in the electrophysiological response of canine ventricular epicardium and endocardium to ischemia: Role of the transient outward current. Circulation 1993;88:2903-2915.

43. Lukas A, Antzelevitch C. Phase 2 reentry as a mechanism of initiation of circus movement reentry in canine epicardium exposed to simulated ischemia. Cardiovasc Res 1996;32:593-603.

44. Lukas A, Antzelevitch C. The contribution of K^+ currents to electrical heterogeneity across the canine ventricular wall under normal and ischemic conditions. InDhalla NS, Pierce GN, Panagia V, ed. Pathophysiology of Heart Failure. Boston, Academic Publishers, 1996, pp 440-456.

45. Sun ZQ, Antzelevitch C. Ionic basis for the electrocardiographic J wave. Circulation 1996;94:I-669.

46. Suzuki J, Tsubone H, Sugano S. Characteristics of ventricular activation and recovery patterns in the rat. J Vet Med Sci 1992;54:711-6.

47. Di Diego JM, Antzelevitch C. High (Ca^{2+})-induced electrical heterogeneity and extrasystolic activity in isolated canine ventricular epicardium: Phase 2 reentry. Circulation 1994;89:1839-1850.

48. Di Diego JM, Antzelevitch C. Pinacidil-induced electrical heterogeneity and extrasystolic activity in canine ventricular tissues: does activation of ATP-regulated potassium current promote phase 2 reentry? Circulation 1993;88:1177-1189.

49. Langer GA, Brady AJ, Tan ST, et al. Correlation of the glucoside response, the force staircase, and the action potential configuration in the neonatal rat heart. Circ Res 1975;36:744-752.

50. Litovsky SH, Antzelevitch C. Transient outward current prominent in canine ventricular epicardium but not endocardium. Circ Res 1988;62:116-126.

51. Liu DW, Gintant GA, Antzelevitch C. Ionic bases for electrophysiological distinctions among epicardial, midmyocardial, and endocardial myocytes from the free wall of the canine left ventricle. Circ Res 1993;72:671-687.

52. Furukawa T, Myerburg RJ, Furukawa N, et al. Differences in transient outward current of feline endocardial and epicardial myocytes. Circ Res 1990;67:1287-1291.

53. Fedida D, Giles WR. Regional variations in action potentials and transient outward current in myocytes isolated from rabbit left ventricle. J Physiol 1991;442:191-209.

54. Clark RB, Bouchard RA, Salinas-Stefanon E, Sanchez-Chapula J, Giles WR. Heterogeneity of action potential waveforms and potassium currents in rat ventricle. Cardiovasc Res 1993;27:1795-9.

55. Wettwer E, Amos GJ, Psoival H, et al. Transient outward current in human ventricular myocytes of subepicaridal and subendocardial origin. Circ Res 1994;75:473-482.

56.   Nabauer M, Beuckelmann DJ, Uberfuhr P, et al. Regional differences in current density and rate-dependent properties of the transient outward current insubepicardial and subendocardial myocytes of human left ventricle. Circulation 1996;93:168-177.
57.   Antzelevitch C, Yan GX, Shimizu W, et al. Electrical heterogeneity, the ECG, and cardiac arrhythmias. In Zipes DP, Jalife J (eds). Cardiac Electrophysiology: From Cell to Bedside. Philadelphia, PA, W.B. Saunders Co., 1995, 1-34.
58.   Antzelevitch C., Sicouri S, Lukas A, et al. Regional differences in the electrophysiology of ventricular cells: Physiological and clinical implications. In Zipes DP, Jalife J (eds). Cardiac Electrophysiology: From Cell to Bedside. Philadelphia, PA, W.B. Saunders Co., 1995, 288-245.
59.   Antzelevitch C, Sicouri S, Litovsky SH, et al. Heterogeneity within the ventricular wall: Electrophysiology and pharmacology of epicardial, endocardial, and M cells. Circ Res 1991;69:1427-1449.
60.   Jeck CD, Boyden PA. Age-related appearance of outward currents may contribute to developmental differences in ventricular repolarization. Circ Res 1992;71:1390-1403.
61.   Antzelevitch C, Shimizu W, Yan G-X, et al.. The M cell: its contribution to the ECG and to normal and abnormal electrical function of the heart. J Cardiovasc Electrophysiol 1999, 10:1124-1152.
62.   Pacioretty LM, Gilmour RF. Developmental changes in the transient outward potassium current in canine epicardium. Am J Physiol 1995;268:H2513-H2521.
63.   Escande D, Loisance D, Planche C, et al. Age-related changes of action potential plateau shape in isolated human atrial fibers. Am J Physiol 1985;249:H843-H850.
64.   Reder RF, Miura DS, Danilo P, et al. The electrophysiological properties of normal neonatal and adult canine cardiac Purkinje fibers. Circ Res 1981;48:658-668.
65.   Kilborn MJ, Fedida D. A study of the developmental changes in outward current of rat ventricular myocytes. J Physiol (Lond) 1990;430:37-60.
66.   Zygmunt AC. Intracellular calcium activates chloride current in canine ventricular myocytes. Am J Physiol 1994;267:H1984-H1995.
67.   Krishnan SC, Antzelevitch C. Flecainide-induced arrhythmia in canine ventricular epicardium: Phase 2 reentry? Circulation 1993;87:562-572.
68.   Litovsky SH, Antzelevitch C. Differences in the electrophysiological response of canine ventricular subendocardium and subepicardium to acetylcholine and isoproterenol. A direct effect of acetylcholine in ventricular myocardium. Circ Res 1990;67:615-627.
69.   Krishnan SC, Antzelevitch C. Sodium channel blockade produces opposite electrophysiologic effects in canine ventricular epicardium and endocardium. Circ Res 1991;69:277-291.
70.   Di Diego JM, Sun ZQ, Antzelevitch C. I_{to} and action potential notch are smaller in left vs. right canine ventricular epicardium. Am J Physiol 1996;271-H548-561.
71.   Di Diego JM, Antzelevitch C. I_{Ca} inhibition and I_{K-ATP} activation induce a transmural dispersion of repolarization resulting in ST segment elevation and arrhythmias. PACE 1997;20:1134 (abst).
72.   Sicouri S., Moro S, Litovsky SH, et al. Chronic amiodarone reduces transmural dispersion of repolarization in the canine heart. J Cardiovasc Electrophysiol 1997;8:1269-1279.
73.   Antzelevitch C, Nesterenko VV, Yan GX. Ionic processes underlying the action potential. In: Liebman J (ed). Electrocardiology '96: from the Cell to the Body Surface. Singapore, World Scientific Publishing Co. Pte. Ltd., 1996, pp 216-229.
74.   Antzelevitch C. Repolarizing currents in ventricular myocardium: Regional differences and similarities. In Vereecke J, van Boagaert P-p, Verdonck F (eds). Potassium Channels in Normal and Pathological Conditions. Belgium, Leuven University Press, 1995, pp 256-259.
75.   Antzelevitch C, Di Diego J, Sicouri S, et al. Selective pharmacological modification ofrepolarizing currents: Antiarrhythmic and proarrhythmic actions of agents that influence repolarization in the heart. In Breithardt G, ed. Antiarrhythmic Drugs. Berlin, Springer-Verlag, 1995, 57-80.
76.   Liu DW, Antzelevitch C. Characteristics of the delayed rectifier current (I_{Kr} and I_{Ks}) in canine ventricular epicardial, midmyocardial and endocardial myocytes: weaker I_{Ks} contributes to longer action potential of the M cell. Circ Res 1995;76:351-365.
77.   Antzelevitch C, Di Diego JM. The role of K^+ channel activators in cardiac electrophysiology and arrhythmias. Circulation 1992;85:1627-1629.
78.   Antzelevitch C, Litovsky SH, Lukas A. Epicardium vs. endocardium: electrophysiology and pharmacology. In Zipes DP, Jalife J, eds. Cardiac Electrophysiology: from Cell to Bedside. Philadelphia, WB Saunders 1990, 386-95.
79.   Matsuo K, Shimizu W, Kurita T, et al. Dynamic changes of 12-lead electrocardiograms in a patient with Brugada syndrome. J Cardiovasc Electrophysiol 1998;9:508-512.
80.   Towbin JA, Vatta M, Wang Z, Bowles NE, Li H. Emerging targets in the long QT syndromes and Brugada syndrome. Emerg Therap Targets 1999;3:423-437.

81. Kasanuki H, Ohnishi S, Ohtuka M, et al. Idiopathic ventricular fibrillation induced with vagal activity in patients without obvious heart disease. Circulation 1997;95:2277-2285.
82. Proclemer A, Facchin D, Feduglio GA, et al. Fibrilazione ventricolare recidivante, blocco di branca destra, persistent sopraslivellamento del tratto ST in V1-V3? G Ital Cardiol 1993;23:1211-1218
83. Kobayashi H, Ohonish O, Momose M, et al. Characteristic findings of I-123 MIBGscintigraphy in patients with Brugada syndrome. Circulation 1997;96:152.
84. Matsuo K, Shimizzu W, Kurita T, et al. Increased dispersion of repolarization time determined by monophasic action potentials in familial ventricular fibrillation. J Cardio Electrophys 1998;9:74-83.
85. Viskin S, Lesh MD, Eldar M, et al. Mode of onset of malignant ventricular arrhythmias in idiopathic ventricular fibrillation. J Cardiovasc Electrophysiol 1997;8:1115-1120.
86. Pertzov AM, Davidenko JM, Salomonsz R, et al. Spiral waves of excitation underlie reentrant activity in isolated cardiac muscle. Circ Res 1993;72:631-650.
87. Asano Y, Davidenko JM, Baxter WT, et al. Optical mapping of drug-induced polymorphic arrhythmias and torsades de pointes in the isolated rabbit heart. J Am Coll Cardiol 1997;29:831-842.
88. Imaizumi Y, Giles WR. Quinidine-induced inhibition of transient outward current in cardiac muscle. Am J Physiol 1987;253:H704-H708.
89. Virag L, Varro A, Papp C. Effect of disopyramide on potassium currents in rabbit ventricular myocytes. Naunyn Schmiedebergs Arch Pharmacol 1998;357:268-275.
90. Yatani A, Wakamori M, Mikala G, et al. Block of transient outward-type cloned cardiac K^+ channel currents by quinidine. Circ Res 1993;73:351-359.
91. Belhassen B, Shapira I, Shoshani D, et al. Idiopathic ventricular fibrillation: inducibility and beneficial effects of Class I antiarrhythmic agents. Circulation 1987;75:809-816.
92. Li GR, Feng J, Yue L, et al. Transmural heterogeneity of action potential and I_{to1} in myocytes isolated from the human right ventricle. Am J Physiol 1998;275:H369-77.
93. Borgers M, Ausma J. Structural aspects of the chronic hibernating myocardium in man. BasicRes Cardiol 1995;90:44-46.
94. Ausma J, Wijffels M, van Eys G, et al. Dedifferentiation of atrial cardiomyocytes as a result of chronic atrial fibrillation. Am J Pathol 1997;151:985-997.
95. Ausma J, Wijffels M, Thone F, et al. Structural changes of atrial myocardium due to sustained atrial fibrillation in the goat. Circulation 1997;96:3157-3163.
96. Chiale PA, Przybylski J, Laino RA, et al. Electrocardiographic changes without manifest myocarditis. Am J Cardiol 1982;49:14-20.
97. Naccarella F. Malignant ventricular arrhythmias in patients with a right bundle-branch block and persistent ST segment elevation in V1-V3 (Editorial). G Ital Cardiol 1993;23:1219-1222.
98. Fontaine G. Familial cardiomyopathy associated with right bundle branch block, ST segment elevation and sudden death (Letter). J Am Coll Cardiol 1996;28:540.
99. Scheinman MM. Is Brugada syndrome a distinct clinical entity? J Cardio Electrophys 1997;8:332-6.
100. Ohe T. Idiopathic ventricular fibrillation of the Brugada type - an atypical form of arrhythmogenic right ventricular cardiomyopathy (Editorial). Intern Med 1996;35:595.
101. Fontaine G, Piot O, Sohal P, et al. Right precordial leads and sudden death. Relation with arrhythmogenic right ventricular dysplasia. Arch Mal Coeur Vaiss 1996;89:1323-9.
102. Morace G, Padeletti L, Porciani MC, et al. Effect of isoproterenol on the early repolarization syndrome. Am Heart J 1979;97:343-347.
103. Lehmann KG, Shandling AH, Yusi AU, et al. Altered ventricular repolarization in central sympathetic dysfunction associated with spinal cord injury. Am J Cardiol 1989;63:1498-1504.
104. Eidelberg EE. Cardiovascular response to spinal cord compression. J Neurosurg 1973;38:326-331.
105. Evans DE, Kobrine AI, Rissoli HV. Cardiac arrhythmias accompanying acute compression of the spinal cord. J Neurosurg 1980;52:52-59.
106. Wang Q, Shen J, Splawski I, et al. SCN5A mutations associated with an inherited cardiac arrhythmia, long QT syndrome. Cell 1995;80:805-811.
107. Bennett PB, Yazawa K, Makita N, et al. Molecular mechanism for an inherited cardiac arrhythmia. Nature 1995;376:683-685.
108. Dumaine R, Wang Q, Keating MT, et al. Multiple mechanisms of sodium channel-linked long QT syndrome. Circ Res 1996;78:916-924.
109. Rampazzo A, Nava A, Danieli GA, et. al. The gene for arrhythmogenic right ventricular cardiomyopathy maps to chromosome 14q23-q24. Hum Mol Genet 1994;3:959-962.
110. Rampazzo A, Nava A, Erne P, et al. A new locus for arrhythmogenic right ventricular cardiomyopathy (ARVD2) maps to chromosome 1q42-q43. Hum Mol Genet 1995;4:2151-2154.
111. Severini GM, Krajinovic M, Pinamonti B, et al. A new locus for arrhythmogenic right ventricular dysplasia on the long arm of chromosome 14. Genomics 1996;31:193-200.

112. Rampazzo A, Nava A, Miorin M, et al. ARVD4, a new locus for arrhythmogenic right ventricular cardiomyopathy, maps to chromosome 2 long arm. Genomics 1997;15:45:259-263.

113. Coonar AS, Protonotarios N, Tsatsopoulou A, et al. Gene for arrhythmogenic right ventricular cardiomyopathy with diffuse nonepidermolytic palmoplantar keratoderma and woolly hair (Naxos disease) maps to 17q21. Circulation 1998;97:2049-2058.

114. Ahmed F, Li D, Karibe A, et al. Localization of a gene responsible for arrhythmogenic right ventricular dysplasia to chromosome 3p23. Circulation 1998;98:2791-2795.

115. Dumaine R, Towbin JA, Brugada P, et al. Ionic mechanisms responsible for the electrocardiographic phenotype of the Brugada syndrome are temperature dependent. Cir Res 1999; In Press.

116. Schott J-J, Alshinawi C, Kyndt F, et al. Cardiac conduction defects associate with mutations in SCN5A. Nat Genet 1999;23:20-21.

117. Wang Q, Li Z, Shen J, et al. Genomic organization of the human SCN5A gene encoding the cardiac sodium channel. Genomics 1996;34:9-16.

118. Wang DW, Yazawa K, George AL Jr, et al. Characterization of human cardiac Na^+ channel mutations in the congenital long QT syndrome. Proc Natl Acad Sci USA 1996; 93:13200-13205.

119. Geisterfer-Lowrance AAT, Kass A, Tanigawa G, et al. A molecular basis for familial hypertrophic cardiomyopathy: A β-cardiac myosin heavy chain gene missense mutation. Cell 1990;62:999-1006.

120. Thierfelder L, Watkins H, MacRae C, et al. α-tropomyosin and cardiac troponin T mutations cause familial hypertrophic cardiomyopathy: A disease of the sarcomere. Cell 1994:77:701-712.

121. Bonne G, Carrier L, Bercovici J, et al. Cardiac myosin binding protein-C gene splice acceptor site mutation is associated with familial hypertrophic cardiomyopathy. Nat Genet 1995;11:438-440.

122. Watkins H, Conner D, Thierfelder L, et al. Mutations in the cardiac myosin binding protein-C gene on chromosome 11 cause familial hypertrophic cardiomyopathy. Nat Genet 1995;11:434-437.

123. Poetter K, Jiang H, Hassanzadeh S, et al. Mutations in either the essential or regulatory light chains are associated with a rare myopathy in human heart and skeletal muscle. Nat Genet 1996;13:63-69.

124. Kimura A, Harada H, Park JE, et al. Mutations in the cardiac troponin I gene associated with hypertrophic cardiomyopathy. Nat Genet 1997;16:379-382.

125. Mogensen J, Klausen IC, Pedersen AK, et al. Cardiac actin is a novel disease gene in familial hypertrophic cardiomyopathy. J Clin Invest 1999;103:R39-R43.

126. Watkins H, Rosenzweig A, Hwang DS, et al. Characteristics and prognostic implications of myosin missense mutations in familial hypertrophic cardiomyopathy. N Engl J Med 1992;326:1108-1114.

127. Watkins H, McKenna WJ, Theirfelder L, et al. Mutations in the genes for cardiac troponin T and α-tropomyosin in hypertrophic cardiomyopathy. N Engl J Med 1995; 332:1058-1064.

128. Towbin JA. The role of cytoskeletal proteins in cardiomyopathies. Curr Opin Biol 1998;10:131-139.

129. Towbin JA, Bowles KR, Bowles NE. Etiologies of cardiomyopathy and heart failure. Evidence for a common final pathway for disorders of the myocardium. Nature Med 1999;5:266-267.

130. Towbin JA, Roberts R. Cardiovascular Diseases Due to Genetic Abnormalities. In: "Hurst's The Heart." Alexander RW, Schlant RC, Fuster V, Eds. McGraw-Hill, Inc., 9th Ed, 1877-1924, 1998.

131. Towbin, JA. Toward an understanding of the cause of mitral valve prolapse. Am J Hum Genet 1999;65:1238-1241.

12
FAMILIAL HYPERTROPHIC CARDIOMYOPATHY GENETICS

Laura M. Bevilacqua, M.D. and Charles I. Berul, M.D.
Department of Cardiology, Children's Hospital • Boston,
Department of Pediatrics, Harvard Medical School, Boston, MA 02115

INTRODUCTION

The familial form of hypertrophic cardiomyopathy (HCM) is an inherited myocardial disease characterized by ventricular hypertrophy and an increased risk of ventricular arrhythmias and sudden death. Recent advances in molecular genetics have allowed the identification of multiple genes responsible for familial HCM. Pathologic examination reveals myocyte hypertrophy with myofibrillar disarray and intercellular fibrosis. This form of inherited cardiomyopathy encompasses a broad range of clinical phenotypes.

PREVALENCE

Maron and colleagues reported the prevalence of HCM based on data obtained from the CARDIA study (Coronary Artery Risk Development in (Young) Athletes) (1). Echocardiograms from young adults ranging in age from 23-35 years selected from the general population were analyzed for HCM. The overall prevalence was 2 cases of HCM per 1000 people (i.e. 0.2%). Subgroup analysis established a prevalence of 0.26% in men, and 0.09% in women. The disease was somewhat more prevalent in Blacks compared to Whites (0.24% vs. 0.10%). As cited by the authors, limitations of the study include the difficulty in finding a truly representative sample. Also, a population of young adults was chosen as the study group; this would overlook those patients who present at an early age with cardiac symptoms or sudden death due to a severe form of the disease, or potentially overestimate disease prevalence in other age groups. The fact that echocardiographic criteria alone were used in the analysis may fail to acknowledge those with milder disease. Overall, however, this estimate is similar to that of other epidemiological studies reporting the prevalence of HCM to be 0.02-0.5% (1,2).

PATHOPHYSIOLOGY

The etiology of the hypertrophy in HCM is postulated to be a compensatory reaction of the myocardium to a hypocontractile sarcomere unit (3,4). In the early phases of the disease, this hypertrophy results in low wall tension and hyperdynamic systolic function. Myocardial ischemia results from increased myocardial oxygen demand, small vessel disease, and coronary wall thickening, with consequent LV remodeling. Histologically there is myocardial fibrosis, necrosis, and disarray. Progressive LV diastolic dysfunction may ensue and cause signs and symptoms of end stage heart failure (3). At the cellular level, hypertrophic myocytes with hyperchromatic, bizarre nuclei are found. Abnormal intercellular connections, with myocytes malaligned in relation to one another, contribute to myocardial hypertrophy and scarring (5-8).

GENETICS/MOLECULAR BIOLOGY

Hypertrophic cardiomyopathy is a heterogeneous disease within and among families. The mode of inheritance is autosomal dominant with variable penetrance. Advances in molecular genetics, such as genetic linkage analysis, have permitted the identification of disease-related genes in the inherited cardiomyopathies. Several single point mutations are implicated in HCM. To date, at least nine genes have been identified (6, 9, 10). All have in common the fact that they encode for sarcomeric structural proteins of cardiac myocytes (Figure 1). Multiple mutations of each gene have been found. It is likely that several more will be identified since those that are known account for only a portion of affected families. *De novo* rather than inherited mutations also account for a significant number of cases (6,11).

The sarcomere consists of multiple proteins with complex protein-protein interactions. Cardiac myosin is the main component that powers the sarcomere. It is an asymmetric molecule consisting of 2 heavy chains and 2 pairs of light chains. Troponin and tropomyosin proteins regulate contraction of the muscle unit (4). The genes affected in HCM encode for the beta-myosin heavy chain, cardiac troponin T, cardiac troponin I, myosin binding protein C, myosin light chain, actin, and titin (6,9,10). Most of the mutations causing HCM are missense mutations or small deletions that lead to the production of stable mutant proteins that become incorporated in the sarcomere, producing a hypofunctional muscle unit.

The beta-myosin heavy chain (beta-MHC) protein is the principal isoform expressed in the adult human ventricular myocardium (4), and is encoded for by a gene located on chromosome 14q11.2-q13 (3). Greater than 70 mutations in various functional domains of the β-MHC gene are associated with HCM (3,6), accounting for as many as 30-40% of all cases (5,12). Different mutations are thought to confer different prognoses (6,11). For instance, analysis of families harboring the Arg403Gln mutation has shown that this defect is associated with high disease penetrance, early age at disease onset, and a particularly high incidence of sudden cardiac death (3,13,14). Similarly, the Arg719Trp and Arg453Cys mutations are linked with a poor prognosis (13). Anan, et al speculated that the malignant β-MHC mutations result in conformational changes in the myosin molecule, which may influence ATP binding and myosin's critical interactions with actin, thereby significantly altering muscle function (13). This may explain why the Arg403Gln mutation, located at the myosin-actin interface (3), heralds a poor prognosis.

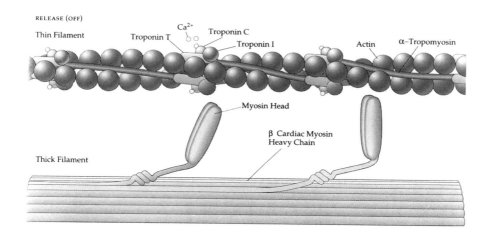

Figure 1. *The structure of the sarcomere.* Known mutations associated with familial hypertrophic cardiomyopathy occur in genes encoding the beta-myosin heavy chain, Troponin T, Troponin I, myosin binding protein C, and myosin light chains. Modified from Seidman and Seidman (15), with permission.

Other mutations in the beta-MHC gene portend a relatively benign prognosis. The Phe513Val (11), Val606Met (6,12,13), and Leu908Val (13) substitutions are three such mutations and are associated with low disease penetrance, a low incidence of sudden death, and a near-normal life expectancy (6,12,13). Anan, et al have suggested that the difference in the phenotypic severity between mutations may be accounted for in part by whether or not charge is conserved by a particular amino acid substitution (13). The malignant mutations described above are all associated with a change in charge, while the known benign mutations are not. The region of the beta-myosin heavy chain affected by the mutation may also influence the phenotype. For instance, the few defects associated with a good prognosis affect the head-rod region of the myosin protein, while none of the malignant defects have been localized to this area (13).

Mutations in the cardiac troponin T (cTnT) gene on chromosome 1q32 (3) account for 15-20% of HCM cases (6) and are associated with early mortality, despite the fact that usually only mild myocardial hypertrophy is seen (3,11). The fact that the degree of ventricular hypertrophy has not been shown to correlate with disease severity (3,4) may indicate that there are other genetic or environmental factors that modify myocardial hypertrophy. Even within families harboring the same mutation, however, there is significant phenotypic heterogeneity (3,6). Known cTnT defects include missense and deletion mutations, all of which share the characteristics of having low disease penetrance, mild myocardial hypertrophy, and a high incidence of sudden death (3,6), particularly in male patients (6).

Many deletions in the gene encoding myosin binding protein C have been described. Defects in this gene account for 10-15% of HCM. Low disease penetrance, mild cardiac hypertrophy, and a low incidence of sudden cardiac death characterize known mutations in this protein (6). The same characteristics pertain to the Asp175Asn mutation in the alpha-tropomyosin gene, located on chromosome 15q2. Alpha-tropomyosin defects (chromosome 15q22) (3) are responsible for fewer than 5% of HCM cases (6). Two other mutations in this gene, Ala63Val and Lys70Thr, result in mild LV hypertrophy, but a high incidence of sudden death (3).

Less commonly, HCM-causing mutations occur in the genes encoding cardiac troponin I or one of the two myosin light chain proteins. Located on chromosomes 3p and 12q respectively, defects in myosin light chains 1 and 2 result in mid-cavitary LV obstruction. As with cardiac troponin I mutations on chromosome 19p13, little is known about their associated risk of sudden death (3,6).

Two additional sarcomeric protein mutations have recently been reported. A specific mutation in the gene encoding titin was recently identified as being associated with hypertrophic cardiomyopathy (9). This mutation, in which there is an arginine to leucine substitution, reportedly changes the binding affinity of titin to alpha-actinin.

Mutations in the alpha cardiac actin gene have also been implicated in HCM (10). Interestingly, mutations in actin also lead to familial dilated cardiomyopathy (see Chapter 13). This appears to be the first identified gene mutation to be involved with two distinct forms of inherited cardiomyopathies. The investigation of genotype-phenotype correlations should further the ability to risk-stratify patients and identify those families at increased risk of sudden cardiac death.

Table 1. Genetic heterogeneity in familial hypertrophic cardiomyopathy. *Modified from* Fananapazir (3), with permission.

Table 1. Genetic Heterogeneity in Hypertrophic Cardiomyopathy (HCM)

Gene [Chromosome Location]	No. of Mutations	Examples of Studied Mutations	
		Mutation (Site in the Molecule)	Clinical Correlates*
Cardiac troponin-T (*TNNT2*) [1q32]	11	...	Low penetrance, mild phenotype but poor prognosis
Essential light chain (*MYL3*) [3p21.2-p21.3]	2	Met149Val	Midcavity HCM, high penetrance, poor prognosis
		Arg154His	Midcavity HCM
Myosin binding protein-C (*MYBPC3*) [11p11.2]	21	Most mutations result in truncated proteins	Low penetrance, mild phenotype, delayed age of onset of symptoms, favorable prognosis
Regulatory light chain (*MYL2*) [12q23-q24.3]	4	Glu22Ly	Mid cavity HCM
β-Myosin heavy chain (*MYH7*) [14q11.2-q13]	>50	Thr124Ile (nucleotide binding pocket)	
		Tyr162Cys (nucleotide binding pocket)	
		Phe244Leu (nucleotide binding pocket)	
		Arg249Gln	Poor prognosis
		Gly256Glu (outer end of the ATP pocket)	Low penetrance, favorable prognosis
		Arg403Gln (myosin-actin interface)	High penetrance, poor prognosis
		Arg453Cys (outer end of the ATP pocket)	Poor prognosis
		Val606Met (50-kd crossover)	High penetrance, poor prognosis in most families
		Arg719Trp (ELC binding site)	High penetrance, moderate prognosis
		Arg663His (moysin-actin interface)	
		Gly716Arg	Poor prognosis
		Arg719Gln (ELC binding interface)	Poor prognosis
		Arg741Gln (ELC binding interface)	
		Lys847Glu (in the rod)	Favorable prognosis
		Arg870His (in the rod)	High penetrance, favorable prognosis
		Leu908Val (in the rod)	Low penetrance, mid-cavity HCM, favorable prognosis
α-Tropomyosin (*TPM1*) [15q22]	4	Asp175Asn	Variable phenotype, favorable prognosis
		Glu180Gly	Mild LV hypertrophy, unclear prognosis
		Ala63Val	Mild LV hypertrophy, heart failure, poor prognosis
		Lys70Thr	Mild LV hypertrophy, heart failure, poor prognosis
Cardiac troponin-I (*TNNI3*) [19p13.2-q13.2]	6	...	...

*LV indicates left ventricular; ellipses, information unavailable.

MOUSE MODEL OF FAMILIAL HYPERTROPHIC CARDIOMYOPATHY

Genetically-manipulated mice have been engineered to express the hypertrophic cardiomyopathy phenotype. The first well-described mouse model of familial hypertrophic cardiomyopathy had an α-myosin heavy chain missense mutation, with a phenotype similar to humans (16,17). The homozygous mutation (α-MHC$^{403/403}$) is uniformly fatal in mice within the first week of life, while the heterozygote mice (α-MHC$^{403/+}$) survive but demonstrate histological and hemodynamic abnormalities characteristic of the human familial HCM phenotype (18). For example, affected mice have experienced sudden death during exercise testing in contrast to their wild-type counterparts (19).

Histologic exam has documented clear gender differences in mice with HCM, with male mice displaying more severe myocyte hypertrophy, cellular disarray, and interstitial fibrosis than their female littermates (18). Gender-specific differences in EP parameters also exist as elucidated by in vivo mouse EP studies, including a higher incidence of sinus node dysfunction, right axis deviation (18), prolonged repolarization, and inducible ventricular tachycardia in male heterozygotes compared to their female counterparts (18,20). These findings are strikingly similar to EP characteristics seen in humans with HCM. Heterogeneity of ventricular repolarization was demonstrated in mutant HCM mice, as in humans with this disease. In contrast to human studies, however, QT dispersion in this murine model did not correlate with arrhythmia inducibility (20). Murine models of HCM also include mutations in other sarcomeric proteins, and phenotypic characterization is currently in progress.

CLINICAL SYMPTOMS

Symptoms in HCM range in severity from nonexistent to severe, including exertional dyspnea, orthopnea, fatigue, angina, and syncope. Congestive symptoms occur in the context of LVOT obstruction, which may be present at baseline or with provocation (e.g. during exercise), or secondary to myocardial ischemia from diastolic dysfunction and impaired coronary perfusion (21). Atrial tachyarrhythmias such as atrial fibrillation may elicit or exacerbate congestive symptoms. No relation between the extent of LV hypertrophy by echocardiography and the degree of symptomatology has been shown. An inverse relationship between age and the degree of LVH has been reported (22).

ELECTROCARDIOGRAPHY

Typical ECG findings include LVH, ST segment abnormalities and T wave inversions. Abnormal Q waves, such as those seen in myocardial infarction, and evidence of atrial enlargement may be present. The ECG may show LVH in the absence of echocardiographic evidence of hypertrophy (7,21,23). The ECG may also be completely normal. Unfortunately, no reliable electrocardiographic marker of increased risk for sudden death has been identified. Patients with certain gene defects causing HCM are more likely to exhibit ECG abnormalities, making this an effective screening tool in some families. While dispersion of refractoriness has been reported by some investigators to correlate with the incidence of ventricular arrhythmias (24), its utility as an effective screening tool has not been established.

ECHOCARDIOGRAPHY

HCM is the most common hereditary structural cardiac disease. The echocardiographic diagnosis of HCM is made when there is a thickened, non-dilated left ventricle without associated disease known to cause left ventricular hypertrophy, such as systemic hypertension or valvular heart disease. In adults, the LV wall thickness equals or exceeds 15mm and may exceed 50mm (22,24). The hypertrophy is usually asymmetric, primarily involving the ventricular septum (7); the right ventricle is variably involved. Significant heterogeneity exists among affected patients.

Hemodynamically, patients may be classified into those with left ventricular outflow tract obstruction and those without. Approximately 25% of HCM patients have some degree of dynamic left ventricular outflow tract obstruction, caused by hypertrophy of the ventricular septum and systolic anterior motion (SAM) of the mitral valve apparatus toward the septum (21,22,26,27). This apposition of the mitral valve and septum may be accompanied by mitral regurgitation secondary to abnormal leaflet coaptation (21,27). Primary structural abnormalities of the mitral valve also occur in association with HCM, including anomalous papillary muscle insertion into the anterior leaflet, leaflet elongation, and mitral valve prolapse (7,21,22). Left ventricular obstruction may be mid-cavitary rather than subaortic if the hypertrophy and obstruction occur at the level of the papillary muscles; this type of hypertrophy is not accompanied by SAM (7).

PACING

The use of dual-chamber pacing to treat symptomatic outflow obstruction in HCM is controversial. Some studies have shown symptomatic improvement, while others have shown unfavorable long-term hemodynamic consequences. The mechanism by which pacing diminishes subaortic obstruction is thought to involve the modification of the ventricular contraction sequence by right ventricular pre-excitation. By altering ventricular activation, the geometry of the LVOT is changed, reducing the obstruction to left ventricular outflow. In this way, systolic anterior motion of the mitral valve, and in turn, mitral regurgitation, may be reduced (28). This requires maintaining a programmed AV delay shorter than the patient's own PR interval, which may be difficult as autonomic tone changes, such as occurs with exercise. Beta-blockers or verapamil may be used in this situation to prolong the patient's intrinsic AV conduction. In some cases, AV nodal ablation has also been used to achieve ventricular pre-excitation with pacing (12).

Chronic benefits of dual chamber pacing have also been reported. By diminishing the outflow gradient with asynchronous ventricular contraction, the stimulus for hypertrophy may be lessened, thereby contributing to ventricular remodeling over time (29). Gadler, et al (30) and Fananapazir, et al (29,31) reported a decrease in LVOT gradient acutely during atrial synchronous ventricular pacing with a short AV delay, and a further decrease in the gradient after long-term pacing therapy. In addition, a decrease in the gradient was noted when pacing was discontinued, suggesting a favorable long-term effect on LV remodeling.

Other investigators have found variable and unpredictable results with pacing, and attribute symptomatic improvement to a placebo effect (32-34). The mechanism of hemodynamic benefit with chronic pacing in HCM is unknown, as is the duration of pacing therapy needed to achieve long-term hemodynamic improvement. Based on available data, pacing therapy should be reserved for patients with severe drug-refractory symptoms, with careful analysis of the effects on each individual patient. It is important to remember that, while dual-chamber pacing may cause symptomatic and/or hemodynamic improvement, there is no evidence that it decreases the risk of sudden death in this disease.

ICD THERAPY

The decision to recommend an implantable cardioverter-defibrillator for patients with HCM and the timing of implantation are made difficult by the fact that sudden death often occurs in asymptomatic individuals. The effect of implantable defibrillators on mortality in HCM has not been systematically evaluated. ICD use has been advocated in patients with a history of cardiac arrest, inducible VT at EP study with or without a history of syncope, and a history of recurrent syncope secondary to myocardial ischemia (29). A potential unwanted side effect of ICD implantation may be inappropriate shocks due to atrial arrhythmias, which are relatively common in HCM patients. New programmable features or dual-chamber devices may allow prevention of this complication.

A low incidence of ICD shocks was reported by Primo and colleagues (35) in a group of patients assumed to be at high risk because of a history of resuscitated sudden death, recurrent syncope, or inducible ventricular arrhythmias. They concluded that ventricular arrhythmias may not be responsible for all cases of syncope or sudden death in HCM. In contrast, other investigators have reported a high incidence (32-57%) of appropriate shocks in HCM patients (36-38). Discrepant findings between investigators may represent differences in the study populations selected. Long-term follow-up of HCM patients who have undergone device implantation is needed before definitive conclusions can be drawn about its effect on mortality in this disease. In the meantime, ICD implantation appears to be a logical measure in those perceived to be at high risk.

ARRHYTHMIAS AND SUDDEN DEATH

The annual mortality rate from sudden death in adults with HCM is estimated at 2-3%. It has been estimated as high as 6% in children and adolescents (39,40). Sudden death may be the first manifestation of the disease, and is most likely attributable to ventricular arrhythmias. It is hypothesized that this may be either a primary arrhythmia, or secondary to ischemia, outflow tract obstruction, hypotension, or rapid conduction of a supraventricular arrhythmia. The finding of ventricular tachycardia during 24 hour ambulatory monitoring, whether sustained or nonsustained, is reported to be an indicator of high risk of sudden death in adults with HCM (41). Bradycardia and heart block also are commonly observed in HCM, and may be responsible for some adverse events.

It is difficult to identify what makes some individuals at particularly high risk for sudden death. In general there is agreement that patients who have survived an episode of ventricular fibrillation, have a history of sustained ventricular arrhythmia by noninvasive monitoring or EP study, or have a malignant family history are at high risk. Clearly specific mutations causing HCM are associated with a poor prognosis, as described above. The onset of symptomatic disease in childhood or adolescence may also portend a worse prognosis (12).

The finding of nonsustained ventricular tachycardia on ambulatory monitoring has been reported to be an indicator of increased sudden death risk in adults with HCM, supporting the notion that the mechanism of sudden death in adults is a primary arrhythmia. McKenna and colleagues (39) studied a group of children and adolescents in an attempt to correlate the incidence of VT and sudden death in a young population. They performed ambulatory ECG monitoring of 53 young patients, ranging from infancy to adolescence, over a period of at least two days. A low incidence of arrhythmias was seen in infants and children: eighteen percent of the adolescents had nonsustained ventricular tachycardia; seven study patients had sudden death events during a follow-up period of one week to seven years. Interestingly, none of the patients with sudden death events had prior evidence of arrhythmias by ambulatory monitoring. There was also no correlation between the degree of LVH and the incidence of arrhythmias. This study raises the question of whether the mechanism of sudden death in young HCM patients is perhaps acute hemodynamic derangement rather than a primary arrhythmia.

WPW in HCM

Patients with HCM have been shown to have both supraventricular and ventricular arrhythmias. Atrial fibrillation occurs in 15-25% of HCM patients, and may exacerbate congestive symptoms, cause embolic complications, and increase morbidity and mortality in this group of patients (42). Another significant supraventricular tachyarrhythmia is atrioventricular reciprocating tachycardia mediated by an accessory pathway in the Wolff-Parkinson-White syndrome. A short PR interval and a delta wave indicative of ventricular pre-excitation characterize the WPW pattern on surface ECG. WPW occurs in approximately 0.015-0.3% of the general population (43), and there are several reports suggesting that WPW is a familial disease. As in HCM, the mode of inheritance appears to be autosomal dominant with incomplete penetrance. MacRae and colleagues (43) studied a large family whose members are affected by WPW, HCM, or both. Using genetic linkage analysis, they found that the gene defect for WPW and HCM in this particular family was located on chromosome 7q3. This represents the first gene locus implicated in WPW and a previously unrecognized locus for familial HCM. Of note, ventricular pre-excitation may be mimicked by the short PR interval and broad QRS complex occasionally seen in HCM due to abnormal activation of the hypertrophied ventricular septum (36), so-called "pseudo-pre-excitation."

ATHLETES' HEART

Athletes may have physiologic left ventricular hypertrophy, which may overlap with the degree of LV wall thickness seen in HCM (7). This problem is concerning since HCM is the most common cause of sudden death in athletes (1,7,44). Other reported cardiac causes of sudden death in athletes include congenital coronary artery abnormalities, aortic stenosis, the long QT syndromes, Marfan syndrome, myocarditis, and dilated cardiomyopathy (25).

Generally, LVH in athletes is mild, allowing its distinction from pathologic hypertrophy. Occasionally a well-trained unaffected athlete may exhibit significant LVH, while an athlete with HCM may have only mild LVH. While there are no strict criteria for distinguishing athlete's heart from HCM, some findings may favor one diagnosis over the other. Deconditioning of the athlete should result in partial reversal of the hypertrophy. Other related factors need to be taken into account, including family history of HCM or sudden death, ECG abnormalities, associated left atrial enlargement, abnormal measures of LV diastolic function, and the level of cardiovascular conditioning of the patient (7). In addition, the pattern of ventricular hypertrophy in HCM tends to be more heterogeneous and asymmetric than in the normal athlete's heart. LV cavity dimension may be dilated in athlete's heart, but is often diminished in HCM. Electrocardiographic evidence of LVH may exist in either condition. Striking Q wave or T wave abnormalities usually support the diagnosis of HCM over athlete's heart.

Though difficult, the distinction is important due to the obvious implications of unnecessarily excluding a competitive athlete from sports participation, or allowing participation by an individual at significant risk. The abnormal echo finding of LVH should be followed into adulthood to avoid the underdiagnosis of HCM that may not reach detectable degrees of hypertrophy until after adolescence (25,44).

THERAPEUTIC OPTIONS

Pharmacological therapy is generally instituted with the onset of symptoms of congestive heart failure, such as fatigue or decreased exercise tolerance. Beta-blockers and verapamil are the most commonly used pharmacological agents used for symptomatic HCM because of their negative inotropic effect. Beta-blockers may also lead to bradycardia, thereby increasing diastolic filling time and reducing myocardial oxygen demand. The use of verapamil may not be advisable in HCM with subaortic obstruction because of the vasodilation it effects, but may decrease symptoms caused by myocardial ischemia in patients with severe diastolic dysfunction from abnormal coronary perfusion. Disopyramide is also used for its negative inotropy to reduce the outflow gradient, though some investigators report that initial symptomatic improvement may diminish over time (12). Beta-blockers may be needed in combination with Disopyramide since the latter enhances AV nodal conduction, causing detriment to patients prone to atrial fibrillation.

Diuretics are prescribed in patients who experience persistent congestive symptoms despite treatment with beta-blocker or verapamil. They should be used judiciously, however, since HCM patients with diastolic dysfunction require high filling pressures. While hemodynamic and symptomatic improvements may result from the use of negative inotropes, there is no evidence that beta-blocker or calcium channel-blocker therapy decreases the risk of sudden death in HCM (12).

While patients with HCM initially exhibit hyperdynamic ventricular function, myocardial performance may deteriorate over time to end-stage ventricular failure and refractory congestive heart failure symptoms. At this point, medical intervention should consist of more conventional CHF therapy, including digoxin, diuretics, and afterload reduction. Patients with severe outflow tract obstruction may be considered for interventions such as pacing or surgical myotomy-myectomy (see below). For patients without obstruction, cardiac transplantation may provide the only effective therapy (12).

Patients with LVOT obstruction represent a minority of HCM patients (approximately 25%). In such patients who fail pharmacological therapy, surgical therapy may be considered. The Morrow procedure, or ventricular septal myotomy-myectomy, involves the resection of muscle from the ventricular septum in an attempt to decrease the outflow tract gradient and decrease LV pressure (26). Surgery should be reserved for those with symptomatic, severe LVOT obstruction refractory to medical therapy. Mitral valve replacement has been performed in place of septal muscle resection in patients with severe mitral regurgitation due to primary mitral valve abnormalities. This includes patients with mid-cavitary obstruction secondary to anomalous papillary muscle insertion into the anterior mitral leaflet. Mitral valvuloplasty has also been performed in addition to myotomy-myectomy for patients with mitral leaflet abnormalities in addition to subaortic obstruction. Operative mortality from this procedure at experienced centers is less than 2%. Reduction of the outflow tract gradient occurs in >90% of cases, with long-term symptomatic improvement in approximately 70% (12).

Percutaneous septal ablation has been performed in some centers as an alternative to surgical myotomy-myectomy. Using intracoronary catheters, ethanol is selectively infused into septal branches of the left coronary artery with the aim of infarcting hypertrophied myocardial tissue, thereby thinning LVOT myocardium in HCM with subaortic obstruction (3,29). While preliminary results of outflow gradient reduction are encouraging, there may be significant morbidity associated with the procedure, such as conduction abnormalities, ventricular arrhythmias, worsening LV function, and death (29). The long-term effects of catheter-based selective ethanol septal ablation are as yet unknown.

SUMMARY

Significant advances in understanding the genetic basis of HCM have been made in the past few years. This will undoubtedly impact upon screening methods in the near future by allowing not only the identification of family members at risk, but also the assessment of individual risk regarding both disease severity and sudden death. Animal models may prove to be a useful tool for extrapolating markers and modifiers of high risk mutations to human patients with familial HCM.

REFERENCES

1.   Maron BJ, Gardin JM, Flack JM, Gidding SS, Kurosaki TT, Bild DE. Prevalence of hypertrophic cardiomyopathy in a general population of young adults. *Circulation* 1995;92:785-789.
2.   Fananapazir L, Epstein ND. Prevalence of hypertrophic cardiomyopathy and limitations of screening methods. *Circulation* 1995;92:700-704.
3.   Fananapazir L. Advances in molecular genetics and management of hypertrophic cardiomyopathy. *JAMA* 1999;281:1746-1752.
4.   Bonne G, Carrier L, Richard P, Hainque, B, Schwartz. Familial hypertrophic cardiomyopathy from mutations to functional defects. *Circ Res* 1998;83:580-593.
5.   Burns J, Camm J, Davies MJ, Peltonen L, Schwartz PJ, Watkins H. The phenotype/genotype relation and the current status of genetic screening in hypertrophic cardiomyopathy, Marfan syndrome, and the long QT syndrome. *Heart* 1997;78:110-116.
6.   Durand JB. Genetic basis of cardiomyopathy. *Curr Opin Cardiol.* 1999;14:225-229.
7.   Posma JL, van der Wall, EE, Blanksma PK, Lie KI. New diagnostic options in hypertrophic cardiomyopathy. *Am Heart J* 1996;132:1031-1041.
8.   Maron BJ. Hypertrophic cardiomyopathy. *Lancet* 1997;350:127-33.
9.   Satoh M, Takahashi M, Sakamoto T, Hiroe M, Marumo F, Kimura A. Structural analysis of the titin gene in hypertrophic cardiomyopathy: identification of a novel disease gene. *Biochem Biophys Res Comm* 1999;262:411-417.
10.   Mogensen J, Klausen IC, Pedersen AK, et al. Alpha-cardiac actin is a novel disease gene in familial hypertrophic cardiomyopathy. *J Clin Invest* 1999;103:R39-43.
11.   Watkins H, Thierfelder L, Hwang DS, McKenna W, Seidman JG, Seidman CE. Sporadic hypertrophic cardiomyopathy due to de novo myosin mutations. *J Clin Invest* 1992;90:1666-1671.
12.   Spirito P, Seidman CE, McKenna WJ, Maron BJ. The management of hypertrophic cardiomyopathy. *N Engl J Med* 1997;336:775-885.
13.   Anan R, Greve G, Thierfelder L, et al. Prognostic implications of novel β cardiac myosin heavy chain gene mutations that cause familial hypertrophic cardiomyopathy. *J Clin Invest* 1994;93:280-5
14.   Watkins H, Rosenzweig A, Hwang D, et al. Characteristics and prognostic implications of myosin missense mutations in familial hypertrophic cardiomyopathy. *N Engl J Med* 1992;326:1108-1114.
15.   Seidman CE and JG Seidman. Gene mutations that cause familial hypertrophic cardiomyopathy. In Molecular Cardiovascular Medicine. Haber, E , ed. 1995. Scientific American: New York. 203.
16.   Geisterfer-Lowrance AA, Christe M, Conner DA, Ingwall JS, Schoen FJ, Seidman CE, Seidman JG. A mouse model of familial hypertrophic cardiomyopathy. *Science* 1996;272:731-734.
17.   Berul CI, Christe ME, Aronovitz MA, Seidman CE, Seidman JG, Mendelsohn ME. Electrophysiological abnormalities and arrhythmias in αMHC mutant familial hypertrophic cardiomyopathy mice. *J Clin Invest* 1997;99:570-576.
18.   Berul CI, Christe ME, Aronovitz MJ, et al. Familial hypertrophic cardiomyopathy mice display gender differences in electrophysiological abnormalities. *J Interv Card Electrophysiol* 1998;2:7-14.
19.   Berul CI, Mendelsohn ME. Molecular biology and genetics of cardiac disease associated with sudden death. In Sudden Cardiac Death in the Athlete. Estes NAM, Salem DN, Wang PJ, eds. 1998. Futura : New York. 465-482.

20. Bevilacqua LM, Maguire CT, Seidman CE, Seidman JG, Berul CI. QT dispersion in αMHC familial hypertrophic cardiomyopathy mice. *Pediatr Res* 1999;45:643-647.
21. Wigle ED, Rakowski H, Kimball BP, Williams, WG. Hypertrophic cardiomyopathy clinical spectrum and treatment. *Circulation* 1995;92:1680-1692.
22. Klues HG, Schiffers A, Maron BJ. Phenotypic spectrum and patterns of left ventricular hypertrophy in hypertrophic cardiomyopathy: Morphologic observations and significance as assessed by two-dimensional echocardiography in 600 patients. *J Am Coll Cardiol.* 1995;26:1699-1708.
23. Ryan MP, Cleland JGF, French JA, et al. The standard electrocardiogram as a screening test for hypertrophic cardiomyopathy. *Am J Cardiol.* 1995;76:689-694.
24. Buja G, Miorelli M, Turrini P, Melacini P, Nava A. Comparison of QT dispersion in hypertrophic cardiomyopathy between patients with and without ventricular arrhythmias and sudden death. *Am J Cardiol* 1993;72:973-976.
25. Maron BJ, Pelliccia A, Spirito P. Insights into methods for distinguishing athlete's heart from structural heart disease, with particular emphasis on hypertrophic cardiomyopathy. *Circulation* 1995;91:1596-1601.
26. Maron BJ. Prevalence of sudden cardiac death during competitive sports activities in Minnesota high school athletics. *J Am Coll Cardiol* 1998;32:1881-1884.
27. Fananapazir L, Cannon RO, Tripodi D, Panza JA. Impact of dual-chamber permanent pacing in patients with obstructive hypertrophic cardiomyopathy with symptoms refractory to verapamil and β-adrenergic blocker therapy. *Circulation* 1992;85:2149-2161.
28. Pavin D, de Place C, Le Breton H, et al. Effects of permanent dual-chamber pacing on mitral regurgitation in hypertrophic obstructive cardiomyopathy. *Eur Heart J* 1999;20:203-210.
29. Fananapazir L, McAreavey D. Therapeutic options in patients with obstructive hypertrophic cardiomyopathy and severe drug-refractory symptoms. *J Am Coll Cardiol.* 1998;31:259-264.
30. Gadler F, Linde C, Juhlin-Dannfelt A, Ribeirot A, Ryden L. Long-term effects of dual chamber pacing in patients with hypertrophic cardiomyopathy without outflow tract obstruction at rest. *Eur Heart J* 1997;18:636-3642.
31. Fananapazir L, Epstein ND, Curiel RV, Panza JA, Tripodi D, McAreavey D. Long-term results of dual-chamber (DDD) pacing in obstructive hypertrophic cardiomyopathy: evidence for progressive symptomatic and hemodynamic improvement and reduction of left ventricular hypertrophy. *Circulation* 1994;90:2731-2742.
32. Maron BJ, Nishimura RA, McKenna WJ, Rakowski H, Josephson ME, Kieval RS. Assessment of permanent dual-chamber pacing as a treatment of drug-refractory symptomatic patients with obstructive hypertrophic cardiomyopathy. *Circulation* 1999;99:2927-2933.
33. Nishimura RA, Trusty JM, Hayes DL, et al. Dual-chamber pacing for hypertrophic cardiomyopathy. *J Am Coll Cardiol* 1997; 29:435-441.
34. Linde C, Gadler F, Kappenberger L, Ryden L. Placebo effect of pacemaker implantation in obstructive cardiomyopathy. *Am J Cardiol* 1999;83:903-907.
35. Primo J, Geelen P, Brugada J, et al. Hypertrophic cardiomyopathy: Role of the implantable cardioverter-defibrillator. *J Am Coll Cardiol* 1998;31:1081-5.
36. Borggrefe M, Beithardt G. Is the implantable defibrillator indicated in patients with hypertrophic cardiomyopathy and aborted sudden death? *J Am Coll Cardiol.* 1998;31:1086-8.
37. Silka MJ, Kron J, Dunnigan A, Dick M. Sudden cardiac death and the use of implantable cardioverter-defibrillator in pediatric patients. *Circulation* 1993;87:800-7.
38. Tripodi D, McAreavey D, Epstein ND, Fananapazir L. Impact of the implantable defibrillator in hypertrophic cardiomyopathy patients of high risk for sudden death. *J Am Coll Cardiol* 1993;21:352A.
39. McKenna WJ, Franklin RCG, Nihoyannopoulos P, et al. Arrhythmia and prognosis in infants, children and adolescents with hypertrophic cardiomyopathy. *J Am Coll Cardiol.* 1988;11:147-53.
40. Schowengerdt KO, Towbin JA. Genetic basis of inherited cardiomyopathies. *Curr Opin Cardiol* 1995;10:312-321.
41. Watson RM, Schwartz JL, Maron BJ, Tucker E, Rosing DR, Josephson ME. Inducible polymorphic ventricular tachycardia and ventricular fibrillation in a subgroup of patients with hypertrophic cardiomyopathy at high risk for sudden death. *J Am Coll Cardiol.* 1987;10:761-74.

42. Robinson K, Frenneaux MP, Stockins B, Karatasakis G, Poloniecki JD, McKenna WJ. Atrial fibrillation in hypertrophic cardiomyopathy: A longitudinal study. *J Am Coll Cardiol* 1990;15:1279-85.

43. MacRae CA, Ghaisas N, Kass S, et al. Familial hypertrophic cardiomyopathy with Wolff-Parkinson-White syndrome maps to a locus on chromosome 7q3. *J Clin Invest* 1995;96:1216-1220.

44. Maron BJ, Isner JM, McKenna WJ. Task force 3: Hypertrophic cardiomyopathy, myocarditis and other myopericardial diseases and mitral valve prolapse. *J Am Coll Cardiol.* 1994;24:845-99.

13

FAMILIAL DILATED CARDIOMYOPATHY

Jeffrey A. Towbin, M.D., and Neil E. Bowles, Ph.D.

Department of Pediatrics (Cardiology), Molecular and Human Genetics, and the Phoebe Willingham Muzzy Pediatric Molecular Cardiology Laboratory, Texas Children's Hospital, Baylor College of Medicine, Houston, Texas

INTRODUCTION

Definition and Classification of Cardiomyopathies

Cardiomyopathies are diseases of the heart muscle. When the term was introduced in 1957, it was used to identify a group of myocardial diseases not attributable to coronary artery disease (1). The definition has been modified since then and now refers to structural or functional abnormalities of the myocardium that are not secondary to hypertension, valvular or congenital heart disease, or pulmonary vascular disease.

From a functional standpoint, cardiomyopathies are classified into three categories: (1) dilated cardiomyopathy, also called congestive cardiomyopathy, in which the left or both ventricles are enlarged and hypocontractile to variable degrees; in general, systolic dysfunction is the main clinical feature, with resultant signs and symptoms of congestive heart failure (CHF); (2) hypertrophic cardiomyopathy, formerly known as *idiopathic hypertrophic subaortic stenosis*, characterized by left ventricular hypertrophy that may be asymmetric; systolic function is usually preserved, and symptoms may result from left ventricular outflow tract (LVOT) obstruction, diastolic dysfunction, or arrhythmias, resulting in sudden death; and (3) restrictive cardiomyopathy, recognized by markedly dilated atria, with generally normal ventricular dimensions and systolic function; diastolic filling is impaired, and symptoms result from pulmonary and right-sided systemic venous congestion; syncope may also be a presenting feature (2).

This chapter reviews the causes, clinical presentation, diagnosis, molecular genetics, management, and long-term outcomes of dilated cardiomyopathy. Other chapters will cover the other forms of myocardial disease.

Incidence and Prevalence of Dilated Cardiomyopathy

Dilated cardiomyopathy (DCM) is reported to be the most common form of cardiomyopathy, with an annual incidence of 2 to 8 cases per 100,000 population in the United States and Europe and an estimated prevalence of 36 affected individuals per 100,000 population (3). Recent reports of adult patients with DCM and CHF demonstrated the most common causes to be idiopathic (47%), myocarditis (12%), coronary artery disease (11%), and other identifiable causes (30%). In two studies of children of varying ages presenting with DCM, 2% to 15%

had biopsy-proven myocarditis, whereas 85% to 90% had no cause identified (4,5). In a group of 24 children who presented with DCM before 2 years of age, Matitiau et al (6) reported that 45% had myocarditis, 25% had endocardial fibroelastosis (EFE), and the remainder had no cause identified. Familial forms of DCM have also been described, with 30% or more of patients having a familial DCM (7-9).

CLINICAL GENETICS OF DILATED CARDIOMYOPATHY

As previously noted, inherited DCM occurs in over 30% of cases. Autosomal dominant transmission is the most common inheritance pattern seen in patients with familial DCM (7-11). However, autosomal recessive, X-linked, and mitochondrial inheritance patterns have been described (10,11) (Figure 1). Autosomal dominant DCM is identified on a pedigree when transmission occurs to approximately 50% of offspring, no skipping of generations occurs, and there is an equal sex distribution. In autosomal recessive DCM, an uncommon form of disease, carrier parents are clinically well and one-quarter of the offspring are affected. This scenario most commonly occurs in consanguineous relationships. Skipped generations are the rule. In X-linked disorders, the affected patients are males and females are carriers of the mutant gene, but are generally asymptomatic and have normal echocardiograms. No male-to-male transmission of the disease-causing gene occurs since the abnormal gene resides on the male X-chromosome but the male passes along only his Y chromosome in the case of a male offspring.

Mitochondrial inheritance is characterized by maternal transmission of the disease (12); this occurs because mitochondrial DNA is found in the egg and not in the sperm. In this form of inheritance, the amount of abnormal mitochondrial DNA versus the amount of normal mitochondrial DNA in any organ defines the clinical phenotype. When little abnormal DNA is noted, the individual is apparently unaffected or mild; individuals with a high percentage of abnormal mitochondria are severely affected. This mixing and matching of mitochondria is called heteroplasmy.

PATHOLOGY

On gross inspection of the heart, the chief morphologic feature seen in DCM is biventricular dilation; the atria may be enlarged to some degree as well.[13] Mural thrombi may be present in the cardiac chambers, particularly the atria. The heart is globular in appearance, and the myocardium is pale and sometimes mottled. The endocardium is usually thin and translucent (13,14); however, focal sclerosis may be seen. The heart weight is usually increased, indicating hypertrophy, and the coronary arteries are by definition, normal.

Histologic features of DCM classically include myocyte hypertrophy and degeneration, and varying degrees of interstitial fibrosis are seen (13,15)(Figure 2). Occasional small clusters of lymphocytes may be present;[16] if lymphocytes are also seen, this disorder must be differentiated from myocarditis in which the lymphocytes are associated with areas of myocyte damage and necrosis (17)(Figure 3). Nonspecific ultrastructural changes in the mitochondria, T tubules, and Z bands have been found in some instances by electron microscopy.

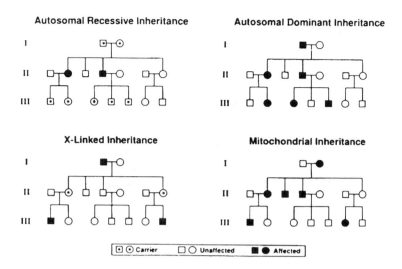

Figure 1. Patterns of inheritance. Autosomal (recessive and dominant), X-linked, and mitochondrial transmission is illustrated using pedigrees. In autosomal recessive inheritance, skipped generations occur. Two abnormal alleles are required to express the disease; carrier state occurs when only one allele is inherited. Autosomal dominant transmission is marked by transmission by either sex, no skipped generations, and when fully penetrant, only one abnormal allele is needed for the disease to occur. X-linked inheritance is identified by female carriers, disease expression in males, and no male-to-male transmission. Skipped generations are seen. Finally, mitochondrial inheritance is maternally transmitted, with all children at risk. However, due to heteroplasmy (i.e., mixture of normal and abnormal mitochondria; the higher the percentage of abnormal mitochondria, the more severe the disease) skipped generations can occur. Males cannot transmit the disease.

PATHOPHYSIOLOGY

Abnormally depressed contractile function manifests as decreased shortening fraction, ejection fraction, cardiac output, and cardiac index. This decline in forward flow parameters results in a pooling of intracavitary blood and a secondary increase in end-diastolic volume, end-diastolic pressure, and ventricular filling pressure (13). To maintain an adequate cardiac output, the ventricles dilate and the myocardium hypertrophies to some degree. The dilation results in increased wall tension, thereby increasing oxygen consumption and decreasing myocardial efficiency. As cardiac output diminishes, renal blood flow decreases. Typically, these features progress slowly and, therefore, increases in atrial and venous compliance result in mild pulmonary edema and systemic venous congestion. In children with acute decompensation, significant pulmonary edema and systemic venous congestion are manifested.

In association with the limitation of ventricular pumping, neurohumoral mechanisms are increasingly activated, particularly the renin-angiotensin system and sympathetic nervous system. Activation of these systems contributes to peripheral vascular changes and the full-blown clinical picture of CHF. Fibrosis of the ventricular myocardium may occur, resulting in irritable foci that cause ventricular arrhythmias (5), systolic and diastolic dysfunction.

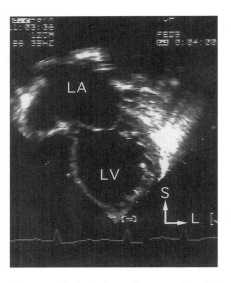

Figure 2. Histologic features of dilated cardiomyopathy. Myocyte hypertrophy and degeneration, interstitial fibrosis, and small clusters of lymphocytes are classically seen.

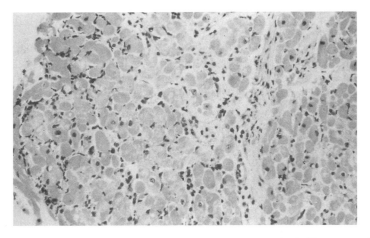

Figure 3. Myocarditis. Histologic features include lymphocytic infiltrate associated with myocytes necrosis.

CLINICAL PRESENTATION OF DILATED CARDIOMYOPATHY
Signs and Symptoms

When an adequate cardiac output cannot be maintained, signs and symptoms of CHF develop (5,18,19). Symptoms and signs may be subtle initially. Older children or parents of young children may notice decreasing exercise tolerance and dyspnea with exertion. In infants, this may be manifested as tachypnea that is more pronounced with feeding, resulting in decreased oral intake and failure to thrive. Palpitations and syncope or near-syncope may be reported in up to 13% of children (5). Obtaining a thorough family history and echocardiograms on first-degree relatives is important to verify whether familial inheritance occurs. Signs and symptoms may be unmasked by a superimposed infectious illness that results in further cardiac decompensation.

Physical Examination

As is seen with symptoms, a wide spectrum of findings can be found on physical examination. Griffin et al (20) reported that 70% to 80% of patients with dilated cardiomyopathy, present with signs of CHF. Tachypnea and tachycardia are frequently present. The skin may be pale. Cyanosis is uncommon unless circulatory collapse is imminent. Peripheral pulses are often weak, with normal to low blood pressure and a narrow pulse pressure. The extremities may be cool with decreased peripheral perfusion. Auscultation of the lungs may reveal diminished breath sounds posteriorly on the left if compression atelectasis from the enlarged heart is present. Occasionally, rales may be heard in this area associated with the atelectasis, but otherwise rales are rare in infants and small children, even in the face of pulmonary edema on chest radiography. Mild to marked intercostal retractions may be present.

Evaluation of the heart usually reveals a displaced apical impulse. The heart sounds may be muffled, and a prominent diastolic filling sound that produces a gallop rhythm (third heart sound) may be heard. Murmurs may be absent, but mitral regurgitation (caused by a dilated mitral valve annulus or papillary muscle dysfunction) may be heard. Tricuspid regurgitation may also be heard, and may be associated with elevated pulmonary vascular resistance.

Examination of the abdomen commonly reveals hepatomegaly. Other signs of systemic venous congestion include neck vein distention and peripheral edema, which are seen more commonly in older children or young adults and are uncommon in infants.

Diagnostic Studies

Radiography. Chest radiographs typically reveal cardiomegaly caused by left atrial and left ventricular enlargement. Pulmonary venous congestion is often present and may progress to frank pulmonary edema (Figure 4). Atelectasis of portions of the left lung may occur because of compression of the left main stem bronchus by the dilated left atrium. Pleural effusions may also be present.

Electrocardiogram and Holter Monitoring. On ECG, most patients have sinus tachycardia. Nonspecific ST segment and T wave changes, left ventricular hypertrophy, right and left atrial enlargement, and right ventricular hypertrophy are common (5,18,19). Arrhythmias are also common. Friedman et al (5) found arrhythmias in 46% of children with DCM who underwent Holter monitoring, with atrial arrhythmias being more common than ventricular arrhythmias. Greenwood et al (18), however, reported ventricular arrhythmias to be more common than atrial arrhythmias. The QT interval may also be prolonged and may lead to ventricular tachyarrhythmias.

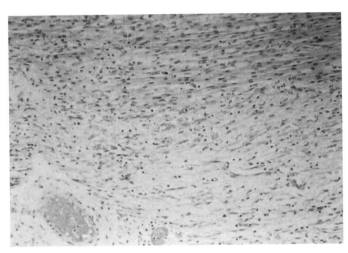

Figure 4. Chest x-ray demonstrating typical features of dilated cardiomyopathy with congestive heart failure, including cardiomegaly and pulmonary edema.

Echocardiogram. Echocardiographic features of DCM most commonly include dilation of the left ventricle and left atrium (Figure 5), with a decreased shortening fraction and ejection fraction (13,21), decreased mean circumferential fiber shortening, and increased ratio of left ventricular pre-ejection period to ejection time (21-23). Pericardial effusion is occasionally seen as well. Doppler and Color Doppler interrogation may identify atrioventricular valve regurgitation.

Cardiac Catheterization and Biopsy. Because DCM can be diagnosed by echocardiography, cardiac catheterization, angiography, and biopsy are deferred in some centers until these patients have been stabilized. Catheterization can be useful to rule out anomalous left coronary artery from the pulmonary artery (ALCAPA) because this may be missed by echocardiography. It may also help to predict cause and prognosis if the biopsy shows myocarditis or metabolic abnormalities, or to evaluate for cardiac transplantation.

Hemodynamic measurements generally reveal elevated left ventricular end diastolic, left atrial, and pulmonary capillary wedge pressures, and cardiac output is usually diminished (13). Angiography often demonstrates left ventricular dilation and reduced ejection fraction, normal coronary artery origins and course, and mitral regurgitation.

In patients with DCM, endomyocardial biopsy typically shows variable degrees of myocyte hypertrophy and fibrosis, usually without significant lymphocytic infiltrate. In some cases, however, mild lymphocytic infiltrate is noted. Biopsies can be useful for detecting myocarditis either by histology (15-17) or by viral-specific polymerase chain reaction (PCR),[24-26] as well as mitochondrial or infiltrative diseases (11,27-30). This may have a significant impact on prognosis and treatment (31).

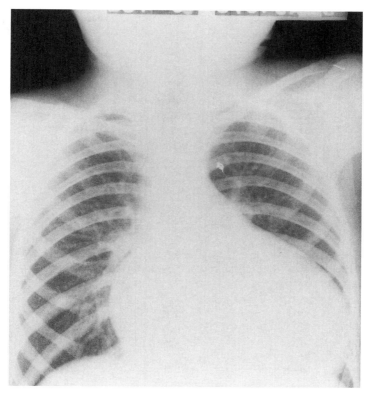

Figure 5. Echocardiographic features of dilated cardiomyopathy including dilated left ventricle and enlarged left atrium. The interventricular septum bulges left to right due to the expanded left ventricular volume. In real-time, systolic dysfunction is seen.

Blood and Urine Studies. Depending on the age at presentation, various studies may be helpful. Urine for organic and amino acids (30,32) may be useful, particularly if 3-methylglutaconic aciduria is found (i.e., Barth syndrome). Blood for lactate, calcium, magnesium, blood urea nitrogen, creatinine, and electrolytes are commonly useful. Molecular analysis for gene mutations may also be diagnostic (10,11,33).

MOLECULAR GENETICS

X-Linked Inheritance
Three forms of X-linked DCM have been reported, including X-linked dilated cardiomyopathy (XLCM), with or without skeletal muscle disease, Barth syndrome, and Emery-Dreifuss muscular dystrophy. In all cases, the gene has been identified.

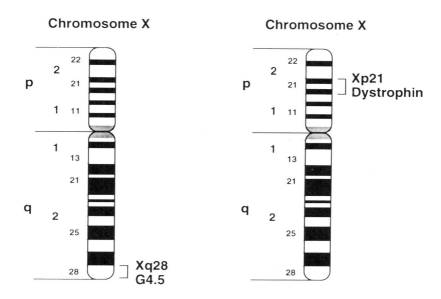

Figure 6. X chromosome. Mapping of the gene for Barth syndrome (*G4.5)* on the long arm (Xq28) and the gene for X-linked dilated cardiomyopathy (dystrophin) on the short arm (Xp21) of the X chromosome.

XLCM: First described in 1987 by Berko and Swift (34), patients with XLCM usually present in the mid-to-late-teen years or early twenties with signs and symptoms of CHF. Rapid progression of cardiac decompensation with associated ventricular tachyarrhythmias commonly leads to death or cardiac transplantation within one to two years of initial diagnosis in these young men. Female carriers may develop clinical disease but onset is typically late (i.e., fifth decade) and progression is slow and relatively easily controlled. Laboratory features are not usually helpful except the serum creatine kinase (CK) which is elevated. Isoform analysis of CK demonstrates essentially all muscle isoform (CK-MM). Despite this biochemical evidence of skeletal myopathy, no clinical skeletal myopathy is observed.

In the early 1990's, my laboratory evaluated this family and others using molecular techniques. Linkage analysis was utilized to map the genetic locus for XLCM to chromosome Xp21.2 with the dystrophin locus (35) (Figure 6). Western blot and Northern blot analysis confirmed dystrophin abnormalities, demonstrating severe reduction of dystrophin in the hearts of these patients using N-terminal and rod domain antibodies to dystrophin, and reduced mRNA within the heart when the

5' portion of the gene was studied (36). This was later confirmed by Muntoni et al (37); in addition, a deletion was found to include the muscle promoter and exon 1 in affected boys. Milasin et al (38) further confirmed the notion initially suggested by Towbin et al (35) that the 5' portion of the gene was at risk, identifying an exon 1-intron 1 splicing mutation. The mutation described by my laboratory in the family initially identified by Berko and Swift (34) was in exon 9, encoding portions of the first hinge of dystrophin (39). Other mutations are known (40-42), including some which are in the 3' portion of the gene. In other cases, abnormalities involving transposons have been reported (43).

Mutations in dystrophin should not be a surprise when considering cardiomyopathic phenotypes. This gene was initially cloned in the mid-1980's and shown to be the cause of Duchenne and Becker muscular dystrophies (44,45). Duchenne muscular dystrophy (DMD) is the more severe form of skeletal myopathy, leading to muscle weakness early in life which requires a wheelchair before age 12 years. Becker muscular dystrophy (BMD) is less severe and these boys do not require wheelchairs until after age 16 years. In both cases, DCM occurs in well over 90% of cases and is a significant cause of death in both groups of patients (46-48). Female carriers develop DCM also albeit later in life. Elevations of MM-CK are hallmarks of DMD and BMD, as well as other muscular dystrophies.

It is important to note that dystrophin complexes with a series of proteins at its N-terminus and C-terminus (49-54), connecting the sarcomere (contractile units of the muscle) to the sarcolemma and extracellular matrix (Figure 7).

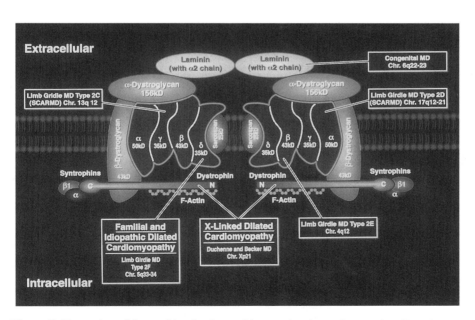

Figure 7. Illustration of dystrophin, the dystrophin-associated protein complex (DAPC), and the extracellular matrix. Mutations in any component leads to skeletal muscle disease with or without dilated cardiomyopathy.

At the C-terminal end of dystrophin, connection with an oligomeric integral membrane complex, the dystrophin-associated protein complex (DAPC), links the sarcolemma with the intracellular region. This DAPC contains a variety of proteins, including the sarcoglycan and dystroglycan subcomplexes, sarcospan, caveolin, and dystrobrevins. These proteins further link the membrane to the extracellular matrix via connections with laminin, merosin, and other proteins (53,54). Disruption of these links to dystrophin tends to lead to abnormalities of cardiac function and skeletal muscle disease (Figure 7), but the severity of disease in each organ system varies widely (53).

Barth syndrome: Initially described by Neustein et al (55) as X-linked cardioskeletal myopathy with neutropenia and abnormal mitochondria, children with this syndrome typically present in significant clinical congestive heart failure. Echocardiographic features of Barth syndrome vary widely and include DCM, hypertrophic dilated cardiomyopathy (HDCM), or LV noncompaction. The histopathology of the myocardium usually includes myocytes hypertrophy and fibrosis, and in many cases, endocardial fibroelastosis may be a prominent feature (55,56)(Figure 8). Abnormalities in mitochondria of the heart and skeletal muscle are notable on electron microscopy (Figure 9). Kelley et al (33) were the first to demonstrate these patients to have 3-methylglutaconic aciduria, a common feature of this disease, which when observed with the cardiac phenotype, neutropenia, and male sex, is essentially diagnostic. Other findings include hypercholesterolemia, lactic acidosis, respiratory chain abnormalities (particularly cytochrome C oxidase/cytochrome C deficiency), and hypoglycemia.

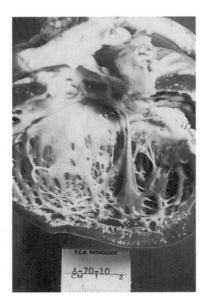

Figure 8. Electron microscopic appearance of abnormal mitochondria with inclusions. In addition, abundant glycogen is notable in this muscle.

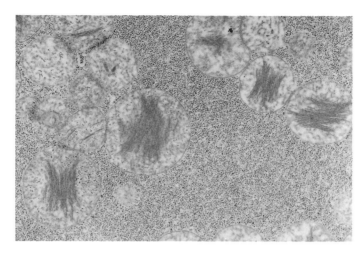

Figure 9. Electron microscopic appearance of abnormal mitochondria with inclusions. In addition, abundant glycogen is notable in this muscle.

The gene for the X-linked inherited disorder was first mapped by Bolhuis et al (57) and localized to the long arm of the X chromosome at Xq28 (57,58)(Figure 6). Bione et al (59) later identified and characterized this gene to be G4.5, a novel gene encoding a novel protein family called tafazzins. The function of the gene is not currently known, although the gene structure is well characterized. The gene consists of 11 exons, two ATG initiation sites and multiple alternative spliced forms of exons 5 to 7 that generate a family of 10 or more mRNAs with tissue-specific distributions. This 6.3 Kb gene encodes a 129-292 amino acid protein of unknown function but, when mutated, results in a wide spectrum of clinical cardiac and systemic disease. A variety of mutations in G4.5 have been identified (59,60), including deletions, point mutations, insertions, and splice-site mutations that introduce a premature stop codon. These mutations result in clinical disorders ranging from classic Barth syndrome to DCM to LV noncompaction (59-63). Mutations in G4.5 are likely to be common in infantile-onset cardiomyopathies in general and probably are responsible for some cases of later-onset disease. Female carriers do not develop clinical disease, probably because of X-inactivation (64).

Left Ventricular Noncompaction (LVNC): Previously called "spongiform myocardium" or "fetal myocardium", these patients most commonly present in the newborn period, although older children and adults are now being recognized (65-67). In some familial cases, the inheritance is X-linked, and in these cases mutations in *G4.5* has been identified (63). In others, autosomal dominant inheritance occurs, but the genes are not yet known (67).

This disorder is recognized by deep trabeculations in the endocardium, giving the appearance of endocardial holes (Figure 10). In many cases, the myocardium is both thick and dilated and LV performance is poor. In some cases, LVNC occurs alone (i.e., isolated LVNC) while other cases include a form of congenital heart disease, such as ventricular septal defects (VSD), pulmonic stenosis (PS), or atrial septal defects (ASDs). In the latter case, this is called nonisolated LVNC (NLVNC) (Figure 11). Therapy is usually based on the physiologic features of these disorders; usually CHF is the predominant feature but occasionally a hypercontractile, hypertrophic left ventricle with diastolic dysfunction predominates.

AUTOSOMAL DOMINANT INHERITANCE

This is the most common form of inherited DCM. To date, ten genes have been mapped to chromosomal loci for the "pure" form of DCM (5 loci) and the DCM associated with conduction abnormalities (4 loci). In the "pure" form of DCM, the affected members have DCM as the predominant disease. Genes have been mapped to chromosomes 1q32, 2q31, 6q23, 9q13-22, 10q21-23, and 15q14 (68-73). In the case of the chromosome 10q21-23 family, mitral valve prolapse was seen in patients with DCM. Two genes have been identified for the "pure" form, including actin (chromosome 15q14) and desmin (chromosome 6q23). When considered with the other known genes causing a DCM phenotype particularly dystrophin, it suggests a "final common pathway" resulting in a dilated, dysfunctional left ventricle (74-77). This pathway appears to involve the cytoskeleton and the result of abnormalities and mechanical stress is DCM.

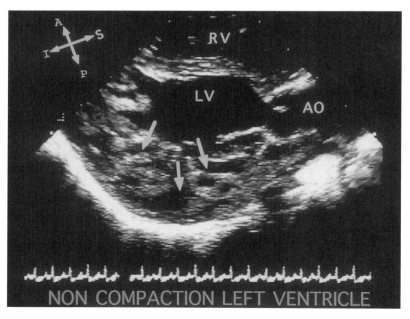

Figure 10. Echocardiogram of a patient with isolated left ventricular noncompaction. Note the deep trabeculations within the endocardium (arrows), the hypertrophic posterior wall and dilated ventricle (with poor systolic function in real-time).

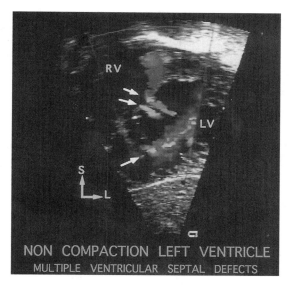

Figure 11. Echocardiogram of a patient with nonisolated left ventricular noncompaction and a ventricular septal defect (VSD). Color Doppler identifies clearly the VSD.

Actin is a sarcomeric protein that is a member of the thin filament, interacting with α-tropomyosin and the troponin complex. Actin also binds to the N-terminus of dystrophin, enabling dystrophin to link the sarcomere with the sarcolemma. Mutations near the dystrophin binding site were shown by Olson et al (73) to cause DCM, while Mogensen et al (78) found that mutations in the sarcomeric end of the protein results in hypertrophic cardiomyopathy (HCM).

Desmin is a cytoskeletal protein that forms intermediate filaments specific for muscle (79). This muscle-specific 53KDa subunit of class III intermediate filaments forms connections between the nuclear and plasma membranes of cardiac, skeletal, and smooth muscle. Desmin is found at the Z lines and intercalated disk and its role is thought to involve attachment or stabilization of the sarcomere. Mutations in this gene appear to cause abnormalities of force and signal transmission (80), similar to that believed for actin (73).

The remaining loci have been identified in families whose initial presentation is primarily one of conduction disturbance which precede cardiac dilation and systolic dysfunction. The initial abnormalities in these patients are usually sinus node dysfunction and/or atrioventricular node dysfunction, resulting in sinus bradycardia, sinus pauses and sinus arrest, first-, second-, or third-degree atrioventricular block, and/or atrial fibrillation. In some cases, mild limb girdle muscular dystrophy (LGMD) is notable. The loci identified include chromosomes 1p1-1q21, 2q14-21, 3p25-22, and 6q23 (81-84). One of these genes was recently identified as encoding lamin A/C on chromosome 1q21 (85). The remainder are still unknown but, since mutations in sarcoglycans have been identified for multiple types of LGMD (86-91), these genes are certainly good candidates.

OTHER CAUSES OF DCM

Other genetic forms of DCM have also been analyzed at the molecular level (10,11,27,32). Deficiencies of enzymes required for efficient myocardial fatty acid β-oxidation, including abnormalities in the plasma membrane carnitine transporter CPTII (carnitine palmitoyl-transferase), carnitine-acylcarnitine translocase, long chain 3-hydroxyacyl-CoA dehydrogenase deficiency, and very long chain acylCoA dehydrogenase deficiency have been described.

"THE FINAL COMMON PATHWAY" HYPOTHESIS

A number of genes have been identified in humans or animal models which could be causes of DCM. The knowledge of these genes and those genes previously described for X-linked and autosomal DCM should enable the genes to be identified for those loci not yet characterized completely. In order to develop a candidate gene approach to successfully identify these genes, we have described the "final common pathway" hypothesis (74-77). This hypothesis is based on the molecular understanding gained from other cardiac disorders. For instance, hypertrophic cardiomyopathy (HCM) is a disease of the sarcomere. Here, all eight genes identified in autosomal dominant HCM are members of the sarcomere, either the thick filament or thin filament. These genes include β-myosin heavy chain, myosin binding protein-C, myosin essential and regulatory light chains, α-tropomyosin, cardiac actin, cardiac troponin T and troponin I (78, 92-97). Mutations in any of the genes encoding sarcomeric proteins result in HCM, albeit with wide clinical variability (98-100)(Figure 12). Similarly, diseases in which ventricular arrhythmias are primary abnormalities, such as long QT syndrome (LQTS) and Brugada syndrome, are caused by mutations in ion channel-encoding genes (101-103). Mutations in potassium channels have been identified in LQTS *(KVLQT1, minK, HERG, MiRP1),* while the cardiac sodium channel has been identified to cause one form of LQTS, as well as Brugada syndrome *(SCN5A)* (101-103). Again, wide clinical heterogeneity exists. Together, these data suggest that mutations in genes encoding a common type of protein result in a specific form of disease phenotype (i.e., ion channelopathy in ventricular arrhythmias; sarcomyopathy in HCM). This information would therefore suggest that the basis of DCM is abnormal cytoskeletal proteins based on the finding that dystrophin, actin, desmin, and lamin A/C mutations result in DCM (Figure 12).

Further support for this is provided by the report by Maeda et al (104) of mutant metavinculin in DCM, as well as the identification of mutations in the DAPC protein adhalin (α-sarcoglycan) and dystroglycans (36,42,105-107). Animal models have been developed which also provide evidence that mutant utrophin (108-109), β,α, and δ sarcoglycan (110-114), and muscle LIM protein (MLP, a protein of the actin cytoskeleton)(115) result in DCM. Further, mutations in DAPC-encoding genes, as well as extracellular matrix proteins-encoding genes, result in forms of muscular dystrophy, with or without DCM and/or conduction disease in humans (116-123). Finally, Badorff et al (124) have shown that infection with coxsackie B3 virus causes myocarditis and via enteroviral protease 2A cleavage of hinge 3 of dystrophin, causes chronic DCM. Hence, this finding suggests myocarditis-induced DCM is an acquired form of XLCM dystrophinopathy.

MODIFIER GENES

Several studies suggest that human leukocyte antigen (HLA)-DR4 and HLA-DQB1 loci on chromosome 6 may be genetic markers for susceptibility to DCM 9125-127). A possible correlation between autoimmunity and the development of cardiomyopathy exists because genetic control of portions of the immune system may be located in that region (128-129). Several immune regulatory abnormalities have been identified in patients with DCM, including humoral and cellular autoimmune reactivity against myocytes, decreased natural killer cell activity, and abnormal suppressor cell activity, thus suggesting that immune defects may be important etiologic factors in the development of DCM (129). Despite the apparent association between HLA loci, the immune system, and DCM, further research is necessary to prove that these are involved in causing some forms of DCM.

In addition, Liggett and colleagues (130,131) have demonstrated that polymorphisms in the β2-adrenergic receptor (β2AR) predispose to poor survival in patients with DCM and CHF. In their studies, the Ile164 polymorphism increases the risk of sudden death in patients with CHF substantially over those with the wild-type Thr164. In addition, they have suggested that β1AR polymorphisms identify β-blocker responders.

Cascade Effectors

The contractile function of cardiomyocytes is regulated in health by a number of mechanisms which may become maladaptive during development of myocardial disease. Generally, contractile function is regulated by changes in calcium flux into and out of the sarcoplasmic reticulum (SR). Increased uptake of calcium into the SR is heralded by activation of β-adrenergic receptors, which leads to calcium pump activity after removal of the tonic inhibitory effect of phospholamban via phosphorylation by cyclic AMP-dependent protein kinase (PKA). In dilated cardiomyopathy, the primary functional disturbance, impaired systolic contractility, is associated with desensitization of β-adrenergic receptors with up-regulation of the β-adrenergic receptor kinase (βARK) (132). Overexpression of the calcium-regulatory protein phospholamban in mice leads to reduced contractility while deficiency of phospholamban halts the progression of CHF and DCM, suggesting a role in the disease state (133,134).

Overexpression of β1-adrenergic receptors (β1AR) and β2-adrenergic receptors (β2AR), or overexpression of $G_s\alpha$ protein (which is coupled to these receptors) demonstrates increased contractile function in mouse models. The same is true when a peptide inhibitor of βARK is overexpressed (135-138). Taken together with the data obtained concerning phospholamban, it seems that β-adrenergic pathways lead to phosphorylation of phospholamban, which reduces its activity and increases ATPase activity in the SR, resulting in normal cardiac function. Dysregulation of this pathway, particularly when cytoskeletal protein abnormalities coexist, is likely to lead to symptomatic DCM with CHF. Disease progression is also affected by biologically active molecules that exert toxic effects on the cardiovascular system, such as tumor necrosis factor (TNF), endothelin, angiotensin II, aldosterone, and norepinephrine (139-144). TNF-α, acting through its receptor, activates apoptotic signals, leading to cell death (145-147). Similarly, p21ras induces c-jun N-terminal kinase leading to apoptosis (148). Other regulators/activators of apoptosis include p38, adenoviral infection, gp130, amongst others (148-150).

Ultimately, these cascade effectors, in addition to the primary abnormality of cytoskeletal proteins, leads to LV remodeling and, the DCM phenotype. It is possible that this further activates pathways which lead to irreversible disease, such as the development of fibrosis. This has been speculated to occur due to activation of matrix metalloproteinases (MMPs), probably by TNF and other cytokines and peptide growth factors expressed in the failing myocardium (151,152).

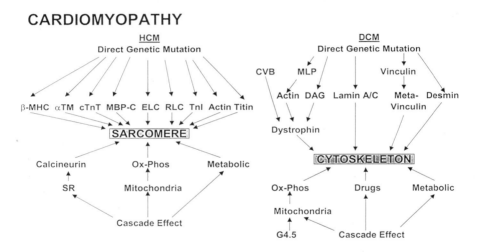

Figure 12. The "final common pathway" of myocardial disease. Note that hypertrophic cardiomyopathy (HCM) is a disease of the sarcomere, with mutations directly affecting genes encoding sarcomeric protein. Cascade pathways also affect the sarcomere resulting in a hypertrophic response. Similarly, dilated cardiomyopathy (DCM) is a disease of the cytoskeleton. HCM, hypertrophic cardiomyopathy; β-MHC, β-myosin heavy chain; α-TM, α-tropomyosin; cTnT, cardiac troponin T; MBP-C, myosin binding protein-C; ELC, essential light chain; RLC, regulatory light chain; TnI, troponin I; SR, sarcoplasmic reticulum; Ox-phos, oxidative phosphorylation; DCM, dilated cardiomyopathy; CVB, Coxsackie B virus; MLP, muscle LIM protein; DAG, dystrophin associated glycoprotein complex.

TREATMENT

Medical

If no identifiable and treatable cause of the DCM is found, therapy typically is supportive and consists of an anticongestive regimen, control of significant arrhythmias, and minimizing the risk for thromboembolic complications. Children who present critically ill frequently require intubation and mechanical ventilation.

Intravenous (IV) inotropic support is used to improve cardiac function and output during episodes of decompensation. The mainstays of therapy have been dobutamine and dopamine (153). Dopamine is begun in renal doses to enhance renal perfusion and diuresis. Myocardial phosphodiesterase inhibitors, such as milirinone (154), possess positive inotropic effects and afterload-reducing properties and improve left ventricular relaxation, They are useful when a combination of these effects is desired. Nitroprusside can also be used for afterload reduction but may have greater blood pressure effects. When these patients are well enough to begin oral medications, digoxin is usually instituted as IV inotropic agents are weaned. Oral captopril or enalapril should also be started as IV afterload-reducing agents are being decreased. β-Adrenergic blocking agents have been used in adults (155) and are becoming useful in children.

Diuretic therapy is used to enhance diuresis and is given intravenously initially to patients requiring inpatient therapy. Electrolytes should be monitored closely because the combination of multiple drugs, poor myocardial function, and electrolyte imbalances may produce significant arrhythmias. Diuretic therapy can be switched to the oral route when signs of pulmonary and systemic venous congestion have decreased and the likelihood of good oral absorption has increased.

Arrhythmias are common in children with DCM (4,5). In some cases, improvement in cardiac function with medical management of CHF and normalizing electrolyte imbalances is all the treatment that is required; however, if significant arrhythmias persist, antiarrhythmic therapy is warranted. Many antiarrhythmic drugs adversely affect ventricular function and may be proarrhythmic. These factors must be taken into account when choosing antiarrhythmic therapy. For maintenance therapy of significant arrhythmias, amiodarone has been shown to be effective and relatively safe in children. If symptomatic bradyarrhythmias occur, temporary pacing may be necessary during the acute phase of illness. Occasionally, permanent pacing may be necessary. Elective pacing to optimize atrioventricular synchrony and ventricular filling is investigational (156). The utility of immunosuppressive agents, including steroids, cyclosporine, and azathioprine, in patients with DCM remains unproven (157,158).

Intracavitary thrombus formation and systemic embolization have been reported in young patients with DCM, and anticoagulation should be considered. If a thrombus is identified, patients are usually anticoagulated with heparin and then switched to warfarin. If a thrombus is not seen, antiplatelet drugs (e.g., aspirin or dipyridamole) may be useful in preventing thrombus formation.

In children with metabolic causes of DCM, careful attention to biochemical derangement is important. Correction of metabolic acidosis and diagnosis of the underlying cause is paramount. Oral feeding should be discontinued until stabilization has occurred. Intravenous fluid and dextrose replacement should be considered to provide energy and reduce the ongoing catabolic process.

In the future, alterations of this treatment strategy may occur due to improved understanding of the molecular basis of DCM and CHF.

Surgical Therapy

Despite maximal medical therapy, some patients continue to deteriorate, and children with acute and severe decompensation may require therapy with a ventricular assist device (VAD), intra-aortic balloon (IAB) counterpropulsion, extracorporeal membrane oxygenator (ECMO), or transplantation. We have used devices (i.e., VADs, IABs) routinely as a bridge to transplantation or to recovery. Recently, the use of implantable VADs has allowed some children to be discharged from the hospital while awaiting transplantation with the VAD in place.

PROGNOSIS

In infants and children presenting with DCM, four possible outcomes may occur: (1) complete resolution, (2) improvement, (3) death, or (4) cardiac transplantation or other surgical option. Review of available studies in children suggests that approximately one-third die, one-third improve but have some residual cardiac dysfunction and one-third recover completely. In children, the 1-year survival rate ranges from 63% to 70%, 5-year survival, 34% to 66%; and 10- to 11-year survival, 50%. Mortality is highest during the first 1-2 years after presentation.

Congestive heart failure is the most common cause of death among patients with DCM, although sudden death also occurs. The time from presentation to approximately 6 months from diagnosis seems most critical in terms of defining outcome. In patients who will recover or improve, signs of improvement are generally seen in the initial 6 months, although continued improvement may be seen for as long as 2 years. The first 6 months are also the time frame in which most of the deaths occur, with chances for survival declining more gradually thereafter.

REFERENCES

1.   Brigden W: Uncommon myocardial diseases: The noncoronary cardiomyopathies. Lancet 1957; 2.1179-1184; 1243-1249.
2.   Richardson P, McKenna WJ, Bristow M, et al. Report of the 1995 World Health Organization/International Society and Federation of Cardiology: Task force on the definition and classification of cardiomyopathy.Circulation 1996; 93:841-842.
3.   Manolio TA, Baughman KL, Rodenheffer R, et al. Prevalence and etiology of idiopathic dilated cardiomyopathy (Summary of a National Heart Lung and Blood Institute workshop). Am J Cardiol 1992; 69:1458-1466.
4.   Wiles HB, McArthur PD, Taylor AB, et al. Prognostic features of children with idiopathic dilated cardiomyopathy. Am J Cardiol 1991; 68:1372-1376.
5.   Friedman RA, Moak JP, Garson A Jr. Clinical course of idiopathic dilated cardiomyopathy in children. J Am Coll Cardiol 1991;18:152-156.
6.   Matitiau A, Perez-Atayde A, Sanders SP, et al. Infantile dilated cardiomyopathy: relation of outcome to left ventricular mechanics, hemodynamics and histology at the time of presentation. Circulation 1994; 90:1310-1318.

7.   Baig MK, Goldman JH, Caforio ALP, et al. Familial dilated cardiomyopathy. Cardiac abnormalities are common in asymptomatic relatives and may represent early disease. J Am Coll Cardiol 1998; 31:195-201.
8.   Michels VV, Moll PP, Miller FA, et al. The frequency of familial dilated cardiomyopathy in a series of patients with idiopathic dilated cardiomyopathy.N Engl J Med 1992; 326:77-82.
9.   Grunig E, Tasman JA, Kucherer H, et al. Frequency and phenotypes of familial dilated cardiomyopathy. J Am Coll Cardiol 1998 31:186-194.
10.   Towbin J. Molecular genetic aspects of cardiomyopathy.Biochem Med Metab Biol 1993; 49:285-320.
11.   Towbin JA, Roberts R. Cardiovascular diseases due to genetic abnormalities. In: Alexander RW Schlant RC, Fuster V (eds): Hurst's The Heart, ed 9. New York, McGraw-Hill, 1998, Chapter 69 pp 1877-1924.
12.   Wallace DC. Mitochondrial genetics: A paradigm for aging and degenerative diseases?Science 1992; 256:628-632.
13.   Gilbert EM, Bristow MR. Idiopathic dilated cardiomyopathy. In: Schlant RC, Alexander RW (eds): Hurst's The Heart, ed 8. New York, McGraw-Hill, 1994, pp 1609-1619.
14.   Doshi R, Lodge KV: Idiopathic cardiomyopathy in infants. ArchDis Child 1973; 48:431-435, 1973.
15.   Lewis AB, Neustein HB, Takahashi M, et al. Findings on endomyocardial biopsy in infants and children with dilated cardiomyopathy. Am J Cardiol 1985 55:143-145.
16.   Tazelaar HD, Billingham ME. Leukocytic infiltrates in idiopathic dilated cardiomyopathy: A source of confusion with active myocarditis. Am JSurg Pathol 1986; 10:405-412.
17.   Aretz HT. Myocarditis: the Dallas criteria. Hum Pathol 1987; 18:619-624.
18.   Greenwood RD, Nadas AS, Fyler DC. The clinical course of primary myocardial disease in infants and children. Am Heart J 1976 92:549-560.
19.   Taliercio CP, Seward JB, Discoll DJ, et al. Idiopathic dilated cardiomyopathy in the young: Clinical profile and natural history.J Am Coll Cardiol 1985; 6:1126-1131.
20.   Griffin ML, Hernandez A, Martin TC, et al. Dilated cardiomyopathy in infants and children. J Am Coll Cardiol 1988 11:39-44.
21.   Mestroni L, Maisch B, McKenna WJ, et al. Guidelines for the study of familial dilated cardiomyopathy. Eur Heart J 1999; 20:93-102.
22.   Ghafour AD, Gutgesell HP. Echocardiographic evaluation of left ventricular function in children with congestive cardiomyopathy. Am J Cardiol 1979 44:1332-1338.
23.   Lewis AB. Prognostic value of echocardiography in children with idiopathic dilated cardiomyopathy. Am Heart J 1994; 128:133-136.
24.   Martin AB, Webber S, Fricker FJ, et al. Acute myocarditis: Rapid diagnosis by PCR in children. Circulation 1994; 90:330-339.
25.   Pauschinger M, Bowles N, Fuentes-Garcia J, et al. Detection of adenoviral genome in the myocardium of adult patients with idiopathic left ventricular dysfunction, Circulation 1999; 99:1348-1354.
26.   Towbin JA. Polymerase chain reaction and its uses as a diagnostic tool for cardiovascular disease. Trends Cardiovasc Med 1995; 5:175-185.
27.   Kohlschutter A, Hausdorf G. Primary (genetic) cardiomyopathies in infancy: A survey of possible disorders and guidelines for diagnosis.Eur J Pediatr 1986; 145:454-459.
28.   Kelly DP, Strauss AW. Inherited cardiomyopathies.N Engl J Med 1993; 330:913-919.
29.   Roberts WC, Ferrans VJ. Pathologic anatomy of the cardiomyopathies: Idiopathic dilated and hypertrophic types, infiltrative types, and endomyocardial disease with and withouteosinophilia. Hum Pathol 1975; 6:287-342.
30.   Schwartz ML, Cox GF, Lin AE, et al. Clinical approach to genetic cardiomyopathy in children. Circulation 1996; 94:2021-2038.
31.   Fenoglio JJ, Ursell PC, Kellogg CE, et al. Diagnosis and classification of myocarditis by endomyocardial biopsy. N Engl J Med 1983 308:12-15.
32.   Strauss AW. Defects of mitochondrial proteins and pediatric heart disease.Prog Pediatr Cardiol 1996; 6:83-90.
33.   Kelley RI, Cheatham JP, Clark BJ, et al. X-linked dilated cardiomyopathy with neutropenia, growth retardation, and 3-methylglutaconicaciduria. J Pediatr 1991; 119:738-747.
34.   Berko BA, Swift M. X-linked dilated cardiomyopathy. N Engl J Med 1987 316:1186-1191.

35.   Towbin JA, Hejtmancik JF, Brink P, et al. X-linked dilated cardiomyopathy: Molecular genetic evidence of linkage to the Duchenne muscular dystrophy (dystrophin) gene at the Xp21 locus. Circulation 1993; 87:1854-1865.

36.   Towbin JA. Biochemical and molecular characterization of X-linked dilated cardiomyopathy (XLCM). Developmental mechanisms of heart disease. Clark EB, Markwald RR, Takao A (Eds), Futura Publishing Co., Inc., New York, 121-132, 1995.

37.   Muntoni F, Cau M, Canau A, et al. Brief report: Deletion of the dystrophin muscle promoter region associated with X-linked dilated cardiomyopathy.N Engl J Med 1993; 329:921-925.

38.   Milasin J, Muntoni F, Severini CM, et al. A point mutation in the 5′ splice site of the dystrophin gene first intron responsible for X-linked dilated cardiomyopathy. Hum Mol Genet 1996 5:73-79.

39.   Ortiz-Lopez R, Su J, Goytia V, et al. Evidence for a dystrophin missense mutation as a cause of X-linked dilated cardiomyopathy (XLCM).Circulation 1997; 95:2434-2440.

40.   Franz WM, Cremer M, Hermann R, et al. X-linked dilated cardiomyopathy. Novel mutation of the dystrophin gene. Ann NY AcadSci 1995; 751:470-491.

41.   Ferlini A, Galie N, Merlini L, et al. A novel Alu-like element rearranged in the dystrophin gene causes a splicing mutation in a family with X-linked dilated cardiomyopathy Am J Hum Genet 1998; 63:436-460.

42.   Bies RD, Maeda M, Roberds SL, et al. A 5′ dystrophin duplication mutation causes membrane deficiency of α-dystroglycan in a family with X-linked cardiomyopathy. J Mol Cell Cardiol 1997; 29:3175-3188.

43.   Yoshida K, Nakamura A, Yazak M, et al. Insertional mutation by transposable element, L1, in the DMD gene results in X-linked dilated cardiomyopathy. HumMolec Med 1998; 7:1129-1132.

44.   Koenig M, Hoffman EP, Bertelson CJ, et al. Complete cloning of the Duchenne muscular dystrophy (DMD) cDNA and preliminary genomic organization of the DMD gene in normal and affected individuals. Cell 1987; 50:509-517.

45.   Hoffman EP, Brown RJ, Kunkel LM. Dystrophin: the protein products of the Duchenne muscular dystrophy locus. Cell 1987; 51:919-928.

46.   Cox GF, Kunkel LM. Dystrophies and heart disease. Curr Opin Cardiol 1997; 12:329-343.

47.   Melacini P, Fanin M, Danieli GA, et al. Myocardial involvement is very frequent among patients affected with subclinical Becker's muscular dystrophy. Circulation 1996 94:3168-3175.

48.   Melacini P, Fanin M, Daniel GA, et al. Cardiac involvement in Becker muscular dystrophy. J Am Coll Cardiol 1993; 22:1927-1934.

49.   Ervasti JM, Ohlendieck K, Kahl SD, et al. Deficiency of a glycoprotein component of the dystrophin complex in dystrophic muscle. Nature 1990 345:315-319.

50.   Ervasti JM, Campbell KP. A role for the dystrophin-glycoprotein complex as a transmembrane linker between laminin and actin. J CellBiol 1993; 122:809-823.

51.   Ervasti JM, Campbell KP. Membrane organization of the dystrophinglycoprotein complex. Cell 1991; 66:1121-1131.

52.   Ozama E, Hagiwara Y, Yoshida M. Creatine kinase cell membrane and Duchenne muscular dystrophy. Mol CellBiochem 1999; 190:143-151.

53.   Ozawa E, Noguchi S, Mizuno Y, et al. From dystrophinopathy to sarcoglycanopathy: evolution of a concept of muscular dystrophy. Muscle Nerve 1998 21:421-438.

54.   Ohlendieck K. Towards an understanding of the dystrophinglycoprotein complex: linkage between the extracellular matrix and the membrane cytoskeleton in muscle fibers. Eur J Cell Biol 1996; 69:1-10.

55.   Neustein HD, Lurie PR, Dahms B, Takahashi M. An X-linked recessive cardiomyopathy with abnormal mitochondria. Pediatrics 1979, 64:24-29.

56.   Barth PG, Scholte HR, Berden JA, et al. An X-linked mitochondrial disease affecting cardiac muscle, skeletal muscle and neutrophil leukocytes. JNeurol Sci 1983; 72:327-355.

57.   Bolhuis PA, Hensels GW, Hulsebos TJ, et al. Mapping of the locus for X-linked cardioskeletal myopathy with neutropenia and abnormal mitochondria (Barth Syndrome) to Xq28. Am J Hum Genet 1991; 48.481-485.

58.   Ades LC, Gedeon AK, Wilson MJ, et al. Barth syndrome: clinical features and confirmation of gene localization to distal Xq28. Am J Med Genet 1993; 45:327-334.

59.   Bione S, D'Adamo P, Maestrini E, et al. A novel X-linked gene G4.5 is responsible for Barth syndrome. Nat Genet 1996; 12:385-389.

60.   Johnston J, Kelley RI, Feigenbaum A, et al. Mutation characterization and genotype-phenotype correlation in Barth syndrome. Am J Hum Genet 1997; 61:1053-1058.

61. D'Adamo P, Fassone L, Gedeon A, et al. The X-linked gene G4.5 is responsible for different infantile dilated cardiomyopathies. Am J Hum Genet 1997, 61:862-867.
62. Bowles KR, Tsubata S, Ortiz-Lopez R, et al. The identification of a *G4.5* mutation in a patient with idiopathic dilated cardiomyopathy. Pediatr Res 1998; 43:18A.
63. Bleyl SB, Mumford BR, Thompson V, et al. Neonatal lethal noncompaction of the left ventricular myocardium is allelic with Barth syndrome. Am J Hum Genet 1997, 61:868-872.
64. Orstavik KH, Orstavik RE, Naumova AK, et al. X chromosome inactivation carriers of Barth syndrome. Am J Hum Genet 1998; 63:1457-1463.
65. Dusek J, Ostadal B, Duskova M. Postnatal persistence of spongy myocardium with embryonic blood supply. Arch Pathol 1975; 99:312-317.
66. Jenni R, Goebel N, Tartini R, et al. Persisting myocardial sinusoids of both ventricles as an isolated anomaly: echocardiographic, angiographic, and pathologic anatomical findings. Cardiovasc Intervent Radiol 1986; 9:127-131.
67. Ichida F, Hamamichi Y, Miyawaki T, et al. Clinical features of isolated noncompaction of the ventricular myocardium. Long-term clinical course, hemodynamic properties, and genetic background. J Am Coll Cardiol 1999; 34:233-240.
68. Durand JB, Bachinski LL, Bieling L, et al. 1995; 92:3387-3389.
69. Siu BL, Nimura H, Osborne JA, et al. Familial dilated cardiomyopathy locus maps to chromosome 2q31. Circulation 1999; 99:1022-1026.
70. Li D, Tapscott T, Gonzalez O, et al. Desmin mutations responsible for idiopathic dilated cardiomyopathy. Circulation 1999; 100:461-464.
71. Krajinovic M, Pinamonti B, Sinagra G, et al. Linkage of familial dilated cardiomyopathy to chromosome 9. Am J Hum Genet 1995; 57:846-852.
72. Bowles KR, Gajarski R, Porter P, et al. Gene mapping of familial autosomal dominant dilated cardiomyopathy to chromosome 10q21-23. J Clin Invest 1996 98:1355.
73. Olson TM, Michels W, Thibodeau SN, et al. Actin mutations in dilated cardiomyopathy, a heritable form of heart failure. Science 1998; 280:750-752.
74. Towbin JA. The role of a cytoskeletal proteins in cardiomyopathies. Curr Opin Cell Biol 1998; 10:131-139.
75. Towbin JA, Bowles KR, Bowles NE. Etiologies of cardiomyopathy and heart failure. Evidence for a final common pathway for disorders of the myocardium. Nature Med 1999; 5:266-267.
76. Towbin JA. Toward an understanding of the cause of mitral valve prolapse. Am J Hum Genet 1999; 65:1238-1241.
77. Towbin JA, Roberts R. Cardiovascular Diseases Due to Genetic Abnormalities. In: 'Hurst's The Heart." Alexander RW, Schlant RC, Fuster V, Eds. McGraw-Hill, Inc., Ninth Edition, Chapter 69, pp. 1877-1924, 1998.
78. Mogensen J, Klausen IC, Pedersen AK, et al. α-cardiac actin is a novel disease gene in familial hypertrophic cardiomyopathy. J Clin Invest 1999 103:R39-R43.
79. Fuchs E, Weber K. Intermediate filaments: structure, dynamics, function, and disease. Annu Rev Biochem 1994; 63:345-382.
80. Goldfarb LG, Park KY, Cerenakova L, et al. Missense mutations in desmin associated with familial cardiac and skeletal myopathy. Nat Genet 1998; 19:402-403.
81. Kass S, MacRae C, Graber HL, et al. A gene defect that causes conduction system disease and dilated cardiomyopathy maps to chromosome1p1-1q1. Nat Genet 1994; 7:546-551.
82. Jung M, Poepping I, Perrot A, et al. Investigation of a family with autosomal dominant dilated cardiomyopathy defines a novel locus on chromosome 2q14-q22. Am J Hum Genet 1999 65:1068-1077.
83. Olson TM, Keating MP. Mapping a cardiomyopathy locus to chromosome 3p22-p25. J Clin Invest 1996; 97:528.
84. Messina DN, Speer MC, Pericak-Vance MA, McNally EM. Linkage of familial dilated cardiomyopathy with conduction defect and muscular dystrophy to chromosome 6q23. Am J Hum Genet 1997; 61:909-917.
85. Fatkin D, MacRae C, Sasaki T, et al. Missense mutations in the rod domain of the lamin A/C gene as causes of dilated cardiomyopathy and conduction disease. N Engl J Med 1999 341:1715-1724.
86. Bonnemann CG, Modi R, Noguchi S, et al. β-sarcoglycan (A3b) mutations cause autosomal recessive muscular dystrophy with loss of the sarcoglycan complex. Nat Genet 1995; 11:266-273.

87.   Lim LE, Duclos F, Broux O, et al. β-sarcoglycan: characterization and role in limb-girdle muscular dystrophy linked to 4q12. Nat Genet 1995 11:257-265.

88.   Nigro V, Moreira ES, Piluso G, et al. The 5q autosomal recessive limb-girdle muscular dystrophy (LGMD2F) is caused by a mutation in the δ-sarcoglycan gene. Nat Genet 1996, 14:195-198.

89.   Vainzof M, Passos-Bueno MR, Canovas M, et al. The sarcoglycan complex in the six autosomal recessive limb-girdle muscular dystrophies. Hum Mol Genet 1996 5:1963-1969.

90.   Noguchi S, McNally EM, Ben Othmane K, et al. Mutations in the dystrophin-associated protein δ-sarcoglycan in chromosome 13 muscular dystrophy. Science 1995 270: 819-822.

91.   Araishi K, Sasaoka T, Imamura M, et al. Loss of the sarcoglycan complex and sarcospan leads to muscular dystrophy in β-sarcoglycan-deficient mice. Hum Mol Genet 1999, 8:1589-1598.

92.   Geisterfer-Lowrance AA, Kass S, Tanigawa C, et al. A β-cardiac myosin heavy chain gene missense mutation Cell 1990, 62:999-1006.

93.   Watkins H, Conner D, Thierfelder LC, et al. Mutations in the cardiac myosin binding protein-C gene on chromosome 11 cause familial hypertrophic cardiomyopathy. Nat Genet 1995 11:434-437.

94.   Bonne G, Carrier L, Bercovici J, et al. Cardiac myosin binding protein-C gene splice acceptor site mutation is associated with familial hypertrophic cardiomyopathy. Nat Genet 1995 11:438-445.

95.   Poetter K, Jiang H, Hassanzadeh S. et al. Mutations in either the essential or regulatory light chains of myosin are associated with a rare myopathy in human heart and skeletal muscle. Nat Genet 1996; 13:63-69.

96.   Thierfelder L, Watkins H, MacRae C, et al. α-Tropomyosin and cardiac troponin T mutations cause familial hypertrophic cardiomyopathy: A disease of the sarcomere. Cell 1994 77:701-712.

97.   Kimura A, Harada H, Park JE, et al. Mutations in the cardiac troponin I gene associated with hypertrophic cardiomyopathy. Nat Genet 1997 16:379-389.

98.   Watkins H, Rosenzweig A, Hwang DW, et al. Characteristics and prognostic implications of myosin missense mutations in familial hypertrophic cardiomyopathy. NEngl J Med 1992, 326:1103.

99.   Watkins H, McKenna WJ, Thierfelder L, et al. Mutations in the genes for cardiac troponin T and α-tropomyosin in hypertrophic cardiomyopathy. N Engl J Med 1995 332:1058-1064.

100.   Nimura H, Bachinski LL, Sangwatanaro JS, et al. Mutations in the gene for cardiac myosin-binding protein C and later onset familial hypertrophic cardiomyopathy. N Engl J Med 1998; 338:1248-1257.

101.   Vincent GM. The molecular genetics of the long QT syndrome: genes causing fainting and sudden death. Annu Rev Med 1998, 49:263-274.

102.   Towbin JA, Vatta M, Wang Z, et al. Emerging targets in long QT syndromes and Brugada syndrome. Emerg Therap Targets 1999, 3:423-437.

103.   Chen Q, Kirsch GE, Zhang D, et al. Genetic Basis and Molecular Mechanisms for Idiopathic Ventricular Fibrillation. Nature 1998, 392:293-296.

104.   Maeda M, Holder E, Lowes B, et al. Dilated cardiomyopathy associated with deficiency of the cytoskeletal protein metavinculin. Circulation 1997, 95:17-20.

105.   Fadic R, Sunada Y, Waclawik AJ, et al. Deficiency of a dystrophin-associated glycoprotein (adhalin) in a patient with muscular dystrophy and cardiomyopathy. N Engl J Med 1996, 334:362-366.

106.   McNally EM, Bonnemann CG, Kunkel LM, et al. Deficiency of adhalin in a patient with muscular dystrophy and cardiomyopathy. N Engl J Med 1996 324:1610-1611.

107.   Ohlendieck K, Matsumura K, Ionasescu VV, et al. Duchenne muscular dystrophy: deficiency of dystrophin-associated proteins in theSarcolemma. Neurology 1993; 43:795-800.

108.   Deconinck AE, Rafael JA, Skinner JA, et al. Utrophin-dystrophin-deficient mice as a model for Duchenne muscular dystrophy. Cell 1997 90:717-727.

109.   Grady RM, Teng H, Nichol MC, et al. Skeletal and cardiac Myopathies in mice lacking utrophin and dystrophin: a model for Duchenne muscular dystrophy. Cell 1997:90:729-738.

110.   Nigro V, Okazaki Y, Belsito A, et al. Identification of the Syrian hamster cardiomyopathy gene. Hum Mol Genet 6:601-607, 1997.

111. Sakamoto A, Ono K, Abe M, et al. Both hypertrophic and dilated cardiomyopathies are caused by mutation of the same gene, δ-sarcoglycan, in hamster: an animal model of disrupted dystrophin-associated glycoprotein complex. Proc Natl Acad Sci USA 1997; 94:13873-13878

112. Hack AA, Ly CT, Jiang F, et al. δ-sarcoglycan deficiency leads to muscle membrane defects and apoptosis independent of dystrophin. J CellBiol 1998; 142:1279-1287.

113. Melacini P, Fanin M, Duggan DJ, et al. Heart involvement in muscular dystrophies due to sarcoglycan gene mutations. Muscle & Nerve 1999, 22:473-477.

114. Araishi K, Sasaoka T, Immamma M, et al. Loss of the sarcoglycan complex and sarcospan leads to muscular dystrophy in β-sarcoglycan-deficient mice. Hum Mol Genet 1999, 8:1589-1598.

115. Arber S, Hunter JJ, Ross J Jr. MLP-deficient mice exhibit a disruption of cardiac cytoarchitectural organization, dilated cardiomyopathy, and heart failure. Cell 1997 88:393-403.

116. Helbling-Leclerc A, Zhang X, Topaloglu H, et al. Mutations in the laminin α2-chain gene (LAMA2) cause merosine deficient congenital muscular dystrophy. Nat Genet 1995 11:216-218.

117. McNally EM, Ly CT, Kunkel LM. Human e-sarcoglycan is highly related to α-sarcoglycan (adhalin) the limb girdle muscular dystrophy type 2D gene. FEBSLett 1998; 422:27-32.

118. Metzinger L, Blake DJ, Squier MV, et al. Dystrobrevin deficiency at the sarcolemma of patients with muscular dystrophy. Hum Mol Genet 1997, 6:1185-1191.

119. Duggan DJ, Gorospe JR, Fanin M, et al. Mutations in the sarcoglycan genes in patients with myopathies. N Engl J Med 1997, 336:618-624.

120. Nogami K, Kusachi S, Nunoyama H, et al. Extracellular matrix components in dilated cardiomyopathy. Immunohistochemical study of endomyocardial biopsy specimens Jpn Heart J 1996; 37:483-494.

121. Philpot J, Sewry C, Pennock J, et al. Clinical phenotype in congenital muscular dystrophy: correlation with expression of merosin in skeletal muscle. Neuromuscul Disorder 1995, 5:301-305.

122. McNally EM, de Sa Moreira E, Duggan DJ, et al. Caveolin-3 in muscular dystrophy. Hum Mol Genet 1998; 7:871-877.

123. Ervasti JM, Campbell KP. A role for the dystrophin-glyprotein complex as a transmembrane linker between laminin and actin. J CellBiol 1993; 122:809-823.

124. Badorff C, Lee G-H, Lamphar BJ, et al. Enteroviral protease 2A cleaves dystrophin: evidence of cytoskeletal disruption in acquired cardiomyopathy. Nature Med 1999 5:320-326.

125. Carlquist JF. Menlove RL, Murray MB, et al. HLA Class II (DR and DQ) antigen associations in idiopathic dilated cardiomyopathy: Validation study and meta-analysis of published HLA association studies. Circulation 1991, 83:515-522.

126. Limas CJ, Limas C. HLA-DR antigen linkage of anti-beta receptor antibodies in idiopathic dilated and ischemic cardiomyopathy. Br Heart J 1992, 67:402405.

127. Limas CJ, Limas C, Boudoulas H. HLA-DQA1 and -DQB1 gene haplotypes in familial cardiomyopathy. Am J Cardiol 1994, 74:510-512.

128. Caforio AL, Keeling PJ, Zachara E, et al. Evidence from family studies for autoimmunity in dilated cardiomyopathy. Lancet 1994, 334:773-777.

129. Kuhl U, Noutsias M, Seeberg B, et al. Immunohistological evidence for a chronic intramyocardial inflammatory dilated cardiomyopathy. Heart 1996 75:295-300.

130. Liggett SB, Wagoner LE, Craft LL, et al. The Ile164 β2-adrenerguc receptor polymorphism adversely affects the outcome of congestive heart failure. J Clin Invest 1998 102:1534-1539.

131. Mason DA, Moore JD, Green SA, et al. A gain-of-function polymorphism in a G-protein coupling domain of the human β1-adrenerguc receptor. J Biol Chem 1999, 274:12670-12674.

132. Bristow MR, Ginsbing R, Minobe W, et al. Decreased catecholamine sensitivity and β-adrenergic receptor density in failing human hearts. N Engl J Med 1982 307:205-211.

133. Kadambi VJ, Ponniah S, Harrer JM, et al. Cardiac-specific overexpression of phospholamban alters calcium kinetics and resultant cardiomyocyte mechanics in transgenic mice. J Clin Invest 1996, 97:533-539.

134. Luo W, Grupp IL, Harrer J, et al. Targeted ablation of the phospholamban gene is associated with markedly enhanced myocardial contractility and loss of β-agonist stimulation. Circ Res 1994; 75:401-409.

135.   Engelhardt S, Hein L, Wiesmann F, Lohse MJ. Progressive hypertrophy and heart failure in β1-adrenergic receptor transgenic mice. Proc Natl Acad Sci USA 1999; 96:7059-7064.

136.   Milano CA, Allen LF, Rockman HA, et al. Enhanced myocardial function in transgenic mice overexpressing the β2-adrenergic receptor. Science 1994; 264:582-586.

137.   Iwase M, Bishop SP, Uechi M, et al. Adverse effects of chronic endogenous sympathetic drive induced by cardiac GSα overexpression. Circ Res 1996; 78:517-524.

138.   Koch WJ, Rockman HA, Samama P, et al. Cardiac function in mice overexpressing the β-adrenergic receptor kinase or a βARK inhibitor. Science 1995; 268:1350-1353.

139.   Hunter JJ, Grace AA, Chien KR. Molecular and cellular biology of cardiac hypertrophy and failure. In: Chien KR, ed. Molecular basis of heart disease: a companion to Braunwald's Heart Disease. Philadelphia: W.B.Saunders, 1999, pp 211-250.

140.   Mann DL. Mechanisms and models in heart failure. A combinatorial approach. Circulation 1999; 100:999-1008.

141.   Boxkurt B, Kribbs S, Clubb FJ Jr, et al. Pathophysiologically relevant concentrations of tumor necrosis factor-α promote progressive left ventricular dysfunction and remodeling in rats. Circulation 1998; 97:1382-1391.

142.   Tan LB, Jalil JE, Pick R, et al. Cardiac myocyte necrosis induced by angiotensin II. Circ Res 1991; 69:1185-1195.

143.   Wolny A, Clozel J-P, Rein J, et al. Functional and biochemical analysis of angiotensin II-forming pathways in the human heart. Circ Res 1997; 80:219-227.

144.   Beuckelman DJ, Nabauer M, Erdmann E. Intracellular calcium1992; 85:1046-1055.

145.   Narula J, Haider N, Virmani R, et al. Apoptosis in myocytes in end-stage heart failure. N Engl J Med 1996; 335:1182-1189.

146.   Olivetti G, Abbi R, Quaini F, Kajstura J, Cheng W, Nitahara JA, Quaini E, Di Loretto C, Beltrami CA, Kratewski S, Reed JC, Anversa P. Apoptosis in the failing human heart. N Engl J Med 1997; 336:1131-1141.

147.   Hirota H, Chen J, Betz UAK. Loss of a gp130 cardiac muscle cell survival pathway is a critical event in the onset of heart failure during biochemical stress. Cell 1999; 97:189-198.

148.   Xia Z, Dickens M, Raingeaud J, et al. Opposing effects of ERK and JNK-p38 MAP kinases on apoptosis. Science 1995; 270:1326-1331.

149.   Wang Y, Huang S, Sah VP, et al. Cardiac muscle cell hypertrophy and apoptosis induced by distinct members of the p38 mitogen-activated protein kinase family. J Biol Chem 1998; 273:2161-2168.

150.   Bowles NE, Towbin JA. Molecular aspects of myocarditis. Curr Opin Cardiol 1998; 13:179-184.

151.   Li YY, Feldman AM, Sun Y, et al. Differential expression of tissue inhibitors of metalloproteinases in the failing human heart. Circulation 1998; 98:1728-1734.

152.   Tyagi SC, Campbell SE, Reddy HK, et al. Matrix metalloproteinase activity expression in infarcted, noninfarcted and dilated cardiomyopathic human hearts. Mol Cell Biochem 1996; 155:13-21.

153.   Om A, Hess ML. Inotrophic therapy of the failing myocardium. Clin Cardiol 1992; 16:5-14.

154.   Konstam MA, Cody RJ. Short-term use of intravenous milrinone for heart failure. Am J Cardiol 1995; 75:822.

155.   Bristow MR. Pathophysiologic and pharmacologic rationales for clinical management of chronic heart failure with beta-blocking agents. Am J Cardiol 1993; 71:12C-22C.

156.   Nishimura RA, Hayes DL, Holmes DR, et al: Mechanism of hemodynamic improvement by dual-chamber pacing for severe left ventricular dysfunction: An acute Doppler and catheterization hemodynamic study. J Am Coll Cardiol 1995; 25:281-288.

157.   Mason JW, O'Connell JB, Herskowitz A, et al: A clinical trial of immunosuppressive therapy for myocarditis. N Engl J Med 1995; 333:269-275.

158.   Parrillo JE, Cunnion RE, Epstein SE, et al: A prospective, randomized controlled trial of prednisone for dilated cardiomyopathy. N Engl J Med 1989; 321:1061-1068.

14
GLYCOGEN STORAGE DISEASES

**Mira Irons M.D., Division of Genetics and Metabolism
and Ellen Roy Elias M.D., Director, Coordinated Care Service**
*Department of Medicine, Children's Hospital • Boston
Department of Pediatrics, Harvard Medical School, Boston, MA 02115*

INTRODUCTION

The glycogen storage diseases are inherited inborn errors of metabolism that affect glycogen metabolism. They are numbered (I-VII) in the order that they were described, although there are several other metabolic disorders that also affect glycogen metabolism (1,2).

Glycogen is the main storage form of glucose in all cells, but is most abundant in cells of the liver and muscle. The body takes up glucose and stores it as glycogen when energy is not needed, and then has the ability to convert the glycogen into glucose during periods of increased energy demand. The different cells in the body utilize glycogen differently. The liver takes up glucose and converts and stores it as glycogen after a meal, and then releases the glycogen as glucose into the bloodstream so that it can be utilized by tissues which cannot make enough themselves during periods of energy demand. Skeletal muscle stores glycogen and then utilizes it as a quickly available short-term fuel source.

The clinical symptoms seen in the various glycogen storage diseases are determined by the tissues affected by the enzyme deficiency (liver, muscle, both) and by the consequence of the biochemical deficiency. Cardiac manifestations are generally seen in the glycogen storage disorders affecting muscle, although cardiac problems secondary to hyperlipidemia can also be seen in GSD I.

GLYCOGEN STORAGE DISEASE I

BACKGROUND/INTRODUCTION

GSD I was the first type of glycogen storage disease described by von Gierke in 1929. Since there are no specific cardiac problems seen in patients with this disorder, only a brief review of its features will be discussed here. For more information, the reader is directed to more detailed reviews (1,2).

There are four subtypes of GSD I. The most common, called GSD Ia, was the form initially described by von Gierke in 1929, and has been also called "von Gierke disease." Patients with this form have deficiency of the enzyme glucose-6-phosphatase which is inherited in an autosomal recessive manner. GSD Ia has an overall frequency of approximately 1 in 100,000 live births.

Later described subtypes include Type Ib which is due to a defect in the microsomal membrane transport system of glucose-6-phosphate, Type Ic which is due to a defect in microsomal phosphate or pyrophosphate transport, and Type Id which is due to a defect in microsomal glucose transport.

CLINICAL PRESENTATION

Patients with GSD I generally present at 3-4 months of age with hepatomegaly and/or hypoglycemia, although there may be a history of hypoglycemia and lactic acidosis in the neonatal period. Physical examination is remarkable for a significantly protuberant abdomen, thin extremities, and full cheeks with a doll-like facial appearance. Other clinical problems include hyperlipidemia, leading to xanthomas of the skin and characteristic retinal changes, enlarged kidneys, and bruising and epistaxis secondary to impaired platelet function. Hypoglycemia with seizures is common after relatively short periods of fasting.

Long-term complications include growth retardation, delayed puberty, gout secondary to hyperuricemia, pancreatitis secondary to the hyperlipidemia, hepatic adenomas, and progresssive renal disease which can lead to renal failure.

Although there are no specific cardiac manifestations of this disorder, there have been three patients identified with pulmonary hypertension who died of progressive heart failure. The first patient had a portacaval shunt performed at age 12, and then developed pulmonary hypertension of the vasoconstrictive type and died suddenly at 16-1/2 years of age (3). The other two patients died at 12 and 16 years of age of progressive cardiac failure and did not have any clinical evidence of portal hypertension, liver cirrhosis, or other disorders that would predispose to pulmonary hypertension. While the pulmonary hypertension was felt to be primary in the first patient, the second patient had a shunt operation between the intestinal vein and inferior vena cava performed at 10 years of age and chronic asymptomatic pulmonary embolism could not be ruled out (4). An additional cardiac risk may be the development of atherosclerosis secondary to long-term hyperlipidemia and hypertriglyceridemia although this has not been reported in this group of patients, since even on nocturnal feedings many patients continue to have low HDL-C, high LDL-C, and high triglyceride levels (5).

Patients with GSD Ib have neutropenia and recurrent bacterial infections in addition to the other symptoms of GSD I. Inflammatory bowel disease has been reported in these patients. Although there have only been a few patients reported with GSD Ic and GSD Id GSD, there is no characteristic clinical presentation and patients have presented with a similar course to that seen in GSD I.

LABORATORY FINDINGS/DIAGNOSIS

The clinical presentation is generally characteristic enough to make one think of this diagnosis. The characteristic laboratory findings include hypoglycemia, hyperuricemia, hyperlipidemia, and elevated lactate levels. Liver transaminases may or may not be elevated. A glucagon stimulation test does not result in elevation of glucose, but does result in elevation of lactate levels. Renal tubular abnormalities can result in hypercalciuria, proteinuria, and aminoaciduria.

Definitive diagnosis depends upon demonstration of deficient enzyme activity in liver. The enzyme cannot be measured in skin fibroblasts or blood cells. Impaired glucose uptake in neutrophils can be seen in patients with GSD Ib.

MANAGEMENT/TREATMENT

Treatment has been directed toward avoidance of fasting and the resultant hypoglycemia by various methods, including frequent feedings, nighttime continuous nasogastric feedings, the administration of uncooked corn starch, and total parenteral nutrition. Intake of fructose and galactose should be restricted since these cannot be converted to free glucose, and allopurinol may be required for treatment of the hyperuricemia.

While portacaval shunts and liver transplantation have been performed, the results of dietary management have been encouraging enough that these therapies should not be necessary. Liver transplantation may still be required to treat malignant transformation of a hepatic adenoma. Renal transplantation may be required to treat renal failure.

Patients with GSD I who require surgery should receive intravenous fluids with glucose, and should not receive Lactated Ringer's solution. They should also have evaluation of their coagulation status, with particular attention to testing bleeding time prior to any surgery.

Granulocyte stimulating factors have been used for patients with GSD Ib.

CLINICAL GENETICS

GSD I is inherited as an autosomal recessive disorder. Carrier testing is possible by molecular mutation testing after identification of mutations in an affected proband in the family. Prenatal diagnosis has been reported by measurement of enzyme activity in fetal liver biopsy and is also possible in at-risk cases by molecular testing described below.

MOLECULAR GENETICS

The gene for this disorder is located on chromosome 17q21, is composed of five exons, and spans 12.5 kb. Multiple mutations have been identified in different populations studied which by expression studies have been shown to abolish or greatly reduce glucose-6-phosphatase activity and are therefore believed to be disease-producing alleles. Lei and colleagues used SSCP analysis and DNA sequencing to characterize the GSD Ia gene and reported sixteen different mutations in 70 patients studied, detecting mutations in all except for 17 alleles (88%). The R83C and Q347X mutations are the most prevalent mutations found in Caucasians, 130X and R83C are the most prevalent in Hispanics, and R83H is the most prevalent mutation in Chinese patients. The Q347X and the 130X appear to be exclusively found in Caucasian and Hispanic patients, respectively (6). Nine mutations were reported in French patients with GSD Ia,with the five mutations, Q347X, R83C, D38V, G188R, and 158delC, accounting for 75% of the mutated alleles (7). The R83C mutation also appears to be commonly found in Jewish patients studied in Israel (8).

In the study by Lei and colleagues, 43% of the mutations identified contained a mutation that altered codon 83, either R83C or R83H. These two mutations occur at a CpG dinucleotide that involves either a C to T transition at nucleotide 326 (R83C) or a G to A transition at nucleotide 327 (R83H). Cytosine methylation at CpG dinucleotides has been shown to cause other genetic disorders. The CpG dinucleotide at codon 83 of the glucose-6-phosphatase gene also appears to be a hotspot for mutations in GSD Ia (6).

Identification of these mutations now allows for non-invasive diagnostic testing, as well as carrier testing, and prenatal testing by means of either amniocentesis or chorionic villus sampling.

GLYCOGEN STORAGE DISEASE II

BACKGROUND/INTRODUCTION

GSD II is the paradigm of lysosomal storage diseases, and is the first human disorder found to be associated with intracellular glycogen storage. The classic form of this disorder was originally described by Pompe in 1932 when he reported a 7 month old girl who died of severe hypertrophic cardiomyopathy (9). He was the first to appreciate that the cardiomegaly in his patient was associated with massive glycogen accumulation in cardiac tissue.

GSD II is an autosomal recessive disorder. The enzymatic defect was discovered in 1963 to be a deficiency in the enzyme acid α-glucosidase, also known as acid maltase. Patients with the infantile form of GSD II (Pompe's disease) have total absence of this enzyme in fibroblasts and muscle, while patients with the childhood and adult forms have a partial enzyme deficiency (10). The gene for α-glucosidase has been mapped to chromosome 17q23.

Glycogen accumulates in all tissues in the infantile form of GSD II, resulting in a multisystem disease that is usually lethal within the first year of life. Following the description of the infantile form, childhood and adult variants of GSD II were also described. The adult form consists of progressive proximal muscle weakness, but is not associated with cardiac pathology. The childhood form is intermediate in severity between the infantile and adult forms, and also usually spares the heart, although rarely cardiac involvement has been reported.

CLINICAL PRESENTATION

Pompe's disease (Infantile GSD II):

Infants with GSD II present in the first 6 months of life, with macroglossia, hepatomegaly, hypotonia, progressive onset of feeding and respiratory issues, progressive congestive heart failure secondary to cardiomyopathy, and usually death secondary to cardiorespiratory failure within the first year of life. The cardiac manifestations of Pompe's disease include progressive biventricular and septal hypertrophy, resulting in loss of ventricular cavity size and outflow tract obstruction (11). Cardiomegaly is apparent on chest radiograph and echocardiogram. EKG changes include large QRS complexes, and a shortened PR interval. Muscle weakness develops proximally, involving skeletal and respiratory muscles to a profound degree. Despite progressive muscle involvement, cognitive development is generally spared.

A variant of the infantile form may present prior to age 6 months, with predominantly skeletal muscle disease, but minimal cardiac involvement, and no hepatomegaly or macroglossia, similar to the childhood onset disease described below. These infants may be misdiagnosed with spinal muscular atrophy (Werdnig-Hoffman disease).

Childhood or Juvenile Onset GSD II

Children with this form usually present with proximal muscle weakness, at some time during later infancy or early childhood. The earlier the presentation, the greater the likelihood that there will be associated cardiac involvement: presentation prior to age 2 years is associated with an 80% chance of cardiomegaly, while children presenting older than age 2 usually have symptoms isolated to the skeletal and respiratory muscles, but do not have cardiac involvement. Hepatomegaly and macroglossia are rarely seen in this group. Death is usually due to respiratory failure and occurs by the end of the second decade. Children with childhood onset GSD II may be misdiagnosed as having muscular dystrophy.

Adult Onset GSD II

Adults with this form present with slowly progressive proximal muscle and respiratory muscle weakness, with no evidence of cardiac disease. Symptoms may start at any time after the second decade, and may be predominantly respiratory, or initially muscular with progressive weakness of the trunk and lower extremities. Deep tendon reflexes are eventually lost. Death ultimately occurs secondary to respiratory failure. Patients may be misdiagnosed with polymyositis.

LABORATORY FINDINGS/DIAGNOSIS

The diagnosis is confirmed by measurement of α-glucosidase enzyme activity in either cultured fibroblasts or muscle in patients who present with clinical symptoms as noted above. Infants with Pompe's disease demonstrate undetectable levels of enzyme activity, while patients with the childhood or adult onset forms have partial enzyme deficiency.

Associated laboratory abnormalities include elevation in serum creatine kinase (CK), which is more pronounced in patients with the infantile form than the other forms. Liver function tests, including AST and LDH, may also be elevated in patients with the infantile form of the disorder.

Microscopic evaluation of muscle biopsy specimens demonstrates intracellular vacuoles which stain positive for glycogen. Patients with the infantile form have increased glycogen content over ten times normal. The glycogen may be present in vacuoles, and also may be dispersed within the cytoplasm of the cell. Patients with the adult form may have variably increased glycogen content, with more severely affected muscles demonstrating a greater degree of glycogen accumulation.

Patients with Pompe's disease have been found at autopsy to have massive glycogen storage in multiple tissue sites, including the heart, eyes, kidneys, skin, smooth muscle and lymphocytes, as well as skeletal muscle. Glycogen deposition also affects the central nervous system, including the spinal cord and brainstem, but appears to spare the cerebral cortex. Patients with the adult-onset form have glycogen storage only in skeletal muscle, sparing these other sites.

Prenatal diagnosis is possible, by measurement of α-glucosidase activity in either chorionic villus biopsy specimens, or cultured amniocytes. Measurement of enzyme activity in amniotic fluid is not reliable, due to the presence of renal neutral α-glucosidase, which interferes with the assay.

DNA mutational analysis can also be offered to families, and used as a tool for heterzygote detection in family members at risk, and for prenatal diagnosis in subsequent pregnancies in couples with a previously affected child with an identified mutation.

MANAGEMENT/TREATMENT

There is no treatment currently available for patients with GSD II, other than palliative intervention. Research into the biochemical and molecular basis of this interesting yet devastating disease may some day yield greater insights into the correlation between genotype and phenotype. Future therapeutic intervention via either enzyme replacement or gene therapy may someday be feasible.

CLINICAL GENETICS

GSD II is inherited as an autosomal recessive disorder. Healthy parents who are obligate heterozygotes have been shown to have diminished α-glucosidase activity. However, there is overlap between enzyme levels of heterozygotes and normal controls, and therefore heterozygote testing is better performed by testing for DNA mutations rather than enzyme activity.

GSD II is usually clinically similar in affected siblings, although some variability has been reported. The gene frequency is different in different ethnic groups. It is particularly common in patients from southern China, where the incidence is approximately 1:50,000, and GSD II (Pompe's) is the most common form of glycogen storage disease. In western countries, the incidence is less than 1: 100,000, and GSD II accounts for only about 15% of GSD cases.

MOLECULAR GENETICS

The gene for GSD II has been mapped to chromosome 17q25.2-q25.3 (12). Reported mutations have been predominantly missense mutations, but nonsense and splice site mutations and deletions have also been described. The structural gene for GSD II is composed of 20 exons. There is conservation of several regions, including the catalytic site of the enzyme, with homology of the coding sequence across multiple species including yeast, rabbit, mouse and human DNA. There is also homology between the human α-glucosidase gene and the genes for human, rabbit and rat sucrase-isomaltase. A majority of the identified α-glucosidase gene mutations are located in these highly conserved regions of DNA (13).

The active site of human α-glucosidase is located in codons 513-524, with an essential Asp 518 necessary for catalytic activity. Mutation at this site has been shown to reduce activity significantly. For example, substitution of either glycine, glutamic acid or asparagine at ASP 518 reduces enzyme activity to between 4-10 percent of normal.

The study of the molecular structure of the α-glucosidase gene has led to a better understanding of the biochemical processing and functioning of its protein. The α-glucosidase protein undergoes extensive post-translational modification including glycosylation and phosphorylation, to allow it to be targeted to the lysosome, its active site. Mutations that alter this modification process have been shown to alter enzyme activity. For example, deletion of codon 233, a known glycosylation site, prevents lysosomal localization and reduces enzyme activity to 20 % of normal.

There are 3 allelic forms of human α-glucosidase, GAAI, GAA2, and GAA4, which represent normal genetic polymorphism. GAA2 is the most rare, and GAA1 the most common. There are also several isoenzymes of α-glucosidase, with limited expression in different tissues (including kidney, lung, intestine and white blood cells), and are linked to different genetic loci. These isoenzymes may occasionally interfere with diagnostic enzyme assays, as noted above for prenatal testing.

There have been insufficient cases where molecular testing has been performed to date, to allow for a correlation between specific gene mutation and clinical phenotype. This correlation may be possible in the future, as novel mutations continue to be identified.

GLYCOGEN STORAGE DISEASE III

BACKGROUND/INTRODUCTION

GSD III is caused by deficiency of the glycogen debrancher enzyme. This enzyme is a protein with both amylo-1,6-glucosidase and 1,4-α-D-glucan 4-α-D-glycosyltransferase activities at two independent catalytic sites. This disorder was first described in 1952, and has also been called "limit dextrinosis", "Cori", or "Forbes" disease. This deficiency results in inability to release glucose from glycogen, but does not affect gluconeogenesis. Patients with both liver and muscle symptomatology have an enzyme deficiency in both tissues, but those with liver disease only have the enzyme deficiency limited to that organ alone. GSD III is inherited by autosomal recessive inheritance.

CLINICAL PRESENTATION

GSD III has been divided into two forms, GSD IIIa and GSD IIIb, on the basis of clinical presentation. Patients with GSD IIIa have both liver and muscle involvement (approximately 85%), while those with GSD IIIb have only liver involvement. In rare cases, selective loss of only one of the two activities has been reported. These rare subtypes have been called GSD IIIc and IIId, for loss of the glucosidase and transferase respectively (14,15). However, clinical variability is seen in this disorder so that there is no single predominant clinical presentation.

Early in life, hepatomegaly, hypoglycemia, hyperlipidemia, and growth retardation are commonly seen. These symptoms are not unlike those seen in GSD I, although they are generally milder in GSD III. The involvement of skeletal and cardiac muscle should make one consider GSD III. While liver symptoms improve with age and have often resolved by puberty, muscle symptoms (progressive weakness, distal muscle wasting) are variable and slowly progress as patients grow older. The timing of development of liver and/or muscle symptoms varies considerably and each can present at different ages, and in a different order. Liver cirrhosis, although rare, has been reported. Age of symptom onset varies from infancy to adulthood.

Cardiac manifestations have included ECG abnormalities indicative of ventricular hypertrophy, cardiomyopathy, and cardiomegaly. Cardiomyopathy is generally asymptomatic and in many cases identifiable only with echocardiography. Labrune and colleagues found no relationship between the skeletal myopathy and cardiomyopathy, and also that serum creatine kinase activity, chest radiography, and ECG were not valuable tools in determining which patients had cardiomyopathy. They stressed the need for echocardiography as a routine diagnostic test that should be performed intermittently, as these patients may become symptomatic during periods of increased cardiac demand (16). Clinical cardiac failure has been reported, associated with elevated glycogen content and decreased debrancher enzyme activity in an endomyocardial biopsy (17).

LABORATORY FINDINGS/DIAGNOSIS

Abnormal laboratory findings include hypoglycemia, hyperlipidemia, and elevated liver transaminases, lactate dehydrogenase, and alkaline phosphatase early in life when hepatic symptoms predominate. These levels normalize with age and as the liver disease improves. Creatine kinase activity is variably elevated, but can be normal, and is generally non-predictive of muscle involvement. Uric acid and lactate levels are usually normal. Nerve conduction velocity may be abnormal, and electromyography shows myopathic changes. Nonspecific ECG abnormalities and changes suggestive of ventricular hypertrophy are also seen.

Liver pathology is notable for increased amounts of glycogen within hepatocytes and fibrosis. The elevated glycogen is also structurally abnormal, characterized by short outer branches.

Diagnosis depends upon demonstration of enzyme deficiency in liver and/or muscle. The enzyme can also be measured in cultured skin fibroblasts, lymphocytes, and erythrocytes in some patients. However, liver and/or muscle tissue are recommended for definitive diagnosis and also to determine which form of the disorder is present.

MANAGEMENT/TREATMENT

Treatment of this form of glycogen storage disease is mainly directed toward treatment of hypoglycemia with continuous feedings at night or uncooked cornstarch. A high protein diet has been suggested in those with the myopathic form of the disorder (18).

CLINICAL GENETICS

GSD III is inherited in an autosomal recessive manner and has been reported in all ethnic backgrounds, although there appears to be a high incidence in non-Ashkenazic Jews of North African ancestry. Heterozygote detection has been reported by enzyme assay in erythrocytes. Prenatal diagnosis is available by measurement of enzyme activity in tissue obtained by either amniocentesis or chorionic villus sampling.

MOLECULAR GENETICS

The gene for this enzyme has been localized to chromosome 1p21 and is encoded by 35 exons spanning at least 85 kb of DNA. Molecular analysis has been performed on patients with both the IIIa and IIIb forms of the disorder. Most patients are compound heterozygotes for two different mutations. While some mutations can be seen in both type IIIa and type IIIb patients, exon three mutations appear to be specific for type IIIb, and therefore may be useful for diagnostic testing and distinguishing these two forms of the disorder. This testing can be useful as well for prenatal or carrier testing, although it is estimated that the mutations identified thus far account for less than 30% of the total mutant alleles in GSD III (19,20).

GLYCOGEN STORAGE DISEASE IV

BACKGROUND/INTRODUCTION

GSD IV is caused by deficiency of the branching enzyme (amylo(1,4 to 1,6) transglucosidase) and was first described in 1956. It has also been called "Andersen disease" or "amylopectinosis". Deficiency of the enzyme results in accumulation of glycogen with unbranched, long outer chains which resemble amylopectin. It is inherited by autosomal recessive inheritance.

CLINICAL PRESENTATION

The classic form of this disorder presents early in life with hepatosplenomegaly and failure to thrive, which generally progresses to liver cirrhosis and early death. Affected patients can also present with signs of myopathy (hypotonia, weakness) and/or peripheral neuropathy (absent or diminished reflexes).

Severe cardiomyopathy has also been reported as the main presenting problem in an older child (21), and in an infant presenting with hypotonia and cardiomyopathy in the neonatal period (22). Two brothers presenting with dilated cardiomyopathy in their teens who presented with heart failure and skeletal myopathy with GSD IV have also been reported (23).

Rare patients have been reported who present later in life with the classic presentation, as well as those whose liver disease does not progress, and others whose symptoms are confined to the nervous system alone.

LABORATORY FINDINGS/DIAGNOSIS

Hypoglycemia may develop as the liver disease progresses and the liver is no longer able to mobilize glucose. Otherwise, there are no other characteristically abnormal laboratory findings.

Pathologic examination of tissues of affected patients reveals deposition of a structurally abnormal glycogen resembling amylopectin. Deposition of this amylopectin-like material is generalized and can be seen in liver, heart, muscle, skin, intestine, brain, spinal cord, and peripheral nerve, and is demonstrated by its distinct staining properties and its electron microscopic appearance. Light microscopy reveals fibrosis, distorted architecture, and cytoplasmic inclusions. Since the condition polysaccharidosis can have similar pathologic findings with normal enzyme activity (24), the diagnosis of GSD IV depends upon demonstration of deficient branching chain activity. Deficiency of the enzyme can be demonstrated in liver, muscle, skin fibroblasts, white blood cells, and erythrocytes.

MANAGEMENT/TREATMENT

There is no specific long-term treatment for this disorder. Maintenance of good nutrition and prevention of hypoglycemia as the liver disease progresses, may retard the progression of the liver or muscle disease.

Liver transplantation has been reported and the results have been mixed. Some patients died after the transplant, while others have survived with improved growth and no progression of neuromuscular or myocardial disease for up to 6 years (25). A decrease in amylopectin deposits in the myocardium has been reported post-liver transplant (26). Since this is a multisystem disorder which varies with time and between patients, it is difficult to predict the long-term efficacy of liver transplantation at this time.

CLINICAL GENETICS

GSD IV is inherited by autosomal recessive inheritance. Carrier detection is available by demonstration of reduced enzyme activity in skin fibroblasts, white blood cells, or erythrocytes. Prenatal diagnosis is available by enzymatic analysis of tissue obtained by either amniocentesis or chorionic villus sampling.

MOLECULAR GENETICS

The human gene for this enzyme has been localized to chromosome 3p12, and the coding sequence contains 2,106 base pairs encoding a protein containing 702 amino acids. Point mutations and deletions causing missense and nonsense mutations have been reported (27). The latter authors feel that all clinical forms of GSD IV are caused by mutations of the same gene, but that some enzyme activity is retained in those presenting with more mild disease.

GLYCOGEN STORAGE DISEASE V

BACKGROUND/INTRODUCTION

GSD V is caused by deficiency of muscle phosphorylase activity and was first recognized in 1951. It is also known as "McArdle disease". It is inherited as an autosomal recessive disorder.

CLINICAL PRESENTATION

Most patients present in the second or third decade with muscle cramps during exercise, as well as other symptoms of exercise intolerance (muscle tenderness, weakness). Some patients also have associated myoglobinuria secondary to rhabdomyolysis. Rare reports of renal failure secondary to severe myoglobinuria have been reported. Symptoms subside with cessation of the activity and rest. Gout and renal calculi have been reported secondary to hyperuricemia.

Since mobilization of glycogen for energy is the major fuel source utilized by muscle during intense exercise and during the early periods of less intense exercise, patients with GSD V have the majority of their symptoms during these periods. They are less symptomatic during sustained exercise of longer duration when energy comes from that mobilized from fatty acids. This explains the "second wind" phenomenon noted in many patients who can resume exercise at a slower pace after the initial symptoms.

While symptoms are less common in childhood, some affected patients do have a history of intermittent myoglobinuria or of fatigue or weakness in childhood. Patients with the classic form of the disorder presenting many years later than the second or third decade have also been reported.

There have been rare variant forms of the disorder characterized by presentation in infancy with severe hypotonia, weakness, respiratory insufficiency, and congenital arthrogryposis. One infant died of severe respiratory insufficiency at twelve weeks of age. She was apparently normal for the first four weeks of life, and then developed hypotonia, weakness, and began to tire easily. She had no evidence of cardiomegaly or heart failure, and died of respiratory insufficiency (28). It is unclear why this severe presentation is so unlike the presentation seen in the more common form of the disorder described above.

There are no specific cardiac manifestations of this disorder.

LABORATORY FINDINGS/DIAGNOSIS

Affected patients often have elevated levels of creatine kinase, ammonia, inosine, hypoxanthine, and uric acid, which rise further following exercise. Muscle pathology may show nonspecific findings and glycogen may be noted between myofibrils.

Elevation of ammonia and lack of elevation of lactate and pyruvate after an ischemic exercise test is seen in GSD V in addition to the other glycogen storage diseases that result in abnormalities of glycogenolysis. Therefore, while this test is abnormal in GSD V, it is not specific. Phosphorus magnetic resonance imaging is also abnormal in affected patients and may be of benefit.

The diagnosis of GSD V is confirmed by demonstration of deficient enzyme activity in muscle.

MANAGEMENT/TREATMENT

There is no specific treatment for this disorder. Most patients learn to adjust their activities and exercise in a manner that does not cause abnormal symptoms.

CLINICAL GENETICS

GSD V is inherited by autosomal recessive inheritance. Enzyme measurement in muscle or phosphorus magnetic resonance imaging can be used for carrier detection.

MOLECULAR GENETICS

The human gene for GSD V has been mapped to chromosome 11q13. Molecular analysis has revealed that the most common mutation is a nonsense mutation that substitutes thymine for cytosine at codon 49 (Arg49Stop), while other missense and nonsense mutations, as well as deletions have been identified (29,30). While many patients are homozygous for the common mutation, others are compound heterozygotes for the common mutation and others, or for two other mutations. It is estimated that molecular testing can be useful for diagnosis in approximately 90% of patients (29). There does not appear to be any specific genotype-phenotype correlation noted at this time.

Rare instances of autosomal dominant transmission have been reported. Molecular testing may be helpful in explaining these rare families, as one family with what appeared to be autosomal dominant transmission of this disorder was actually found to have three different mutations present in the same family (29).

GLYCOGEN STORAGE DISEASE VI

BACKGROUND/INTRODUCTION

GSD VI is due to decreased activity of the hepatic phosphorylase system which actually represents a group of enzymatic reactions stimulated by glucagon. This system is the rate-limiting system of glycogenolysis. At the present time, GSD VI is comprised of a defect in liver phosphorylase alone or of one of the four subunits of phosphorylase kinase. Phosphorylase kinase deficiency can be divided into several subtypes based on the tissues affected (liver, blood, muscle, heart, or some combination of these) and the mode of inheritance (autosomal recessive vs. X-linked recessive). In the past, the autosomal recessive form of phosphorylase kinase deficiency had been called GSD IX, but is now generally classified as a form of GSD VI.

CLINICAL PRESENTATION/LABORATORY

Because GSD VI is made up of a group of different enzymatic defects with different tissue specificity, there is no one characteristic clinic presentation. The clinical and laboratory findings will be addressed together in this section.

Patients with liver phosphorylase deficiency present with a benign disorder characterized by hepatomegaly and growth retardation first noted in childhood. Some patients may have hypoglycemia, ketosis, and hyperlipidemia, although usually mild. In contrast to GSD I lactate and uric acid levels are generally normal. Mild developmental delay has been noted early in life, which resolves with age. The hepatomegaly resolves with age and usually disappears by puberty. There are no muscle or cardiac manifestations. This disorder is inherited by autosomal recessive inheritance and has been called "Hers disease".

The most common form of GSD VI is due to the X-linked recessive deficiency of liver phosphorylase kinase. Affected patients present in childhood with hepatomegaly, growth retardation, and variable hypoglycemia, hyperlipidemia, and elevation of the liver transaminases. These findings resolve with age with most affected adults having no clinical problems, so that this is generally considered to be a benign disorder. Most patients attain a normal adult height. Histologic examination of the liver reveals increased amounts of glycogen. Fibrous septal formation and inflammatory changes have also been reported. Decreased enzyme activity can be demonstrated in liver, red and white blood cells, and skin fibroblasts, but not in muscle.

Patients with phosphorylase kinase deficiency that affects both liver and muscle have also been reported. These patients present with hypotonia and other muscle symptomatology in addition to the clinical presentation described in the preceding paragraph. Decreased enzyme activity in muscle has been shown in some affected patients. This is presumed to be inherited by autosomal recessive inheritance.

Patients with phosphorylase kinase deficiency confined to muscle alone and presenting with symptoms of muscle disease alone have also been reported. Clinical presentation is not unlike that of GSD V. Patients present in the second or third decade of life with muscle cramps and myoglobinuria with exercise, along with a history of muscle weakness and atrophy. Muscle biopsies reveal glycogen deposition and deficient enzyme activity. Enzyme activity is normal in liver and blood cells. This is presumed to be inherited by autosomal recessive inheritance.

Rare cases of phosphorylase kinase deficiency confined to the heart presenting in infancy have been reported. Servidei and colleagues reported an infant who presented in cardiac failure and died suddenly of cardiac arrest at four months of age (31). Echocardiogram prior to death revealed a massive hypertrophic cardiomyopathy and endocardial fibroelastosis of the left ventricle. Post-mortem studies revealed greater than a ten-fold increase of glycogen in the heart, with no increase in glycogen in skeletal muscle or liver. The activity of phosphorylase kinase was undetectable in heart, but normal in muscle, liver, and kidney. This patient was similar to two previously reported patients (32,33). This disorder is presumed to be due to an autosomal recessive deficiency of phosphorylase kinase which affects a heart-specific subunit of the enzyme.

DIAGNOSIS

Elevated glycogen content can be noted by histologic examination of the tissues involved (liver, skeletal muscle, or heart). Since the enzyme deficiency can be isolated to a specific tissue, definitive diagnosis depends upon demonstration of the enzyme deficiency in the specific tissue involved.

MANAGEMENT/TREATMENT

Treatment of the hepatic form of the disorder is generally not necessary since it is benign and tends to improve over time. If hypoglycemia is present, treatment with frequent feedings and/or a diet high in carbohydrate has been used. Prolonged fasting should be avoided. There is no treatment for the forms of the disorder that affect skeletal or cardiac muscle.

CLINICAL GENETICS

All forms other than the X-linked form of liver phosphorylase deficiency are inherited by autosomal recessive inheritance. The liver phosphorylase gene has been mapped to human chromosome 14, while the X-linked phosphorylase kinase gene has been mapped to Xp22. Carriers have been noted to have intermediate enzyme activities for some of these disorders.

MOLECULAR GENETICS

The gene for liver phosphorylase has been mapped to human chromosome 14 (14q21-q22). Several splice site and missense mutations have been identified in affected patients (34). A splice site abnormality in a Mennonite family was identified which is estimated to be present in 3% of the Mennonite population and can be used for disease and carrier detection in this population (35).

The gene for the X-linked form of phosphorylase kinase deficiency has been mapped to human chromosome Xp22.1-22.2. There is no molecular testing available for the cardiac specific form of phosphorylase kinase deficiency.

GLYCOGEN STORAGE DISEASE VII

BACKGROUND/INTRODUCTION

GSD VII was first described in 1965 and is caused by deficiency of phosphofructokinase. Phosphofructokinase is a tetrameric enzyme with M (muscle), L (liver), and P (platelet) subunits. Muscle expresses only the M subunit, while red cells express both the M- and L-subunits. This disorder is inherited by autosomal recessive inheritance and has also been called "Tarui disease."

CLINICAL PRESENTATION

Patients with GSD VII have a similar clinical presentation to those with GSD V, and generally present with exercise-induced fatigue and muscle cramps/pain and myoglobinuria. These symptoms may start in childhood and are more severe than those in patients with GSD V and may be associated with nausea and vomiting. Symptoms are also more severe after a high-carbohydrate diet and may be due to inhibition of lipolysis by glucose with resultant deficiency of an available energy source (36). Affected patients can also present with jaundice secondary to a hemolytic anemia due to abnormality of red cell phosphofructokinase isozyme. A later-onset variant has also been described which presents later in adult life and has a course characterized more by muscle weakness. Gout has been reported in some patients secondary to prolonged hyperuricemia.

A fatal, multisystem infantile variant of this disorder has been described by several authors characterized by a rapidly progressive myopathy and neurologic symptoms (37,38). Cardiomyopathy has been reported in this form of the disorder (39).

LABORATORY FINDINGS/DIAGNOSIS

Elevated bilirubin levels, reticulocyte counts, creatine kinase, and uric acid levels are seen in affected patients, which increase with exercise. Excessive elevation of uric acid, inosine, hypoxanthine, and ammonia with no rise in lactate and pyruvate are seen during the ischemic exercise test.

Muscle histology reveals the presence of an abnormal polysaccharide that resembles amylopectin that can also be seen in GSD IV.

Definitive diagnosis is established by demonstration of the enzyme deficiency in muscle. Patients with the classical form of the disorder have a genetic defect of the M-subunit of the enzyme which results in deficiency of the enzyme in muscle and approximately 50% activity in red blood cells which also express the L-subunit. Patients with the later-onset form have both M-and L-subunits in their red blood cells.

MANAGEMENT/TREATMENT

The only form of treatment of this disorder is avoidance of sudden, strenuous exercise. Glucose-induced exertional fatigue has been reported in affected patients and may have some therapeutic implications (36). There is no treatment for the severe infantile form of this disorder.

CLINICAL GENETICS

The gene for this disorder has been localized to human chromosome 12q13.3 and it is inherited by autosomal recessive inheritance. Carriers have been reported to have decreased enzyme activity.

MOLECULAR GENETICS

Multiple mutations have been reported in patients with GSD VII. Many patients are compound heterozygotes for the various mutations. Raben and Sherman reported 15 mutations and several polymorphisms in individuals of Ashkenazi Jewish descent. A splice site defect of exon 5 accounted for 2/3 of the mutant alleles in this ethnic group (40).

CONCLUSIONS

While much has been learned about this group of disorders since the original description of GSD I by von Gierke in 1929, new information regarding the clinical problems encountered by patients affected with these conditions continues to accumulate. As treatment for these disorders leads to longer life expectancy, the long-term complications secondary to the disease itself as well as to our treatment are now being identified and reported. Since molecular testing for these disorders is still in its infancy, genotype-phenotype correlations are still unknown. As many of these disorders affect muscle and others cause hyperlipidemia, cardiac complications may easily occur and should be suspected.

REFERENCES

1. Chen YT, Burchell Y. Glycogen storage diseases. In The Metabolic and Molecular Bases of Inherited Disease. C.R. Scriver, A.L. Beaudet, W.S. Sly, and D. Valle, editors. McGraw-Hill, Inc., New York. 1995:935-966.

2. Fernandes J, Chen YT. Glycogen storage diseases. *In:* Inborn Metabolic Diseases. 2nd ed. Fernandes J, Saudubray JM, van den Berghe G, editors. Springer-Verlag, Berlin. 1996:71-86.

3. Pizzo C. Type I glycogen storage disease with focal nodular hyperplasia of the liver and vasoconstructive pulmonary hypertension. *Pediatrics* 1980;65:341-343.

4. Hamaoka K, Nakagawa M, Furukawa N, Sawada T. Pulmonary hypertension in Type I glycogen storage disease. *Pediatr Cardiol.* 1990;11:54-56.

5. Levy E, Thibault A, Roy CC,Bendayan M, Lepage G, Letarte J. Circulating lipids and lipoproteins in glycogen storage disease type I with nocturnal intragastric feeding. *J Lipid Research* 1988;29:215-226.

6. Lei KJ, Chen YT, Chen H, Wong LC, Liu J,McConkie-Rosell A, Van Hove J,Ou H, Yeh NJ, Pan LY, Chou JY. Genetic basis of glycogen storage disease type Ia: Prevalent mutations at the glucose-6-phosphatase locus. *Am J Hum Genet.* 1995;57:766-771.

7. Chevalier-Porst F, Bozon D, Bonardot A, Bruni N, Mithieux G, Mathieu M, Maire I. Mutation analysis in 24 French patients with glycogen storage disease type Ia. *J Med Genet* 1996;33:358-60.

8. Parvari R, Lei KJ, Bashan N, Hershkovitz E, Korman SH, Barash V, Lerman-Sagie T, Mandel H, Chou JY, Moses SW. Glycogen storage disease type Ia in Israel. *Am J Med Genet* 1997;72:286-90.

9. Pompe J-C. Over idiopatische hypertrophie van het hart. *Ned Tijdshr Geneeskd* 1932;76:304-312.

10. Hirschhorn R. Glycogen storage disease type II: Acidα-glucosidase (Acid maltase) deficiency. *In:* The Metabolic and Molecular Basis of Inherited Disease. Scriver C, Beaudet AL, Sly WS,Valle D, eds. McGraw-Hill, New York. 2443-2465.

11. Metzl JC, Elias ER, Berul CI. An interesting case of sudden death: severe hypertrophic cardiomyopathy in Pompe's disease. *PACE* 1999;22:821-822.

12. Solomon E, Swallow D, Burgess S, Evans L. Assignment of the human acid alpha-glucosidase gene to chromosome 17 using somatic cell hybrids. *Ann Hum Genet* 1979;42:273-281.

13. Huie ML, Tsujino S, Sklower-Brooks S, Elias E, Bonthron DT, Bessley C, Shanske S, DiMauro S, Goto YI, Hirschhorn R. Glycogen storage disease type II: identification of four novel missense mutations (D645N, G648S, R672W, R672Q) and two insertions/deletions in the acidα-glucosidase locus of patients of differing phenotype. 1998 *Biochem Biophys Res Commun.* 921-927.

14. Van Hoof F, Hers HG. The subgroups of type III glycogenosis. *Eur J Biochem.* 1967;2:265-270.

15. Ding JH, de Barsy T, Brown BI, Coleman RA, Chen YT. Immunoblot analyses of glycogen debranching enzyme in different subtypes of glycogen storage disease type III. *J Pediatr.* 1990;116:95-100.

16. Labrune P, Huguet P, Odievre M. Cardiomyopathy in glycogen-storage diseasetype III: clinical and echographic study of 18 patients. *Pediatr Cardiol.* 1991;12:161-163.

17. Olson LJ, Reeder GS, Noller KL, Edwards WD, Howell RR, Michels VV. Cardiac involvement in glycogen storage disease III: Morphologic and biochemical characterization with endomyocardial biopsy. *Am J Cardiol.* 1984;53:980-981.

18. Slonim AE, Weisberg C, Benke P, Evans OB, Burr IM. Reversal of debrancher deficiency myopathy by the use of high-protein nutrition. *Ann Neurol* 1982;11:420-422.

19. Shen J, Bao Y, Liu HM, Lee P, Leonard JV, Chen YT. Mutations in exon 3 of the glycogen debranching enzyme gene are associated with glycogen storage disease type III that is differentially expressed in liver and muscle. *J Clin Invest.* 1996;98:352-357.

20. Shen J, Liu HM, Bao Y, Chen YT. Polymorphic markers of the glycogen debrnaching enzyme gene allowing linkage analysis in families with glycogen storage disease type III. *J Med Genet* 1997;34:34-38.

21. Servidei S, Riepe RE, Langston C, Tani LY, Bricker JT, Crisp-Lindgren N, Travers H, Armstrong D, DiMauro S. Severe cardiopathy in branching enzyme deficiency. *J Pediatr.* 1987;111:51-56.

22. Tang TT, Segura AD, Chen YT, Ricci LM, Franciosi RA, Splaingard ML, Lubinsky MS. Neonatal hypotonia and cardiomyopathy secondary to type IV glycogenosis. *Acta Neuropath.* 1994;87:531-6.

23. Nase S, Kunze KP, Sigmund M, Schroeder JM, Shin Y, Hanrath P. A new variant of type IV glycogenosis with primary cardiac manifestation and complete branching enzyme deficiency. In vivo detection by heart muscle biopsy. *Eur Heart J.* 1995;16:1698-1704.

24. Greene GM, Weldon DC, Ferrans VJ, Cheatham JP, McComb RD, Gumbiner BI, Vanderhoff JA, Itkin PG, McManus BM. Juvenile polysaccharidosis with cardioskeletal myopathy. *Arch Path Lab Med.* 1987;111:977-982.

25. Selby R, Starzl TE, Yunis E, Brown BI, Kendall RS, Tzakis A. Liver transplantation for type IV glycogen storage disease. *New Engl J Med.* 1991;324:39-42.

26. Starzl TE, Demetris AJ, Trucco M, Ricordi C, Ildstad S, Terasaki PI, Murase N, Kendall RS, Kocova M, Rudert WA, Zeevi A, Van Thiel D. Chimerism after liver transplantation for type IV glycogen storage disease and type I Gaucher's disease. *New Engl J Med* 1993;328:745-749.

27. Bao Y, Kishnani P, Wu JY, Chen YT. Hepatic and neuromuscular forms of glycogen storage disease type IV caused by mutations in the same glycogen-branching enzyme gene. *J Clin Invest.* 1996;97:941-948.

28. DiMauro S, Hartlage PL. Fatal infantile form of muscle phosphorylase deficiency. *Neurology* 1978;28:1124-1129.

29. Tsujino S, Shanske S, DiMauro S. Molecular genetic heterogeneity of myophosphorylase deficiency (McArdle's disease). *N Engl J Med.* 1993;329:241-245.

30. Vorgerd M, Kubisch C, Burwinkel B, Reichmann H, Mortier W, Tettenborn B, Pongratz D, Lindemuth R, Tegenthoff M, Malin JP, Kilimann MW. Mutation analysis in myophosphorylase deficiency (McArdle's disease). *Ann Neurol.* 1998;43:326-331.

31. Servidei S, Metlay LA, Chodosh J, DiMauro S. Fatal infantile cardiopathy caused by phosphorylase b kinase deficiency. *J Pediatr.* 1988;113:82-85.

32. Mizuta K, Kashimoto E, Tsutou A, Eishi Y, Takemura T, Narisawa K, Yamamura H. A new type of glycogen storage disease caused by deficiency of cardiac phosphorylase kinase. *Biochem Biophys Res Commun.* 1984;119:582-587.

33. Eishi Y, Takemua T, Sone R, Yamamura H, Narisawa K, Ichinohasama R, Tanaka M, Hatakeyama S. Glycogen storage disease confined to the heart with deficient activity of cardiacphosphorylase kinase: a new type of glycogen storage disease. *Hum Pathol.* 1985;16:193-197.

34. Burwinkel B, Bakker HD, Herschkovitz E, Moses SW, Shin YS, Kilimann MW. Mutations in the liver glycogen phosphorylase gene (PYGL) underlyingglycogenosis type VI (Hers diseaese). *Am J Hum Genet.* 1998;62:785-791.

35. Chang S, Rosenberg MJ, Morton H, Francomano CA,Biesecker LG. Identification of a mutation in liver glycogen phosphorylase in glycogen storage disease VI. *Hum Mol Genet* 1998;7:865-870.

36. Haller RG, Lewis SF. Glucose-induced exertional fatigue in muscle phosphofructokinase deficiency. *N Engl J Med* 1991;324:364-369.

37. Servidei S, Bonilla E, Diedrick RG, Kornfeld M, Oates JD, Davidson M, Vora S, DiMauro S. Fatal infantile form of muscle phosphofructokinase deficiency. *Neurology* 1986;36:1465-1470.

38. Danon MJ, Carpenter S, Manaligod JR, Schliselfeld LH. Fatal infantile glycogen storage disease: deficiency of phosphofructokinase and phosphorylase β kinase. *Neurology* 1981;31:1303-1307.

39. Amit R, Bashan N, Abarbanel JM, Shapira Y, Sofer S, Moses S. Fatal familial infantile glycogen storage disease: multisystem phosphofructokinase deficiency. *Musc Nerve* 1992;15:455-458.

40. Raben N, Sherman JB. Mutations in muscle phosphofructokinase gene. *Hum Mutat* 1995;6:1-6.

15

ARRHYTHMOGENIC RIGHT VENTRICULAR DYSPLASIA/CARDIOMYOPATHY

Frank I. Marcus, M.D., and Peter Ott, M.D.
University of Arizona College of Medicine
Tucson, Arizona

INTRODUCTION

Arrhythmogenic right ventricular dysplasia/cardiomyopathy (ARVD/C) is a disease characterized by fatty replacement of the right ventricular muscle (1). The residual myocardial fibers are often embedded in fibrous tissue. This substrate is conducive to right ventricular re-entrant arrhythmias. Initially this condition was called dysplasia because it was thought to represent an abnormality of development of the right ventricle. Subsequently it has been classified as a cardiomyopathy since the right ventricular myocardium may be normal at birth with fatty replacement progressive after birth. Since the pathogenesis of this disease is not exactly clear, the two terms are frequently combined as ARVD/C.

DIAGNOSIS OF ARVD/C

The diagnosis of ARVD/C is based upon identification of electrical, anatomical and functional abnormalities that predominately affect the right ventricle in a person usually having associated ventricular arrhythmias (Table 1) (2).

Patients with ARVD/C usually present with ventricular arrhythmias between ages of 12-45 years. There is a predominance of males (3). Clinical manifestations of the disease are rare before puberty. The ventricular arrhythmias consist of premature ventricular beats, almost always of left bundle branch block configuration or transient or sustained ventricular tachycardia. Sudden death may sometimes be the first manifestation of this condition. These arrhythmias are more likely to occur during exercise. Three to four percent of sudden deaths during sports appear to be due to ARVD/C (4, 5). Later in the course of the disease, right or bi-ventricular failure may develop. In fact, 4-5% of patients undergoing cardiac transplantation have this disease at pathological examination, having been misdiagnosed as having idiopathic dilated cardiomyopathy (6). Pathological evidence for ARVD/C should be carefully investigated in individuals who die suddenly and unexpectedly.

ELECTRICAL ABNORMALITIES

During sinus rhythm there are abnormalities of the QRS configuration that are due to slow conduction of electrical activity in the Purkinje system of the right ventricular free wall (7). This is called parietal block. There may be abnormalities of repolarization secondary to the underlying abnormal anatomy of the right ventricular free wall and enlargement of this chamber.

These abnormalities consist of:

1.   A) QRS duration in V_1 >110 msec (7)

B) QRS duration in $V_1 + V_2 + V_3 > V_4 + V_{5+} V_6$ by a ratio of 1.2 (8). These represent alterations of conduction delay predominately affecting the right ventricular free wall, the last portion of the heart to be depolarized.

2.   Epsilon waves: These are small electrical potentials that occur immediately after the QRS complex (9). They may also be present as jagged alterations of the terminal part of the QRS complex, and represent delayed depolarization of the right ventricle. The electrical abnormalities listed above appear to correlate with the extent of right ventricular involvement; in turn, this is associated with increased right ventricular size and volume. Thus these findings are usually present in patients with the more advanced forms of the disease and their presence is helpful in diagnoses since the specificity is excellent. However, the sensitivity of these findings in patients with minimal involvement, as in family members is unknown.

3.   Presence of late potentials by signal averaged ECG. These represent delayed depolarization of the right ventricle due to the abnormal substrate. The presence of late potentials are most closely correlated with decreased right ventricular ejection fraction. (10). In addition, a decreased voltage of the terminal 40 msec at 25 H_z is an independent factor for the occurrence of sustained ventricular arrhythmias.

4.   T wave inversion beyond lead V_1 in an individual over the age of 12 years. The extent of T wave inversion beyond lead V_1 has been correlated with the extent of right ventricular involvement and increase in right ventricular size in one study (11) but not in another (12). In a study of 74 patients with ARVD who presented with symptomatic tachycardia and were followed for a mean of 9.5 ± 3.2 years, the prevalence of T wave inversion in V_1-V_3 increased from 50% at initial examination to 98% (13).

5.   The ventricular arrhythmias are almost always of left bundle branch block configuration, since they arise from the right ventricular free wall. The septum is usually unaffected. The frontal plane QRS axis of the ventricular arrhythmias provides information regarding the site and origin of the ventricular ectopy. For example, left bundle branch block with an inferior QRS axis and a negative QRS in aVL indicates that the origin of the ectopy is from the right ventricular outflow tract.

Table 1: Criteria for Diagnosis of Right Ventricular Dysplasia

I. Global and/or Regional Dysfunction and Structural Alterations*

• Major

Severe dilatation and reduction of right ventricular ejection fraction with no (or only mild) LV impairment.

Localized right ventricular aneurysms (akinetic or dyskinetic areas with diastolic bulging).

Severe segmental dilatation of the right ventricle.

• Minor

Mild global right ventricular dilatation and/or ejection fraction reduction with normal left ventricle.

Mild segmental dilatation of the right ventricle.

Regional right ventricular hypokinesia.

II. Tissue Characterization of Wall

• Major

Fibrofatty replacement of myocardium on endomyocardial biopsy.

III. Repolarization Abnormalities

• Minor

Inverted T waves in right precordial leads (V_2 and V_3) (people aged >12 years, in absence of right bundle branch block).

IV. Depolarization/Conduction Abnormalities

• Major

Epsilon waves or localized prolongation (>110 ms) of the QRS complex in right precordial leads (V_1 - V_3).

• Minor

Late potentials (signal-averaged ECG).

V. Arrhythmias

• Minor

Left bundle branch block type ventricular tachycardia (sustained and nonsustained) on ECG, Holter monitor, or exercise test.

Frequent ventricular extrasystoles (>1000/24 hours) on Holter monitor.

VI. Family History

• Major

Familial disease confirmed at necropsy or surgery.

• Minor

Family history of premature sudden death (<35 years) due to suspected right ventricular dysplasia.

Familial history (clinical diagnosis based on present criteria).

*Detected by echocardiography, angiography, magnetic resonance imaging, or radionuclide scintigraphy. ECG = electrocardiogram; LV = left ventricle. From McKenna et al. (2). The diagnosis of ARVD would be fulfilled by the presence of 2 major, or 1 major plus 2 minor criteria or 4 minor criteria from different group.

STRUCTURAL CHANGES

In contrast to the left ventricle that has relatively smooth endocardium with a symmetrical shape and contraction pattern, the right ventricle has a highly trabeculated endocardial surface and the shape of this chamber is quite irregular. This provides a challenge to assess normal size and function. The structural changes in the right ventricle due to ARVD/C consists of increased chamber size, deep fissuring and trabeculation of the right ventricular outflow tract and there may be localized akinetic or dyskinetic bulges or outpouchings, particularly at the infundibulum at the apex and the posterior sub-tricuspid areas (14). There may be localized thinning of the right ventricular wall. Since the right ventricular wall is not uniform and is only 3-5 mm in thickness (15), it may be extremely difficult to be certain whether or not there is thinning or fatty penetration of the right ventricular wall (Figure 1).

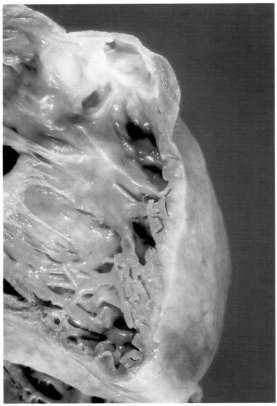

Figure 1: Heart from a 16 year-old boy who died suddenly. This is a view showing the right ventricle and right ventricular outflow tract. The tricuspid valve is at the left, and the pulmonary valve in superior. There is transmural fat in the right ventricular outflow tract.

The various methods used to assess right ventricular structure and function are as follows:

A) Echocardiogram. 2D echocardiography when properly performed by focusing attention on the right ventricular function and wall motion abnormalities, as suggested by Foale et al (16), is an excellent way to screen for ARVD/C. It is important to visualize the posterior and inferior wall of the right ventricular inflow tract under the tricuspid valve, since this is the most frequently affected area. This may be best seen in the parasternal long axis view with the probe angled toward the inferior vena cava or the liver. The apical right ventricular 2 chamber view with the probe angled toward the right ventricle by 20-30° is another projection to visualize this area as well as the right ventricular apex (17).

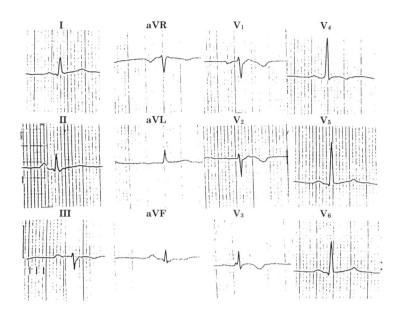

Figure 2: Electrocardiogram from a patient with ARVD/C. Note that the T waves are inverted in V_1-V_4. There are epsilon waves at the end of the QRS complex in V_1 and V_2.

B. Angiography. The right ventricular angiogram remains the gold standard to substantiate abnormalities of right ventricular function and anatomy for the diagnosis of ARVD/C, (14, 18) but its diagnostic accuracy is also dependent on the protocol used. The following views should be obtained: 1) a 60° LAO view with a 25-30° caudal-cranial tilt; 2) a 30° RAO view with a 15-20° caudal-cranial tilt; and 3) PA and lateral views. A pigtail catheter should be inserted into the right ventricular inflow tract, deep enough in the right ventricle to opacify the right ventricular apex. Low toxicity contrast dye is injected at a velocity not to exceed 10-12 ml/sec, with effort made to avoid inducing premature beats during the injection.

C. Magnetic resonance imaging. The diagnostic role of the MRI is controversial. When a patient has the overt manifestations of the disease including evident right ventricular abnormalities, the MRI can be confirmatory by its unique ability to identify and characterize fatty tissue infiltration in the right ventricular free wall (19, 20, 21). However, in patients with ventricular arrhythmias of left bundle branch block morphology who have minimal anatomic abnormalities of the right ventricle, the sensitivity and specificity of the MRI may not be sufficient to distinguish normals from ARVD/C (22). In addition, there may be variable degrees of penetration of epicardial fat extending to the medial layer of the right ventricle in normal individuals. Since the right ventricular free wall is only 3-5 mm thick, the resolution of the MRI to detect thinning of several millimeters is questionable. Most radiologists have limited experience in the diagnosis of ARVD/C by MRI. Until these issues are clarified, we should be cautious not to solely rely on the MRI to determine whether there are anatomic or functional changes diagnostic of ARVD/C.

It is because of the difficulty in evaluation of the right ventricular function and structure, that criteria have been proposed to confirm the diagnosis based on a variety of tests, including depolarization and conduction abnormalities, presence of arrhythmias, family history, global and regional dysfunction of the right ventricular and tissue characterization of the right ventricular wall (Table 1). It should be cautioned that the accuracy of this algorithm depends upon the diagnostic quality of the information applied to this scheme. For example, conclusions obtained from an inadequate echocardiographic examination will render this approach useless.

DIFFERENTIAL DIAGNOSIS

The major condition that needs to be differentiated from ARVD/C is right ventricular outflow tract (RVOT) tachycardia (23). This is the most common condition in young people that causes similar ventricular arrhythmias such as premature ventricular beats, transient or sustained ventricular tachycardia. As in ARVD/C, the arrhythmias may be exercise-induced (24). This condition enters into the differential diagnosis if the ventricular ectopy has a left bundle branch block configuration and an inferior QRS axis with a negative QRS in lead aVL indicating an origin from the right ventricular outflow tract. Since the infundibulum is one of the regions that is frequently affected in ARVD/C, the ventricular arrhythmias may have a similar morphology in both conditions. The electrical abnormalities described for ARVD/C are found less frequently in patients with RVOT tachycardia (25) (Table 2). As previously mentioned, the specificity of electrical abnormalities is good, but their sensitivity may be limited. The presence of right precordial QRS prolongation, epsilon potentials or late potentials are highly specific for ARVD and may be helpful to distinguish ARVD from idiopathic RVOT tachycardia (25). Therefore, the presence of one or more electrical abnormalities favors the diagnosis of ARVD/C but their absence does not exclude this diagnosis.

Other entities that need to be considered in the differential diagnosis of ARVD/C are abnormalities that primarily affect the right side of the heart such as atrial septal defect, anomalous pulmonary venous return and Ebstein's malformation. Uncommonly myocarditis can predominately affect the right side of the heart and sarcoidosis must be included in the differential diagnosis.

Table 2: Differentiation of ARVD/C from RVOT Tachycardia on Surface ECG

	ARVC	RVO-VT	Control
T-wave inversion > V_2	54.3%*	33.0%	1.4%
max. QRS duration (V_{1-3})	114±19 ms*	104±13 ms	98±11 ms
max QRS >110 ms (V_{1-3})	51.7%*	21.0%	12.9%
Epsilon potential	22.5%*	2.8%	0%
Late potentials (25 Hz)	41.4%*	11.7%	3.0%
QRS dispersion	40±13 ms*	34±10 ms	33±9 ms
QT dispersion	54±21 ms	47±16 ms	40±13 ms

* =p<0.001 for ARVD/C vs. RVOT Tachycardia and Control

PATHOLOGY

The most striking morphological feature of ARVD/C is fatty replacement of the epicardium and mid-myocardium of the right ventricular free wall. The endocardium is usually spared as is the septum (26). As the disease progresses, the left ventricle may become involved, particularly, the epicardium of the left ventricle (27). The right ventricular wall thickness is usually normal, but in there may be focal thinning of the right ventricle, especially in the pulmonary infundibulum, in the diaphragmatic inferior wall or at the apex. Histology shows severe myocardial atrophy with residual myocytes interspersed with fibro-fatty tissue. Evidence of patchy and acute inflammation with myocyte death and focal round cell infiltrates, mostly lymphocytes are present in 2/3 of the cases. It is not known whether this inflammation represents evidence of viral myocarditis or is the response to the process that causes destruction of the myocardium (28, 29). The diagnosis of ARVD/C may be unclear if there is fat interspersed with myocardial cells in the right ventricle in the absence of fibrosis or an active inflammatory response (30). It is now recognized that fatty infiltration of the free wall of the right ventricle may be found at autopsy in a sizable number of "normals" whose death was not attributable to ARVD/C. Myocardial biopsy can be useful to obtain pathological material if the biopsy is obtained at the junction of the posterior septum and myocardial free wall rather than in the usual septal location (31). However, most physicians are reluctant to biopsy this site because of concern of myocardial perforation.

GENETICS

A family history of ARVD/C is present in 30-50% of cases. With the exception of a variant of the disease found in Naxos, Greece, with a recessive mode of transmission, the disease is transmitted in an autosomal dominant pattern with various degrees of clinical expression. The autosomal dominant form of ARVD has been shown to be genetically heterogeneous, with six genes for a pure form of ARVD mapped to chromosomes shown in Table 3 (32-37). A seventh gene mapped for Naxos disease, a complex disorder consisting of ARVD/C, diffuse nonepidermolytic palmoplantar keratoderma and woolly hair identified in individuals from Naxos, Greece has been localized to chromosome 17q21 (38). The gene(s) for ARVD/C have not yet been identified. There is evidence that there may be different phenotypic expressions of the different genes. For example, it has been observed that there is a higher incidence of sudden cardiac death in patients who have gene localized to chromosome 1q42.3 (39). These patients have exercise induced polymorphic ventricular tachycardia, normal ECGs and apical aneurysms.

Table 3: Chromosomal Loci in Families with ARVD by Linkage Analysis

Locus #	# Families	Locus	Ref #
1	6	14q24.3	32
2	4	1q42//3	33
3	3	14q12-q22	34
4	4	2q32.1-q32.3	35
5	1	3p23	36
6	1	10p12-14	37
7	9	17q21	38

Locus 1-6 = Autosomal Dominant Transmission
Locus 7 = Autosomal Recessive

There is a high incidence of ARVD/C in Northern Italy, but the disease has been observed in a variety of races, including Japanese, and has been recently reported in a Native American Indian (40).

IDENTIFICATION OF THE DISEASE IN FAMILY MEMBERS AND RISK FACTORS FOR ARRHYTHMIC DEATH

Since it is now known that ARVD/C may be genetically transmitted and that there is a risk of arrhythmic death in affected individuals, it is advised that first degree relatives of the probands undergo testing to see if they have the disease. The sensitivity and specificity of the tests to determine electrical and morphological changes of the right ventricle to confirm the presence of ARVD/C in minimally affected individuals is unknown. It is advised that family members have an ECG, signal averaged ECG, a 24-hour ambulatory ECG, stress testing and echocardiogram with special attention to assess right ventricular size and regional wall abnormalities. Scognomolio et al found that, if the echocardiogram in a family member was normal at the first examination, there was only a 3% chance of the development of ventricular arrhythmias during an 8 year follow up and no sudden deaths in this group of 142 individuals (41). In contrast, if the family member was one of 74 subjects who had an abnormal echo at first examination, the incidence of developing arrhythmias was 90% and 54% showed progressive involvement of the right ventricle. As previously mentioned, the role of the MRI for diagnosis of ARVD/C in family members is unclear at this time because of the unknown specificity and sensitivity of this test. It is also not clear whether to recommend that family members with possible abnormalities of the right ventricle undergo right ventricular angiography to confirm the diagnosis. At present, individual circumstances such as the desire to engage in competitive sports may influence this decision since individuals who are affected are advised not to do so. This is based on the observation that sudden cardiac death in ARVD/C is more likely to occur during sports activities (42). In addition, it has been observed that the clinical manifestations of the disease appear at a younger age in athletic individuals (43).

The clinical profile of the individual with ARVD/C likely to have a fatal arrhythmia is incomplete. Among risk factors for sudden cardiac death appear to be a history of syncope (44). Patients with ARVD/C who have been resuscitated from sudden cardiac death generally have the overt manifestations of the disease including the typical ECG findings and echocardiographic abnormalities. As previously mentioned, there is a higher incidence of sudden cardiac death in patients with chromosome 1q42.3 (39). This variant may be recognized by exercise induced polymorphic ventricular tachycardia. In addition, the echocardiographic findings are those of localized apical aneurysms. The ECG may be normal in these patients.

THERAPY

Medical therapy consists of antiarrhythmic drugs to suppress ventricular arrhythmias (45). There has not been a prospective study of antiarrhythmic drugs to determine optimal and safe therapy. A wide variety of antiarrhythmic drugs have been prescribed including propafenone, flecainide, amiodarone and sotalol. The latter drug is most commonly used. Although sotalol seems to be effective in prevention of recurrence of sustained ventricular tachycardia, it is not known if it is effective in preventing sudden cardiac death, even if it is prescribed based on the results of programmed electrical stimulation.

Catheter ablation of ventricular tachycardia is feasible in selected patients with ARVD/C (46). However, recurrences of ventricular tachycardia after ablation are not uncommon during long term follow up (47) since ARVD/C is a progressive disease and new ventricular arrhythmias can develop later despite apparently successful ablation.

The implanted cardioverter defibrillator (ICD) is recommended for patients who have had cardiac arrest or are judged to be at high risk due to history of syncope or who appear to have polymorphic ventricular tachycardia. The low amplitude of the endocardial signals due to the diseased right ventricle may be a problem in lead placement (48). It is not known whether patients who do not have the overt manifestation of the disease and spontaneous monomorphic sustained ventricular tachycardia should have this device implanted. Emotional factors may play a role as to whether to advise implantation of an ICD in an affected family member where the sibling has died suddenly with this disease.

UNANSWERED QUESTIONS

Although the disease has been known for 23 years, there are many unanswered questions. Most pressing for the clinician are methods to accurately diagnose patients who may be minimally affected since the diagnosis carries the concern of being susceptible to arrhythmic death, possible changes in lifestyle to avoid competitive sports and the recommendation to take antiarrhythmic drugs for an indefinite period and possibly implantation of an ICD. Proper therapy to prevent arrhythmic death also needs to be investigated by prospective studies. The ultimate goal is to localize the gene(s) that could be decisive in directing further investigation to understand the genetic defect(s) upon which to focus definitive treatment. Towards this end, an international registry has been established (49). Physicians are encouraged to advise their patients to enroll in this registry. Among other goals, the registry will serve to channel patients to laboratories that are investigating the genetics of the disease.

REFERENCES

1.	Marcus FI, Fontaine G. Arrhythmogenic right ventricular dysplasia/cardiomyopathy: A review: PACE 1995;18:1298-1314.
2.	McKenna WJ, Thiene G, Nava A, Fontaliran F, Blomstrom-Lundqvist C, Fontaine F, Camerini F. Diagnosis of arrhythmogenic right ventricular dysplasia/cardiomyopathy. Br Heart J 1994;71:215-218.
3.	Marcus FI, Fontaine GH, Guiraudon G, Frank R, Laurenceau JL, Malergue C, Grosgogeat Y. Right ventricular dysplasia: A report of 24 adult cases. Circulation 1982;65:384-398
4.	Marcus FI. Right ventricular dysplasia: Evaluation and management in relation to sports activities. In: Estes NAM Salem DN, Wang PJ (eds) Sudden Cardiac Death in the Athlete, pg 277-284. Futura Publishing Co., Inc., Armonk NY 1998.
5.	Maron BJ, Shirani J, Poliac LC, Mathenge R, Roberts WC, Mueller FO. Sudden death in young competitive athletes. JAMA 1996;276:199-204.
6.	Nemec J, Edwards BS, Osborn MJ, Edwards WD. Arrhythmogenic right ventricular dysplasia masquerading as dilated cardiomyopathy. Am J Cardiol 1999;84:237-238.
7.	Fontaine G, Umemura J, DiDonna P, Tsezana R, Cannat JJ, Frank R. La duree des complexes QRS dans la dysplasie ventriculaire droite arythmogene. Ann Cardiol Angeiol 1993;42:399-405.
8.	Peters S, Gotting B, Peters H. Localized right precordial QRS prolongation as the basic ECG finding in arrhythmogenic right ventricular dysplasia cardiomyopathy. A.N.E. 1999;4:4-9
9.	Fontaine G, Fontaliran F, Hebert JL, Chemla D, Zenati O, Lecarpentier Y, Frank R. Arrhythmogenic right ventricular dysplasia. Annu Rev Med 1999:50:17-35.
10.	Turrini P, Angelini A, Thiene G, Buja G, Daliento L, Rizzoli G, Nava A. Late potentials and ventricular arrhythmias in arrhythmogenic right ventricular cardiomyopathy. Am J Cardiol 1999;83:1214-1219.
11.	Nava A, Canciani B, Buja G, Martini B, Daliento L, Scognamiglio R, Thiene G. Electrovectorcardiographic study of negative T waves on precordial leads in arrhythmogenic right ventricular dysplasia: Relationship with right ventricular volumes. Journal of Electrocardiology 1988;21:239-245.
12.	Metzger JT, de Chillou C, Cheriex E, Rodriguez LM, Smeets JLRM, Wellens HJJ. Value of the 12-lead electrocardiogram in arrhythmogenic right ventricular dysplasia, and absence of correlation with echocardiographic findings. Am J Cardiol 1993;72:964-967.
13.	Jaoude SA, Leclercq JF, Coumel P. Progressive ECG changes in arrhythmogenic right ventricular disease. Eur Heart J 1996;17:1717-1722.
14.	Daliento L, Rizzoli G, Thiene G, Nava A, Rinuncini M, Chioin R, Dalla Volta S. Diagnostic accuracy of right ventriculography in arrhythmogenic right ventricular cardiomyopathy. Am J Cardiol 1990;60:741-745.
15.	Burke AP, Farb A, Tashko G, Virmani R. Arrhythmogenic right ventricular cardiomyopathy and fatty replacement of the right ventricular myocardium. Are they different diseases? Circulation 1998;97:1571-1580.

16. Foale RA, Nihoyannopoulos P, Ribeiro P, McKenna WJ, Oakley CM, Krikler DM, Rowland E. Right ventricular abnormalities in ventricular tachycardia of right ventricular origin: Relation to electrophysiological abnormalities. Br Heart J 1986:56:45-54.

17. Villanova C. Arrhythmogenic right ventricular cardiomyopathy/dysplasia: Echocardiographic features and criteria. Thesis Universita Degli Studi Di Padova Padua Italy December 1998.

18. Daubert JC, Descaves C, Foulgoc JL, Bourdonnec C, Laurent M, Gouffault J. Critical analysis of cineangiographic criteria for diagnosis of arrhythmogenic right ventricular dysplasia. Am Heart J 1988;115;448-459.

19. Blake LM, Scheinman MM, Higgins CB. MR features of arrhythmogenic right ventricular dysplasia. Am J Radiol 1994:162:809-812.

20. Auffermann W, Wichter T, Breithardt G, Joachimsen K, Peters PE. Arrhythmogenic right ventricular disease: MR imaging versus angiography. Am J Radiol 1993;161:549-555.

21. Wichter T, Lentschig MG, Reimer P, Borggrefe M, Breithardt G. Magnetic resonance imaging. In: Nava A, Rossi L, Thiene G (eds.): Arrhythmogenic right ventricular cardiomyopathy/dysplasia. Amsterdam, Elsevier Science BV 1997:269-284.

22. Marcus FI. Problems in the clinical recognition and documentation of arrhythmogenic right ventricular dysplasia/cardiomyopathy. Morie Sekiguchi, M.D. (ed) In: Arrhythmogenic Right Ventricular Cardiomyopathy. Springer-Verlag Tokyo, in press.

23. Marcus FI. Is arrhythmogenic right ventricular dysplasia, Uhl's anomaly and right ventricular outflow tract tachycardia: a spectrum of the same disease? Cardiology in Review 1997:5:25-29.

24. Lerman BB, Stein KM, Markowitz SM. Idiopathic right ventricular outflow tract tachycardia: A clinical approach. PACE 1996;19:2120-2137.

25. Wichter T, Wilke K, Haverkamp W, Breithardt G, Broggrefe M. Identification of arrhythmogenic right ventricular cardiomyopathy from surface the ECG: parameters for discrimination from idiopathic right ventricular tachycardia. PACE 1999;22:A69(abs).

26. Basso C, Corrado D, Rossi L, Thiene G. Morbid anatomy. In:Nava, A, Rossi L, Thiene G (eds) Arrhythmogenic right ventricular cardiomyopathy/dysplasia.Elsevier Science BV, Amsterdam, The Netherlands 1997:71-86.

27. Corrado D, Basso C, Thiene G, McKenna WJ, Davies MJ, Fontaliran F, Nava A, Silvestri F, Blomstrom-Lundqvist C, Wlodarska EK, Fontaine G, Camerini F. Spectrum of clinicopathologic manifestations of arrhythmogenic right ventricular cardiomyopathy/dysplasia: A multicenter study. J Am Coll Cardiol 1997;30:1512-1520.

28. Thiene G, Corrado D, Nava A, Rossi L, Poletti A, Boffa GM, Daliento L, Pennelli N. Right ventricular cardiomyopathy: Is there evidence of an inflammatory aetiology? Eur Heart J 1991;12:22-25.

29. Fontaine G, Fontaliran F, Zenati O, Guzman CE, Rigoulet J, Berthier JL, Frank R. Fat in the heart: A feature unique to the human species? Observational reflections on an unsolved problem. Acta Cardiol 1999:54:189-194.

30. Fontaine G, Fontaliran F, Andrade FR, Velazquez E, Tonet J, Jouven X, Fujioka Y, Frank R. The arrhythmogenic right ventricle. Dysplasia versus cardiomyopathy. Heart Vessels 1995;10:227-235.

31. Angelini A, Thiene G, Boffa GM, Calliaris I, Daliento L, Valente M, Chioin R, Nava A, Dalla Volta S. Endomyocardial biopsy in right ventricular cardiomyopathy. International Journal of Cardiology 1993;40:273-282.

32. Rampazzo A, Nava A, Danieli GA, Buja G, Daliento L, Fasoli G, Scognamiglio R, Corrado D, Thiene G. The gene for arrhythmogenic right ventricular cardiomyopathy maps to chromosome 14q23-q24. Hum Mol Genet 1994;3:959-962.

33. Rampazzo A, Nava A, Erne P, Eberhard M, Vian E, Slomp P, Tisa N, Thiene G, Danieli GA. A new locus for arrhythmogenic right ventricular cardiomyopathy (ARVD2) maps to chromosome 1q42-q43. Hum Mol Genet 1995;4:2151-2154.

34. Severini GM, Krajinovic M, Pinamonti B, Sinagra G, Fioretti P, Brunazzi MC, Falaschi A, Camerini F, Giacca M, Mestroni L. A new locus for arrhythmogenic right ventricular dysplasia on the long arm of chromosome 14. Genomics 1996;31:193-200.

35. Rampazzo A, Nava A, Miorin M, Fonderice P, Pope B, Tisa N, Livolsi B, Zimbello R, Thiene G, Danieli GA. ARVD4, a new locus for arrhythmogenic right ventricular cardiomyopathy, maps to chromosome 2 long arm. Genomics 1997;45:259-263.

36.	Ahmad F, Li D, Karibe A, Gonzalez O, Tapscott T, Hill R, Weilbaecher D, Blackie P, Furey M, Gardner M, Bachinski LL, Roberts R. Localization of a gene responsible for arrhythmogenic right ventricular dysplasia to chromosome 3p23. Circulation 1998;98:2791-2795.

37.	Li D, Ahmad F, Gardner MJ, Hill R, Conzalez O, Tapscol TL, Sharratt GP, Killam IW, Bachinski LL, Roberts R. A novel locus responsible for arrhythmogenic right ventricular dysplasia maps to chromosome 10p12-p14. Circulation 1999;100:I-216 (abst).

38.	Coonar AS, Protonotarios N, Tsatsopoulou A, Needham EWA, Houlston RS, Cliff S, Otter MI, Nurday VA, Mattu RK, McKenna WJ. Gene for arrhythmogenic right ventricular cardiomyopathy with diffuse nonepidermolytic palmoplantar keratoderma and woolly hair (Naxos disease) maps to 17q21. Circulation 1998;97:2049-2058.

39.	Bauce B, Nava A, Rampazzo A, Daliento L, Muriago M, Basso C, Thiene G, Danieli GA. Familial effort polymorphic ventricular arrhythmias in arrhythmogenic right ventricular cardiomyopathy map to chromosome 1q42-q43. Am J Cardiol; in press

40.	Galloway JM, Koepke L, Ott P, Marcus FI. Arrhythmogenic right ventricular dysplasia in American Indian woman. PACE 1999;22:1093-1096.

41.	Scognamiglio R, Rahimtoola SH, Thiene G, Nava A, Fasoli G, Daliento L, Buja GF, Nistri S, Palisi M, Marin M, Dalla-Volta S. Concealed phase of familial arrhythmogenic right ventricular cardiomyopathy (ARVC): Early recognition and long-term follow-up. J Am Coll Cardiol 1997;29:194A.

42.	Corrado D, Basso C, Thiene G. Does sports activity enhance the risk of sudden death in young people? Eur Heart J 1999;20:444.

43.	Daubert C, Vauthier M, Carre F, Laurent M, Leclercq C, Mabo P. Influence of exercise and sport activity on functional symptoms and ventricular arrhythmias in arrhythmogenic right ventricular disease. J Am Coll Cardiol 1994;34A:847-864.

44.	Marcus FI, Fontaine GH, Gallagher FR, Reiter JJ, Long term follow up in patients with arrhythmogenic right ventricular disease. Eur Heart J 1989;10(Supplement D):68-73.

45.	Wichter T, Borggrefe M, Haverkamp W, Chen X, Breithardt G. Efficacy of antiarrhythmic drugs in patients with arrhythmogenic right ventricular disease: Results in patients with inducible and noninducible ventricular tachycardia. Circulation 1992;86:29-37.

46.	Ellison KE, Friedman PL, Ganz LI, Stevenson WG. Entrainment mapping and radiofrequency catheter ablation of ventricular tachycardia in right ventricular dysplasia. J Am Coll Cardiol 1998;32:724-8.

47.	Wichter T, Hindricks G, Kottkamp H, Breithardt G, Borggrefe M. Catheter ablation of ventricular tachycardia. In: Nava, A, Rossi L, Thiene G (eds.) Arrhythmogenic right ventricular cardiomyopathy/dysplasia. Elsevier Science BV Amsterdam, The Netherlands 1997:376-391

48.	Link MS, Wang PJ, Haugh CJ, Homoud MK, Foote CB, Costeas XB, Estes MA III. Arrhythmogenic right ventricular dysplasia: Clinical results with implantable cardioverter defibrillators. J Intervent Card Electrophysiol 1997;1:41-48.

49.	Corrado D, Fontaine G, Marcus FI, McKenna WJ, Nava A, Thiene G, Wichter T. Arrhythmogenic right ventricular dysplasia/cardiomyopathy. The need for an international registry. Circulation, 2000, in press

16

CARDIAC DISEASE IN DUCHENNE AND BECKER MUSCULAR DYSTROPHIES: THE DYSTROPHINOPATHIES

Leslie B. Smoot M.D. and Gerald Cox M.D.

Department of Cardiology, Children's Hospital • Boston,
Department of Pediatrics, Harvard Medical School, Boston, MA 02115

INTRODUCTION

The muscular dystrophies are a clinically and genetically heterogeneous group of skeletal muscle wasting diseases that differ widely in their frequency and pattern of cardiac involvement. Clinically, muscular dystrophies are characterized by progressive muscle weakness and atrophy. Pathologically, muscle histology reveals fiber size variability, central nuclei, as well as muscle necrosis with fatty replacement and fibrosis (1,2). Their pattern of muscle involvement, severity, mode of inheritance, unique clinical features, and primary gene defect distinguish individual types of muscular dystrophy (3).

Duchenne muscular dystrophy is one of the most common and severe hereditary diseases of muscle. Duchenne muscular dystrophy (DMD), Becker muscular dystrophy (BMD) and X-linked dilated cardiomyopathy (XLDCM) are allelic disorders caused by different types of mutations in the dystrophin gene (4-5). These diseases are therefore frequently referred to as dystrophinopathies.

Myocardial disease manifesting predominantly as cardiomyopathy and congestive heart failure is characteristic of Duchenne and Becker muscular dystrophy and X-linked dilated cardiomyopathy. Myocardial involvement in the form of cardiomyopathy and congestive heart failure play a major role in the clinical course of these and other related myopathies. Primary cardiac involvement in muscular dystrophy is not surprising, given structural and physiological similarities between skeletal and cardiac muscle. What is perhaps surprising is the wide variability observed in the incidence and pattern of cardiac involvement in different types of muscular dystrophy (6,7). Discordance between the degree of skeletal and cardiac pathology is common, influenced in part by tissue-specific protein expression and the presence or absence of compensatory proteins (8,9). Increasing knowledge as to the identity and function of proteins participating in the dystrophin -associated – glycoprotein complex (DAP complex) is providing new clues into the mechanisms underlying disease specific pathophysiology (11-14).

Muscular dystrophy may also preferentially affect the myocardium or conduction tissue in a disease specific manner. Myocardial involvement may take the form of structural or functional changes in cardiac muscle, which lead to cardiomyopathy and subsequent heart failure (15,16). When cardiac conduction tissue is affected primarily the cardiac phenotype may include decreased automaticity, heart block, malignant arrythmia or sudden death. The presence of two distinct patterns of cardiac disease in selected muscular dystrophies suggests that at least two cellular processes may be involved; one involving mechanical stabilization of the plasma membrane and the other involving signal transduction (17,18).

As the building blocks of the dystrophin glycoprotein complex are uncovered, along with their partners who influence diverse cell functions, a clearer picture is emerging to explain the spectrum of pathophysiology seen in muscular dystrophy and related cardiomyopathies (19,20).

I.   Duchenne and Becker Muscular Dystrophy

Duchenne muscular dystrophy (DMD) is the most common and severe form of muscular dystrophy in childhood, accounting for more than ¾ of all cases of muscular dystrophy. Duchenne dystrophy occurs with a frequency of approximately one in 3500 male births. Becker dystrophy occurs $1/10^{th}$ as often as DMD and is associated with a milder and more variable clinical course. Because Duchenne and Becker dystrophies are inherited as X-linked recessive conditions; almost all affected individuals are male. De novo mutations are responsible for approximately one third of cases (3).

Female carriers of dystrophin mutations may manifest overt disease when the normal paternal X chromosome fails to be expressed   (as in Turners syndrome (46XO), skewed X-inactivation, etc)(21-23). An estimated 8% of DMD carriers manifest mild to moderate myopathy. Many asymptomatic DMD carriers have elevated serum creatine kinase (CK) levels and all show some abnormality in dystrophin immunostaining of skeletal muscle (24,25).

Duchenne dystrophy is associated with a marked reduction or absence of dystrophin. Becker muscular dystrophy (BMD) is associated with a reduced amount of dystrophin or a dystrophin of abnormal size. It is generally believed that the amount of residual dystrophin in muscle is important in determining clinical severity of the disease (26).

Dystrophin –the gene and the proteins
The dystrophin gene is among the largest known, spanning 2.4 megabases of DNA and comprising about 1% of the entire X chromosome. The dystrophin gene is made up of 79 coding exons and numerous large introns (27). The dystrophin protein is a rod shaped cytoskeletal protein found along the inner surface of the plasma membrane in skeletal, cardiac and smooth muscle where it exists as part of a much

larger protein complex (28). In cardiac muscle it is also localized at the transverse tubules (29).

Dystrophin is divided into four domains: an amino terminal actin-binding domain, a central rod domain containing multiple spectrin-like repeats, a cysteine rich domain and a unique carboxy-terminal domain. Mutations involving separate regions of the dystrophin gene produce distinct phenotypic disorders characterized by their effect on specific functional domains of the dystrophin molecule. Five different cell type-specific dystrophin transcripts, each with its own promoter have been identified to date (30,31). Alternate splicing of specific exons provides additional diversity and complexity. Increased understanding of dystrophin's tissue specific expression and its distinct functional domains has made genotype-phenotype correlation possible in muscular dystrophy and X-linked cardiomyopathy (32,33).

Much has been learned in recent years about the role of dystrophin and its associated glycoprotein complex. This glycoprotein complex includes the sarcoglygans, dystroglycans (*a,b*) syntrophins (*a,b*) , sarcospan, and dystrobrevin. These proteins in association with dystrophin appear to cooperate in forming a transmembrane link between the intracellular actin-based cytoskeleton and the extracellular matrix. (Figure 1 DAPcomplex) Abnormalities of individual proteins within the complex have been associated with a disease phenotype, predominantly forms of limb-girdle muscular dystrophy (11,12,34). Mutations in selected members of the sarcoglycan complex have also been associated with a cardiomyopathy phenotype in human and/or animal models, reinforcing the importance of tissue specific roles for individual proteins within this syncitium (35).

The primary role of the dystrophin protein complex has long been thought to involve stabilizing the sarcolemma and protecting muscle from contraction-induced cell damage. Abnormalities in the dystrophin protein resulting from primary mutation or secondary perturbation have been shown to result in disruption of the sarcolemma, leading to increased membrane permeability, subsequent myocyte dysfunction and eventual cell death (36).

Recently, animal models have demonstrated that absence of one of the dystrophin associated proteins, *a*lpha-dystrobrevin, is associated with impairment in nitric oxide mediated signaling (37). This, along with other evidence, supports the theory that the dystrophin associated glycoprotein complex has a significant role in cell signaling in addition to its structural role in maintaining cell integrity.

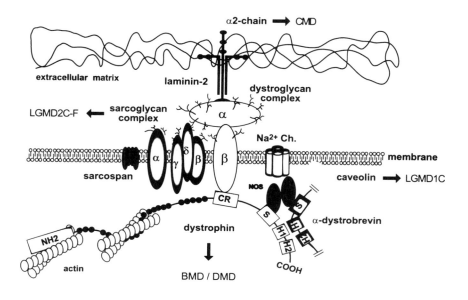

Figure 1- Dystrophin associated protein (DAP) complex

The dystrophin associated protein complex.
Dystrophin links the actin cytoskeleton to the extracellular matrix (laminin, α2-chain) via the dystroglycans (α,β). Transmembrane components of the complex include $\alpha,\beta,\gamma,\delta$ −sarcoglycan and sarcospan. Intracellular interacting proteins include the syntrophins (α,β), dystrobrevin. Arrows depict the various muscular dystrophies associated with mutations in individual proteins within the complex. Dystrophin shown depicting specific binding domains (actin binding domain, cysteine rich (CR) region binding β-dystroglycan, syntrophin binding region (S) and region binding dystrobrevin via helical repeat structures (H1,H2). The syntrophins may interact with nitric oxide synthase (NOS) and voltage gated sodium channels, both of which involve signal transduction. Congenital muscular dystrophy (CMD), Limb-girdle muscular dystrophy (LGMD) of various types, Duchenne (DMD) and Becker (BMD) muscular dystrophy.

Clinical features of dystrophinopathies- DMD, BMD, XLDCM

Clinical features of DMD

DMD generally presents with signs/symptoms of skeletal muscle weakness between 3 and 6 years of age, however growth failure, especially short stature, may be present prior to this. Proximal skeletal muscle weakness appears initially, with progressive weakness leading to loss of ambulation usually before the teenage years. Lumbar lordosis with waddling gait and positive Gowers' sign (mode of rising from the ground using the arms to assist in raising the torso) may be the first outward signs of underlying dystrophy. Pseudohypertrophy of the calves and other muscle groups is common. Deep tendon reflexes are lost in the weak muscles. In the second decade of life, after ambulation is lost there is progressive weakness resulting in kyphoscoliosis, respiratory insufficiency and eventual respiratory failure. Death usually occurs in the third decade (2).

The primary cause of death for individuals with DMD is respiratory failure due to diaphragm muscle weakness (affecting an estimated 40% of individuals with DMD). Cardiac failure is estimated to be the primary cause of death in 10-40%. Coexistent congestive heart failure or complications of low cardiac output (such as pulmonary embolus, etc.) may hasten respiratory failure.

Cardiac Findings in Duchenne dystrophy

Cardiac involvement in DMD develops insidiously during the first decade of life at a time when skeletal muscle weakness is already significant. Sinus tachycardia is present in most patients after age 5 and persists throughout life (3). The classic ECG of advanced cardiac disease in DMD exhibits tall R waves in V1 and right precordial leads and deep, narrow Q waves in the left precordial and limb leads (anterior QRS pattern). Pathological studies have suggested this ECG pattern reflect selective atrophy and scarring of the posterobasal region and adjacent lateral wall of the left ventricle, rather than actual right ventricular hypertrophy (38).

In a series of DMD patients studied over a ten year period, 62% of patients showed conduction abnormalities by age 10; consisting of a shortened PQ segment, prolonged QT interval, and/or an increased QT:PQ ratio (termed "cardiomyopathic index"). During the second decade of life there developed conduction system abnormalities (atrio-ventricular and intraventricular conduction delays as well as arrhythmias) and overt echocardiographic signs of cardiomyopathy (hypertrophic and dilated). Whereas the incidence of conduction defects remained relatively constant throughout life (6--13%), the incidence of clinical cardiac involvement, predominantly cardiomyopathy, rose steadily throughout the teenage years, affecting roughly 1/3 of patients by age 14, 1/2 of patients by age 18, and all patients over age 18 (39).

Dilated cardiomyopathy is the predominant type of heart disease at all ages. In DMD patients followed prospectively over several years, progressive dilation developed after a period of hypertrophy in some individuals. Despite the high incidence of cardiac involvement, many patients with DMD remain asymptomatic despite their underlying cardiomyopathy. Cardiac symptoms were present in only 28% of patients under age 18 with overt cardiac involvement (11/39) and in 57% (12/21) thereafter (39). The lack of cardiac symptomatology has been attributed to a reduced cardiac workload in the non-ambulatory state.

Coronary vascular pathology in Duchenne dystrophy demonstrates hypertrophy of medial smooth muscle with associated focal narrowing of the vascular lumen (40). (Figure 2) This smooth muscle hypertrophy is in striking contrast to the degeneration and necrosis seen in striated muscle of DMD patients. It is not known what contribution this obstructive vasculopathy plays in initiating or perpetuating the cardiomyopathy of DMD, but its role may be substantial. Recent studies in genetically engineered mice deficient in one of the dystrophin-associated-proteins (delta-sarcoglycan) demonstrate similar coronary vascular pathology. In this model the vascular pathology clearly precedes signs of myocardial necrosis, suggesting that secondary ischemia may play a causative role in the degenerative process of skeletal and/or cardiac muscle seen in some dystrophies (41).

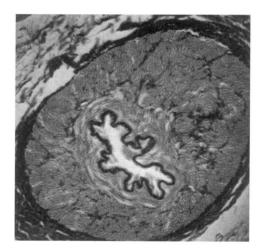

Figure 2- Coronary vessel in Duchenne dystrophy

Gomori-Trichrome staining elastin/ coronary vessel from patient with DMD.
Demonstrates severe smooth muscle hypertrophy resulting in narrowing of vessel lumen. Role of obstructive vasculopathy contributing to ischemic myocyte damage in dystrophinopathy may be significant.

Ultrastructural and biochemical evidence support the theory that dystrophin plays a major role in maintaining integrity and mechanical properties of the plasma cell membrane. Its disruption would be anticipated to have severe consequences, particularly in contractile tissue faced with constant mechanical stress. Simultaneously the dystrophin-associated complex appears central to the maintenance of membrane and cytoskeletal homeostasis via its cell signaling functions. Abnormalities such as those previously described, in addition to vascular pathology associated with smooth muscle dysfunction, may act in concert to produce the cardiac phenotype(s) seen in the spectrum of dystrophinopathies.

Clinical Findings in Becker dystrophy
Becker muscular dystrophy was described in 1953 with the observation of a 'benign' X-linked variant of DMD. This was confirmed following the identification of dystrophin, when both Duchenne and Becker muscular dystrophy patients were found to have dystrophin gene mutations. DMD patients were lacking any detectable dystrophin in skeletal muscle, correlating with mutations causing disruption of the reading frame or creating premature stop codons. Skeletal muscle from individuals with Becker dystrophy demonstrated dystrophin to be present in reduced amounts or of altered size, usually secondary to deletions which maintained an open reading frame for the protein.

Clinically, individuals with Becker muscular dystrophy may have no symptoms other than muscle cramping or myalgias. Becker muscular dystrophy may present with an asymptomatic CK elevation, myoglobinuria with exercise, or mild limb girdle or proximal muscle weakness. Loss of ambulation has occurred in BMD patients anywhere between 10 and 80 years of age, illustrating the wide variability in symptom severity.

Cardiac findings in BMD
Several studies have demonstrated that patients with BMD show a high incidence of clinical cardiac involvement despite their milder skeletal muscle disease (42-44). In fact, patients with BMD have presented with cardiomyopathy severe enough to require cardiac transplantation and/or with insufficient skeletal involvement to be diagnosed at time of transplantation (45). Although BMD patients may be asymptomatic for long periods of time, the most common cause of death in BMD is heart failure. In a series of 68 BMD patients studied from 1976--1993 whose diagnosis was confirmed by dystrophin testing, all showed preclinical or clinical cardiac involvement by 30 years of age (42). Overall, two thirds of patients had overt signs of cardiac disease: 44% had cardiomyopathy; 15% displayed regional wall motion abnormalities or ECG evidence of myocardial damage; and 7% had arrhythmias. Cardiomyopathy was rarely identified in patients under age 16, but rose steadily throughout adulthood, and was present in approximately 70% of patients above age 40. As in DMD, dilated cardiomyopathy (40%) appeared more commonly than hypertrophic cardiomyopathy (4%). Clinical cardiac disease was seen more frequently in individuals with advanced myopathy who remained ambulatory (80%) than in those with either mild myopathy or those who were non-

ambulatory. As has with DMD, a reduced cardiac workload may be responsible for the improved cardiac status of wheelchair-bound BMD patients.

Separate studies have demonstrated significant myocardial dysfunction among BMD patients classified as having subclinical muscle disease or mild weakness. It should be noted that some patients could be described as falling within the spectrum of XLDCM given an absence of clinical skeletal muscle abnormalities. Right ventricular dysfunction, as measured by end-diastolic diameter and ejection fraction, was more prevalent than left ventricular impairment (64% vs. 28%). Left ventricular dysfunction has been observed to correlate directly with age in most individuals with BMD. In this patient group (those with mild myopathy and significant cardiac involvement) there appears to be a clustering of dystrophin gene deletions involving exons 47 through 49 (43,46). A previous survey of 84 BMD patients found that deletions in this region were also associated with a higher frequency of severe cardiac involvement than deletions elsewhere in the dystrophin gene (47). These exons encode the middle portion of the rod domain of dystrophin, and fall within one of two deletion "hotspots" (exons 2--19 and 44--54) within dystrophin (30).

At least one study comparing the cardiac function BMD and DMD patients concluded that the progression of heart disease in BMD differs from that in DMD (47). In BMD patients, the most common ECG pattern included decreased R wave amplitude or prominent Q wave in leads I, aVL, and V6, (90%), whereas DMD patients most commonly exhibited prominent R wave amplitude in lead V1 (88%). There was considerable overlap of the ECG patterns between the two groups. BMD patients had a significantly higher PEP:ET ratio (pre-ejection period to ejection time) than DMD patients, even at the same level of muscle weakness. BMD patients also had a significantly larger left ventricular end diastolic dimension and mitral valve annular size, and a higher incidence of mitral regurgitation than DMD patients, all of which were progressive with age. It has been suggested that the slow progression of skeletal muscle weakness in typical BMD patients permit a prolonged workload on an impaired myocardium, eventually resulting in progressive ventricular dilatation and mitral regurgitation.

X- Linked Dilated Cardiomyopathy (XLDCM)
XLDCM typically presents as congestive heart failure in adolescent to young adult males and as atypical chest pain in middle-aged female carriers, neither of which display clinical muscle weakness. In males, the disease course may be progressive and result in cardiac transplantation or death within 1 to 2 years of presentation. Heart failure in carrier females may present later in life and progress over a number of years. The serum CK level has been elevated in most patients with XLDCM identified to date. (33) Like BMD patients, most individuals with XLDCM are asymtomatic but may demonstrate evidence of subclinical skeletal muscle disease.

The molecular basis for the selective cardiac involvement in numerous families with XLDCM has been successfully determined (49-53). Unlike those with Duchenne or Becker muscular dystrophy, individuals in these families failed to exhibit signs of skeletal involvement. An understanding of the complexity of dystrophin's genomic organization and transcriptional control is important to understanding the cardio-specific phenotype of XLDCM (Figure 3).

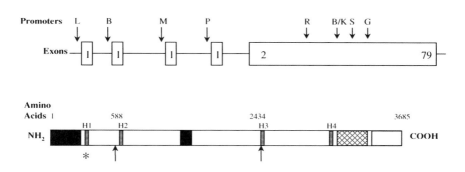

Figure 3. Dystrophin genomic organization and cDNA

A. Dystrophin gene organization.
The dystrophin gene is under intricate transcriptional control, utilizing eight different promoters for tissue-specific expression. Four full-length isoforms (L-lymphocyte, B-brain, M-muscle, P-Perkinje cerebellar cell) and four truncated isoforms (R-retinal [Dp116], B/K-brain/kidney [Dp140], S-Schwann cell [Dp116] and G-general [Dp71])
Full-length dystrophin isofoms contain a unique exon 1 that is spliced into exons 2-79. Isoforms depicted here demonstrate differential expression in some cases of XLDCM, due to mutations involving the muscle specific promoter and/or exon 1.
B.Dystrophin protein- schematic.
Dystrophin protein illustrating actin binding domain, rod domain, cystiene rich domain , and caboxy- terminal domain . Four hinge regions (H1,H2,H3,H4)   also shown. XLDCM mutation described affecting H1 (*) and sites of cleavage by enteroviral protease 2A (arrows). Findings suggest importance of hinge regions in maintaining myocyte integrity.

In several families with dilated cardiomyopathy, linkage was initially demonstrated to the dystrophin gene on Xp21. Mutations initially identified in families with XLDCM involved disruption of the 5' end of the dystrophin gene, including the muscle promoter and exon 1 (49,52). Rearrangement of Alu-like repetitive elements in the downstream portion of dystrophin (intron 11) has been described, resulting in a truncated transcript (54). These mutations result in loss of the full-length muscle isoform of dystrophin (M-Dp427) that is normally expressed in cardiac and skeletal muscle.

The presence of dystrophin immunostaining with carboxy-terminal but not amino-terminal antibodies in heart biopsies from patients with XLDCM may be explained by the presence of DP71, a small carboxy--terminal isoform of dystrophin that is normally expressed in all tissues except skeletal muscle. DP71 cannot fully replace the function of full-length dystrophin, supported by the results of transgenic mouse studies in which overexpression of the shortened isoform (Dp71) does not prevent the dystrophic phenotype in mdx mice, the mouse model of DMD (8,9).

Individuals with XLDCM have been shown to have upregulated transcription of the full-length brain (B--Dp427) and cerebellar Purkinje cell (P--Dp427) isoforms of dystrophin in skeletal muscle, but show no such upregulation of these transcripts in cardiac muscle. Dystrophin levels in the skeletal muscle of XLDCM patients appear reduced compared to normal control muscle, possibly explaining the mild myopathic features (52). Alternatively, the non-muscle isoforms may not be able to completely replace the function of the muscle isoform.

Identification of a missense mutation in exon 9, resulting in a change in polarity of an amino acid in the highly conserved first hinge region (H1; see Fig 3), demonstrated new insight into the production of cardiac-specific phenotypes related to dystrophin (53). Interestingly, disruption in two other hinge regions of dystrophin (H2 and H3) (see Fig 3) caused by action of enteroviral protease 2A (a product of Coxsackievirus) has been demonstrated in association with a dilated cardiomyopathy phenotype (36). These studies provide clues into the unique function of the dystrophins in cardiac muscle and further illustrate the complexity of tissue specific phenotypes seen in mutations involving dystrophin.

While most patients affected with a dystrophinopathy can be classified into one of three groups (DMD, BMD,) providing utility in predicting clinical prognosis, these diagnoses should be viewed as a continuum of disease expression. In particular, BMD shows great variability in the degree of skeletal and cardiac muscle involvement between individuals. Others referred to as having "atypical" or "subclinical" BMD do not have muscle weakness per se, but show mild skeletal muscle involvement with an elevated serum creatine phosphokinase (CPK), cramping or exertional myalgias, episodic myoglobinuria, or calf pseudohypertrophy. When these atypical patients develop severe cardiomyopathy, the distinction between BMD and XLDCM is blurred.

Cardiac disease in female carriers of DMD/BMD

Despite being an X--linked disorder, DMD and BMD female carriers show a surprisingly high incidence of cardiac involvement that progresses with age (Figure 1), manifesting primarily as cardiomyopathy. A ten year study of 152 DMD and 45 BMD carriers that found preclinical or clinical cardiac involvement in 55% of carriers under age 16 and in 90% after age 16. (23,24) Arrhythmias were rare at all ages (0-6%). Under age 16, 15% of females had detectable cardiomyopathy (12% hypertrophic, 3% dilated) compared to 41% over age 16 (30% hypertrophic, 11% dilated). Whereas dilated cardiomyopathy is more common in affected males, interestingly, hypertrophic cardiomyopathy was more common in carriers. Approximately 8% of carriers showed clinical signs of skeletal muscle disease.

As in skeletal muscle biopsies, cardiac muscle biopsies of DMD and BMD carriers showed a mosaic pattern of absent (DMD) or reduced (BMD) dystrophin immunoreactivity. In female carriers, the number of dystrophin-negative fibers is typically higher in cardiac muscle than in skeletal muscle. Unlike cardiac myocytes, skeletal muscle fibers may become progressively dystrophin-positive over time, presumably due the replacement of dystrophin-negative fibers with dystrophin-positive myoblasts (genetic normalization) and/or the intracellular diffusion of dystrophin from dystrophin-positive nuclei along the muscle fiber syncitium (biochemical normalization) (24).

Molecular Diagnosis

Characteristic clinical features and a dystrophic skeletal muscle biopsy in a male are strongly suggestive of DMD or BMD, but standard clinical practice is to confirm the diagnosis at the molecular level. Molecular testing can yield important information regarding prognosis and recurrence risk. Deletions in the dystrophin gene account for 65% of the mutations in DMD and 85% of the mutations in BMD, with duplications adding another 5% to each. A PCR--based assay performed on a sample of blood detects 98% of these deletion mutations (55,56). The reading frame hypothesis predicts with greater than 90% accuracy whether a mutation will result in a DMD or a BMD phenotype (57,58). Typically, a mutation that alters the reading frame of the dystrophin transcript causes a severe DMD phenotype, whereas mutations that preserve the reading frame are associated with a milder BMD phenotype. In general, frameshift and nonsense mutations that produce an unstable, truncated dystrophin protein that lacks its carboxy-terminus cause DMD, whereas those that preserve the carboxy-terminus of dystrophin cause BMD. The identification of point mutations or other small mutations is a formidable task given the large size of the dystrophin gene, but several have been documented using techniques such as single-stranded conformation polymorphism and the protein truncation test (58). Given recent data demonstrating critical regions of dystrophin potentially associated with isolated cardiomyopathy, exclusion of dystrophin mutations in dilated cardiomyopathy becomes increasingly important.

If no deletion or duplication is detected, dystrophin analysis is usually performed on skeletal muscle by immunocytochemistry and/or Western blotting. DMD is characterized by an absence or marked reduction in dystrophin using both techniques, whereas BMD is characterized by patchy staining of the plasma membrane by immunocytochemistry and dystrophin that has an abnormal size and/or is reduced in amount by Western blotting. A decreased amount of normal size dystrophin is not specific to BMD, as this pattern is also seen in several patients with autosomal recessive LGMD due to primary sarcoglycan deficiency (60-62).

Because manifesting female carriers of DMD and BMD have one normal and one abnormal dystrophin gene, detection of deletions by PCR or Southern blotting requires precise quantitation, which makes the interpretation of results more difficult. Dystrophin analysis in a muscle biopsy is generally more informative. Since only one X chromosome within each nucleus is active, carriers exhibit a mosaic pattern of normal and abnormal dystrophin immunostaining in skeletal and cardiac myocytes. In DMD carriers, dystrophin immunoreactivity is absent from a subpopulation of cells, whereas in BMD carriers, some cells show patchy or reduced dystrophin immunoreactivity.

A useful starting point in the evaluation of a dystrophinopathy as the cause of idiopathic DCM is a serum CPK level and a PCR assay for dystrophin gene deletions. Male patients with BMD (7,42) and female carriers with DMD (23) may initially present with DCM without symptoms of muscle weakness or elevated serum CPK, exertional myalgias or calf pseudohypertrophy. Since the standard PCR assay described above does not include the 5'-most end of the dystrophin gene where several mutations that cause XLDCM have been localized (32,33,50,53), primers that amplify muscle exon 1 should be included the analysis. At the protein level, immunocytochemistry and/or Western blotting using antibodies directed to different sites on dystrophin may determine whether dystrophin is present, absent, or abnormal in cardiac and/or skeletal muscle. That a deficiency of full-length dystrophin in cardiac muscle will always be due to mutations in the dystrophin gene may be premature, as primary deficiencies in dystrophin-associated proteins could result in a secondary loss of cardiac dystrophin. Previous attempts to screen for a dystrophinopathy in groups of patients with idiopathic cardiomyopathy have not been successful (59), which suggests that age, elevated CPK, and muscle involvement may be important discriminating variables. Should a patient's serum CPK be elevated and the analysis of dystrophin be normal, other myopathies or muscular dystrophies with primary cardiac involvement should be considered.

Future Directions

One of the challenges in the future will be to develop a unifying concept for understanding the molecular pathophysiology of muscular dystrophy. Identification of several disease genes and characterization of their protein products has revealed new cellular processes and biochemical pathways that are involved in the dystrophic process (60-65). Decreased mechanical stability of the plasma membrane as a final common pathway remains an attractive hypothesis given the primary involvement of the dystrophin-glycoprotein complex in several forms of muscular dystrophy, but undoubtedly represents an oversimplification of its function. Alternatively, it now appears that the dystrophin-associated glycoprotein complex serves other critical functions, e.g. in signal transduction and the regulation of intracellular calcium levels, distinct from any role as a mechanical stabilizer of the plasma membrane. Further investigations into protein expression and function should shed light on why certain muscular dystrophies preferentially target the myocardium or specialized cardiac tissue. Natural animal models of muscular dystrophy, in conjunction with laboratory engineered transgenic and knockout mice, continue to be important in vivo tools for studying the functions of individual proteins and evaluating parameters for future gene therapy. Caution must be used in extrapolating results of these animal models to humans, particularly in predicting genotype-phenotype correlations (66).

The demand for molecular genetic testing of the muscular dystrophies will continue to increase as physicians and patients become better educated as to how these results can influence patient care and family planning decisions. The most immediate benefits will be to confirm disease diagnosis for patients, identify presymptomatic family members, screen individuals with idiopathic cardiac conduction disturbances and cardiomyopathy, and prenatal diagnosis. Unfortunately, interpretation of an abnormal result, i.e. prediction of disease severity based on mutation analysis, may be clear for some disorders but not others. Additional genetic and non-genetic factors undoubtedly modify the disease phenotype in different families or in different members of the same family, making prognostic predictions unreliable and potentially dangerous. Several of the disease genes causing muscular dystrophy have only recently been identified, and the continued characterization of individual mutations and their phenotypes is necessary to establish clinically meaningful correlations.

Treatment for the muscular dystrophies continues to be symptomatic and supportive, but with further understanding of disease specific pathophysiology there is hope that the application of genetic approaches will have some therapeutic application. Promising results have been obtained using gene therapy to correct the dystrophic phenotype of the mdx mouse model of DMD, including myoblast transfer (67). Replacement of dystrophin via expression of recombinant dystrophin "minigenes" (smaller dystrophin genes that contain internal in-frame deletions associated with a mild BMD phenotype) (68,69), have been performed in animals. Only myoblast transfer has been attempted in humans, and the results of recent clinical trials have thus far been disappointing (70). Newer viral-based gene delivery systems are being developed which can accommodate the extremely large 14 kilobase dystrophin cDNA. Undoubtedly, a more complete understanding of the unique role of dystrophin and the dystrophin associated proteins in the heart will be necessary before any comprehensive therapeutic strategies can be successfully employed.

REFERENCES

1. Dubowitz V: Muscle Biopsy: A Practical Approach. In The Muscular Dystrophies, London: Baillière Tindall; 1985:289-404.
2. Engel AG, Yamamoto M, Fischbeck KH: Dystrophinopathies. In Myology, 2nd ed. Engel AG, Franzini-Armstrong C, eds. New York: McGraw Hill; 1994:1133-1187
3. Cox GF, Kunkel LM: Dystrophies and heart disease. Curr Opin Cardiol 1997;12:329-343.
4. Koenig M, Beggs AH, Moyer M, et al.: The molecular basis for Duchenne versus Becker muscular dystrophy: Correlation of severity with type of deletion. Am J Hum Genet 1989,45:498-506.
5. Koenig M, Hoffman EP, Bertelson CJ, Monaco AP, Feener C, Kunkel LM: Complete cloning of the Duchenne muscular dystrophy (DMD) cDNA and preliminary genomic organization of the DMD gene in normal and affected individuals. Cell 1987;50:509-517.
6. Monaco AP, Bertelson CJ, Liechti GS, Moser H, Kunkel LM: An explanation for the phenotypic differences between patients bearing partial deletions of the DMD locus. Genomics 1988;2:90-95.
7. Yoshida K, Ikeda S, Nakamura A, et al: Molecular analysis of the Duchenne muscular dystrophy gene in patients with Becker muscular dystrophy presenting with dilated cardiomyopathy. Muscle Nerve 1993;16:1161-1166.
8. Cox GA, Sunada Y, Campbell KP, Chamberlain JS: Dp71 can restore the dystrophin-associated glycoprotein complex in muscle but fails to prevent dystrophy. Nature Genet 1994;8:333-339.
9. Greenberg DS, Sunada Y, Campbell KP, Yaffe D, Nudel U: Exogenous Dp71 restores the levels of dystrophin associated proteins but does not alleviate muscle damage inmdx mice. Nature Genet 1994;8:340-344.
10. Worton R: Muscular dystrophies: diseases of the dystrophin-glycoprotein complex. Science 1995;270:755-756.
11. Bönnemann CG, McNally EM, Kunkel LM: Beyond dystrophin: current progress in the muscular dystrophies. Curr Opin Pediatr 1997;8:569-582.
12. Vainzof M, Passos-Bueno MR, Moreira ES, et al.: The sarcoglycan complex in the six autosomal recessive limb-girdle muscular dystrophies. Hum Molec Genet 1996;5:1963-1969.
13. Ervasti JM, Campbell KP: A role for the dystrophin-glycoprotein complex as a transmembrane linker between laminin and actin. J Cell Biol 1993;122:809-823.
14. Carlson, George C: The Dystrophinopathies: An Alternative to the Structural Hypothesis. Neurobiol Dis 1998;5:3-15.
15. Politano L, Nigro V, Nigro G, et al: Development of cardiomyopathy in female carriers of Duchenne and Becker muscular dystrophies. JAMA 1996;275:1335-1338.
16. Nigro G, Comi LI, Politano L, et al.: Evaluation of the cardiomyopathy in Becker muscular dystrophy. Muscle Nerve 1995;18:283-291.
17. Song KS, Scherer PE, Tang Z, et al: Expression of caveolin-3 in skeletal, cardiac, and smooth muscle cells. Caveolin-3 is a component of thesarcolemma and co-fractionates with dystrophin and dystrophin-associated glycoproteins. J Biol Chem 1996;271:15160-15165.
18. Bredt DS. Knocking signaling out of the dystrophin complex. Nature Cell Biology 1999;1:E89-91.
19. Fadic R, Sunada Y, Waclawik AJ, et al: Deficiency of a dystrophin-associated glycoprotein (adhalin) in a patient with muscular dystrophy and cardiomyopathy. N Engl J Med 1996;334:362-6.
20. Roberds SL, Ervasti JM, Anderson RD, et al: Disruption of the dystrophin-glycoprotein complex in the cardiomyopathic hamster. J Biol Chem 1993;268:11469-11499.
21. Hoffman EP, Arahata K, Minetti C, Bonilla E, Rowland LP: Dystrophinopathy in isolated cases of myopathy in females. Neurology 1992;42:967-975.
22. Lyon MF: X-chromosome inactivation and developmental patterns in mammals. Biol Rev 1972;47:1-35.
23. Mirabella M, Servidei S, Manfredi G, et al: Cardiomyopathy may be the only clinical manifestation in female carriers of Duchenne muscular dystrophy. Neurology 1993;43:2342-2345.
24. Clerk A, Rodillo E, Heckmatt JZ, Dubowitz, V, Strong PN, Sewry CA. Characterisation of dystrophin in carriers of Duchenne muscular dystrophy. J Neurol Sci 1991;102:197-205.

25. Kunkel LM, Snyder JR, Beggs AH, Boyce FM, Feener CA: Searching for dystrophin gene deletions in patients with atypical presentations. In Etiology of Human Disease at the DNA level. Lindsten J, Ed. Raven Press; 1991:51-59.

26. Petrof BJ, Shrager JB, Stedman HH, Kelly AM, Sweeney HL: Dystrophin protects the sarcolemma from stresss developed during muscle contraction. Proc Nat Acad Sci 1993;90:3710-3714.

27. Hoffman EP, Brown RJ, Kunkel LM: Dystrophin: the protein product of the Duchenne muscular dystrophy locus. Cell 1987;51:919-928.

28. Koenig M, Monaco AP, Kunkel LM: The complete sequence of dystrophin predicts a rod-shaped cytoskeletal protein. Cell 1988;53:219-226.

29. Meng H, Leddy J, Frank J, Holland P, Tuana B: The Association of Cardiac Dystrophin with Myofibrils/Z-disk Regions in Cardiac Muscle Suggests a Novel Role in the Contractile Apparatus. J Biol Chem 1996;271:12364-12371.

30. Sadoulet-Puccio HM, Kunkel LM: Dystrophin and its isoforms. Brain Pathology 1996;6:25-35.

31. Ahn AH, Kunkel LM: The structural and functional diversity of dystrophin. Nat Genet 1993;3:283-291.

32. Muntoni F, Wilson L, Marrosu G, et al: A mutation in the dystrophin gene selectively affecting dystrophin expression in heart. J Clin Invest 1995;96:693-699.

33. Milasin J, Muntoni F, Severini M, et al.: A point mutation in the 5' splice site of the dystrophin gene first intron responsible for X-linked dilated cardiomyopathy. Hum Molec Genet 1996;5:73-79.

34. Ozawa E, Yoshida M, Hagiwara Y, Suzuki A, Mizuno Y, Noguchi S: Dystrophin-associated proteins in muscular dystrophy. Hum Molec Genet 1995;4:1711-1716.

35. Nigro V, Okazaki Y, Belsito A, et al.: Identification of the Syrian hamster cardiomyopathy gene. Hum Molec Genet 1997;6:601-607.

36. Badorf C, Lee G-H, Lamphear BJ, Martone ME, Campbell KP, Rhoads RE, Knowlton KU. Enteroviral protease 2A cleaves dystrophin:Evidence of cytoskeletal disruption in an acquired cardiomyopathy. Nat Med 1999;5:320-326.

37. Grady RM, Grange RW, Lau KS, et al. Role for alpha-dystrobrevin in the pathogenesis of dystrophin-dependent muscular dystrophies. Nat Cell Biol 1999;1:215-220.

38. Perloff JK, Roberts WC, de Leon Jr AC, O'Doherty D: The distinctive electrocardiogram of Duchenne's progressive muscular dystrophy. Am J Medicine 1967;42:179-188.

39. Nigro G, Comi LI, Politano L, Bain RJI: The incidence and evolution of cardiomyopathy in Duchenne muscular dystrophy. Int J Cardiol 1990;26:271-277.

40. Perloff, JK: Cardiac Manifestations of Neuromuscular Disease. Atlas of Heart Disease-Cardiomyopathies, myocarditis and pericardial disease. Philadelphia: Curr Medicine;1995:6.2-6.19.

41. Coral-Vasquez R, Cohn RD, Moore SA, et al: Disruption of the sarcoglycan-sarcospan complex in vascular smooth muscle: a novel mechanism for cardiomyopathy and muscular dystrophy. Cell 1999;98:465-474.

42. Melacini P, Fanin M, Danieli GA, et al.: Myocardial involvement is very frequent among patients affected with subclinical Becker's muscular dystrophy. Circulation 1996;94:3168-3175.

43. Saito M, Kawai H, Akaike M, Adachi K, Nishida Y, Saito S: Cardiac dysfunction in Becker muscular dystrophy. Am Heart J 1996;132:642-647.

44. Nigro G, Comi LI, Politano L, et al.: Evaluation of the cardiomyopathy in Becker muscular dystrophy. Muscle Nerve 1995;18:283-291.

45. Quinlivan RM, Dubowitz V: Cardiac transplantation in Becker muscular dystrophy. Neuromusc Dis 1992;2:165-167.

46. Beggs AH, Hoffman EP, Snyder JR, et al: Exploring the molecular basis for variability among patients with Becker muscular dystrophy: dystrophin gene and protein studies. Am J Hum Genet 1991;49

47. Nigro G, Politano L, Nigro V, Petratta VR, Comi LI: Mutation of the dystrophin gene and cardiomyopathy. Neuromusc Dis 1994;4:371-379.

48. Muntoni F, Melis M, Ganau A, Dubowitz V: Transcription of the dystrophin gene in normal tissues and in skeletal muscle of a family with X-linked dilated cardiomyopathy. Am J Hum Genet 1995;56:151-157.

49. Towbin JA, Hejtmancik JF, Brink P, et al: X-linked dilated cardiomyopathy: molecular genetic evidence of linkage to the Duchenne muscular dystrophy (dystrophin) gene at the Xp21 locus. Circulation 1993;87:1854-1993.

50. Muntoni F, Cau M, Ganau A, et al: Deletion of the dystrophin muscle-promoter region associated with X-linked dilated cardiomyopathy. N Engl J Med 1993;329:921-925.

51. Franz WM, Cremer M, Herrmann R, et al: X-linked dilated cardiomyopathy.Novel mutation of the dystrophin gene. Ann New York Acad Sci 1996;752:470-491.

52. Klamut HJ, Bosnoyan-Collins LO, Worton RG, Ray PN, Davis HL: Identification of a transcriptional enhancer within muscle intron 1 of the human dystrophin gene. HumMolec Genet 1996;5:1599-1606.

53. Ortiz-Lopez R, Li H, Su J, Goytia V, Towbin JA. Evidence for a dystrophin missense mutation as a cause of x-linked dilated cardiomyopathy. Circulation 1997;95:2434-2440.

54. Ferlini A, Galie N, Merlini L, Sewry C, Branzi A, Mutoni F. A novel Alu-like element rearranged in the dystrophin gene causes a splicing mutation in a family with X-linked dilated cardiomyopathy. Am J Hum Genet 1996;63:436-46.

55. Beggs AH, Kunkel LM: Improved diagnosis of Duchenne/Becker muscular dystrophy. J Clin Invest 1990;85:613-619.

56. Chamberlain JS, Gibbs RA, Ranier JE, Caskey CT: Multiplex PCR for the diagnosis of Duchenne muscular dystrophy. In PCR protocols: a guide to methods and applications, New York, Academic Press; 1990:272-281.

57. Koenig M, Beggs AH, Moyer M, et al.: The molecular basis for Duchenne versus Becker muscular dystrophy: Correlation of severity with type of deletion. Am J Hum Genet 1989;45:498-506.

58. Gardner RJ, Bobrow M, Roberts RM: The identification of point mutations in Duchenne muscular dystrophy patients by using reverse-transcription PCR and the protein-truncation test. Am J Hum Genet 1995;57:311-320.

59. Michels VV, Pastores GM, Moll PP, et al.: Dystrophin analysis in idiopathic dilated cardiomyopathy. J Med Genet 1993;30:955-957.

60. Tinsley JM, Blake DJ, Zuellig RA, Davies KE: Increasing complexity of the dystrophin-associated protein complex. Proc Nat Acad Sci 1994;91:8307-8313.

61. Bönnemann CG, Modi R, Noguchi S, et al.: Beta-sarcoglycan (A3b) mutations cause autosomal recessive muscular dystrophy with loss of the sarcoglycan complex. Nat Genet 1995;11:266-273.

62. Nigro V, de Sa Moriera E, Piluso G, et al: The 5q autosomal recessive limb-girdle muscular dystrophy (LGMD 2F) is caused by a mutation in the sarcoglycan gene. Nat Genet 1996;14:195-98.

63. Helbling-Leclerc A, Zhang X, Topaloglu H, et al.: Mutations in the laminin alpha 2-chain gene (LAMA2) cause merosin-deficient congenital muscular dystrophy. Nat Genet 1995;11:216-218.

64. Munoz-Mármol AM, Strasser G, Isamat M, et al: A dysfunctional desmin mutation in a patient with severe generalized myopathy. Proc Natl Acad Sci USA 1998;96:11312-11317.

65. Mizuno Y, Noguchi S, Yamamoto H, et al.: Selective defect of sarcoglycan complex in severe childhood autosomal recessive muscular dystrophy muscle. Biochem Biophys Res Comm 1994;203:979-983.

66. Sakamoto A, Ono K, Abe M, et al: Both hypertrophic and dilated cardiomyopathies are caused by mutation of the same gene, d-sarcoglycan, in hamster: An animal model of disrupted dystrophin-associated glycoprotein complex. Proc Natl Acad Sci USA 1997;94:13873-13878.

67. Partridge TA, Morgan JE, Coulton GR, Hoffman EP, Kunkel LM: Conversion of mdx myofibers from dystrophin negative to positive by injection of normal myoblasts. Nature 1989;337:176-179.

68. Phelps SF, Hauser MA, Cole NM, et al: Expression of full-length and truncated dystrophin mini-genes in transgenic mdx mice. Hum Molec Genet 1995;4:1251-1258.

69. Wells DJ, Wells KE, Asante EA, et al: Expression of human full-length and minidystrophin in transgenic mdx mice: implications for gene therapy of Duchenne muscular dystrophy. HumMolec Genet 1995;4:1245-1250.

70. Mendell JR, Kissel JT, Amato AA, et al.: Myoblast transfer in the treatment of Duchenne Muscular Dystrophy. New Engl J Med 1995;333:832-838.

17
MYOTONIC MUSCULAR DYSTROPHY GENETICS AND CARDIAC SEQUELAE

Sita Reddy, Ph.D. and Charles I. Berul, M.D.

The University of Southern California, Los Angeles, CA
Children's Hospital • Boston, Harvard Medical School, Boston, MA

INTRODUCTION

Myotonic dystrophy [DM] (Steinert's disease) is the most common adult onset muscular dystrophy in humans. DM is a progressive, multi-system disorder which manifests as a highly variable pathological phenotype of the skeletal muscle, smooth muscle, heart, brain, glucose metabolism, lens and testicular function (1,2,3). The phenotypic variability in DM is compounded by clinical anticipation, a phenomenon in which the severity of the symptoms increase, while the age of disease onset decreases, with each successive generation within a disease pedigree (4). Thus the spectrum of DM symptoms can vary from mild, where cataracts develop late in adult life, to a severe congenital form associated with skeletal muscle hypotonia, often resulting in respiratory arrest and mortality. An intermediate adult-onset form of DM can manifest with one or more characteristic features of DM including myotonia, or abnormal muscle membrane depolarization which results in abnormally elongated muscle relaxation time, skeletal muscle weakness and wasting, cardiac conduction system disease, cataracts, endocrine dysfunction, frontal balding, epithiliomas and mental retardation (2,3).

Adult-onset DM
Table 1 summarizes the major systemic changes observed in DM patients. Some or all of the changes may be found with one or more system being affected (1,2,3).

Skeletal muscle
A brief review of skeletal muscle pathology in DM is provided as extensive histological and electrophysiological studies have been conducted on skeletal muscle when compared to cardiac tissue. These studies can therefore provide a framework for understanding cardiac pathology in DM. Although a range of skeletal muscles can be affected in DM, fast twitch muscles are usually more severely affected than slow twitch muscles. During the course of the disease it is not uncommon to find the early involvement of facial and neck muscles, including the temporalis, masseter, and sternomastoid while the extensor forearm muscles and anterior tibial muscles, and muscles of the hands and feet usually show significant changes later during disease progression. Skeletal muscle symptoms include myotonia, muscle weakness and dystrophy (5,6). Myotonia is the abnormal depolarization of muscle which results in delayed muscle relaxation after a strong contraction. Percussion myotonia is often elicited in DM patients by a mechanical stimulus applied directly to the muscle. Electrical myotonia is usually irregularly distributed about the skeletal muscles (7). Myotonia usually manifests early in disease progression often preceding dystrophy and can diminish as muscle wasting becomes significant (3).

Table 1: Systemic Involvement in DM System Pathology	
1. Skeletal muscle	Weakness, myotonia and dystrophy are predominantly observed in facial, neck and distal limb muscles
2. Heart	Conduction disorders more prominent than overt cardiomyopathy
3. Smooth muscle	Widespread involvement of pharynx, esophagus, colon and uterus. Delayed relaxation, abnormal peristalsis
4. Eye	Cataracts and decreased vision independent of cataracts
5. Endocrine system	Abnormal carbohydrate metabolism and gonadal atrophy
6. Brain	Mental retardation and hypersomnolence
7. Skeletal system	Cranial and facial abnormalities, talipes
8. Lungs	Hypoventilation
9. Skin	Premature balding and calcifying epithelioma

Muscle wasting is slow and 10-30 years of progressive loss may be required before significant changes in muscle mass are observed in DM. The histological changes are variably manifested and depend on the muscle biopsied and stage of the disease. Some or all of the following changes have been reported in DM muscle biopsies: variation in fiber size, fibrosis, central nuclei, nuclear chains, ringed fibers, sarcoplasmic masses (homogenous areas of disorganized intermyofibrillary material), atrophy of type 1 fibers and increased arborization of terminal enervations. Less prominent features include small angular fibers, moth-eaten fibers and hypertrophy of type 2 fibers (8-10). Ultrastructural changes of the Z line, A band, T tubules and sarcoplasmic reticulum changes are seen in DM (11,12). Skeletal muscle weakness can be profound and in several cases be disproportionate to the dystrophic changes (2,3) observed in the muscle. This may suggest that a functional abnormality may contribute to the muscle weakness manifested.

Abnormalities of ion channels and pumps in DM
The etiology of the myotonia and muscle weakness in DM is poorly understood. However one or more steps in the established series of events elicited in normal muscle by the binding of acetylcholine to acetylcholine receptors may be abnormal.

Depolarization commences with the inflow of potassium ions through inward rectifier channels. Once depolarization proceeds beyond a threshold value, voltage dependent sodium channels open to allow the influx of sodium ions which allows extensive depolarization. Repolarization begins with an outward potassium ion conductance occurring through a transient outward potassium channel immediately followed by the opening of voltage gated calcium channels (both L-type DHPRs and T-type) allowing the inflow of calcium ions. Repolarization is completed by the outflow of potassium ions through the voltage-gated delayed rectifier channels.

Calcium influx in muscle cells facilitates excitation-contraction coupling by allowing the calcium gated ryanodine receptors on the sarcoplasmic reticulum to release internal sarcoplasmic reticulum stores of calcium into the cytoplasm which subsequently results in muscle contraction. Muscle relaxation and membrane repolarization occur when calcium is pumped back into the sarcoplasmic reticulum by SR-Calcium pumps. In addition, membrane repolarization proceeds with the exchange of two sodium ions for three potassium ions occurring via the Na^+/K^+ pump (Reviewed in 13). Several of these basic steps are altered in myotonic dystrophy and could contribute to myotonia and muscle weakness of the skeletal muscle observed in DM. There is significant variability in the electrophysiological studies carried out in DM patients. This may be a reflection of the variability in the pathology observed (5). However some features of interest are discussed below.

Muscle fibers from DM patients have been reported to show increased sodium conductance of sodium channels (14-16) and reduced Na/K-ATPase activity (17). These changes may be responsible for the increased intracellular sodium ion concentration (18) and the decrease in resting membrane potential reported in DM muscles (19-21). This decrease in resting membrane potentials could in turn lead to abnormal activity of voltage gated channels such as the L-type calcium channels which may be active under conditions in which they normally inactive (22).

In this regard, it is of interest to note that intracellular calcium concentrations are higher in DM muscles (18,22,23). Thus the more negative potentials observed may allow calcium to be drawn in more rapidly through L-type calcium channels. It is unclear if L-type channel dysfunction occurs indirectly as a consequence of the less negative membrane potentials generated by abnormal sodium conductance and/or directly due to altered phosphorylation of the DHP receptors (24).

Furthermore, activity and content of SR-calcium ATPase has been reported to be reduced 35-40% in DM muscle (25). As the specific activity of the SR-calcium ATPases is not altered, the total number of SR-calcium ATPases is predicted to be lower in DM muscles. This defect may underlie both the increased intracellular calcium ion concentrations reported and the smaller amounts of calcium that are released from the SR when DM muscles are stimulated with acetylcholine (22). In the latter event the slower rates of calcium removal from the cytoplasm to the SR may result decreased SR calcium stores which in turn may reduce the magnitude of calcium outflow from the SR in a second round of depolarization. Such a decrease in acetylcholine mediated outflow of calcium from the SR may be responsible for the decrease in the absolute force generated, while the delayed kinetics of the abnormal calcium ion removal from the cytoplasm could underlie the prolonged contraction /myotonia associated with DM. In this regard it is of interest to note that SR-calcium ATPases are far more abundant in skeletal fast twitch muscles, which show greater pathology in DM patients, compared to slow twitch muscles (26).

In addition to the abnormal recruitment of sodium and calcium channels, calcium-dependent potassium currents, which can be experimentally blocked by apamin, have been hypothesized to contribute to DM associated myotonia (27). Apamin sensitive calcium-dependent potassium channels are absent in normal adult muscle and are highly expressed in myotubes and denervated muscles (28). Blockade of axonal flow has been shown to induce an increase in apamin channels (29). In such muscles abnormal repetitive electrical discharges and prolonged relaxation time, occurring due to potassium induced depolarization of the T-tubule membranes, has been observed (29). Importantly, intramuscular injection of apamin has been shown to sharply decrease myotonia specifically in DM patients but not in myotonia congenita patients, where myotonia has been shown to occur as a consequence of abnormal chloride ion conductance (27). Apamin sensitive channels are increased in fast twitch muscles which are more affected in DM patients, and decrease with age, thus appearing to parallel the more severe pathology of fast-twitch muscles and the age-related decrease in myotonia reported in DM patients (30). Parallel defects in cardiac muscle and the brain may underlie the cardiac conduction defects and the cognitive deficits observed in DM patients.

Cardiac defects in DM

Sudden death occurs with high incidence (15-30%) in DM patients when compared to the general population (31). Although the underlying reasons for sudden death in DM are potentially numerous, progressive deterioration of cardiac function has been shown to play a major contributing role (32-36). The overall incidence of cardiac abnormality is very high (~80%) in DM patients being approximately four fold higher when compared with age matched normal controls (19%) (p<0.001) (37,38,39). Cardiac abnormalities are primarily conduction disorders which occur in 45-80% of DM patients and the increased incidence of sudden cardiac death occurs from either complete atrioventricular (AV) block or ventricular arrhythmias (3,31-39). Disorders of impulse formation in the sinus node are also observed and a significant proportion of patients exhibit sinus bradycardia (39). The mechanism of arrhythmogenesis in DM is shown in Table 2.

Table 2: Electrocardiographic Abnormalities in DM Patients

1. Disorder of Impulse formation
       Sinus bradycardia
       Prolonged SA recovery time
       SA node dysfunction (3)
2. Disorders of Impulse Conduction
       Atrioventricular Block (Intermittent/Stable 1°, 2°, 3° A-V block)
       Intraventricular conduction defects (fascicular block, bundle branch block)
3. Arrhythmias
       Premature atrial beats, atrial flutter, atrial fibrillation
       Premature ventricular beats, ventricular tachycardia
       Q waves and repolarization abnormalities
       More common with severe neuromuscular disease (35,39-41)
4. Combined Electrophysiological Disorders

Progression in the severity of cardiac conduction defects in DM

Most DM patients show a gradual but predictable increase the severity of the conduction disorders. One study in which 56 DM patients, exhibiting three different grades of neuromuscular disease, were followed for 52 months, suggested frequent and severe conduction abnormalities, which could not always be predicted (40). Progression often appears to occur from intermittent to stable first degree A-V block followed by more serious intraventricular block including HV prolongation, bundle branch blocks, ventricular late potentials and ventricular arrhythmias and pathological Q waves (35,40,41). Thus, although intermittent or stable A-V block is usually not a pathological finding in the general population, it should be regarded with caution in DM patients, as it often represents an early presymptomatic marker of developing more severe conduction defects.

As most of these abnormalities reflect A-V-His Purkinje disease which can culminate in fatal Stokes-Adams episodes unless treated by pacemaker implantation, it is useful to define parameters which have predictive value in the possible rate of deterioration and/or progression to possibly fatal conduction disorders in DM. Although a rough correlation exists between the severity of the neuromuscular disease and progression of cardiac disease in DM, other studies suggest that the PR interval duration is a better predictor of both the rate of deterioration and the severity of the conduction blocks which may develop (36). In a six year study of 37 DM patients in which the PR interval (191+ 30 to 208+31msec) increased with time in 90% of the patients and QRS interval (92+14 to 105+20 msec) increased in 74% of the patients, demonstrated that the rate of change was gradual, with the PR interval increasing by 1.5% and the QRS by 2.5% per year. However the maximal individual change per year (5.3% for the PR interval and 11% for QRS) corresponded to individual patients showing the longest baseline PR interval. In addition, most patients diagnosed with long PR intervals tended to have HV expansions and were prone to complete heart block and sudden death (36). Therefore, serial ECGs and the determination of baseline PR intervals may predict sudden death or complete heart block presenting as syncope better than the progression of other neurological involvement including muscle weakness.

Echocardiographic abnormalities reported in DM patients
Unlike Freidrich's ataxia, DM is less frequently associated with overt cardiac failure and cardiomegaly (42,43). Coronary artery disease incidence is not increased in DM (3). However as abnormal Q waves with normal coronary arteries have been reported in DM patients regional myocardial dystrophy may be indicated (44). Mitral valve prolapse (17-32%) (37,45,46,47) and systolic dysfunction (28%) (37,48,49) are reported at a low frequency in DM patients. Systolic dysfunction includes wall motion abnormalities which when further evaluated by Doppler echocardiography have revealed depressed left ventricular systolic function including reductions in ejection fraction, fractional shortening and reduced stroke volume in DM patients when compared to normal controls (37). However in contrast to characteristic incidence of myotonia in skeletal muscle (1-3), diastolic abnormalities are not consistently reported (39,48,50). Although the conduction system is the primary cardiac tissue affected in DM, myocardial abnormalities may contribute to the overall pathology. Echocardiographic abnormalities are usually more prevalent in older patients who show severe neuromuscular symptoms.

Structural alterations in the conduction system may produce pathology
The etiology of cardiac disease in DM is unknown. However both structural and functional abnormalities in the heart may contribute to the pathology. The conduction system normally is comprised of neuromyocardium embedded in fibro-elastic tissue. For proper conduction to be maintained, the components of the conduction system should be contiguous and also maintain extensive connections with the myocardium. In DM patients, the non-specific structural changes observed in the conduction system and in the myocardium could serve to disrupt the continuity of electrical impulses being propagated. Structural changes contributing to abnormal signal generation or conduction may be a result of atrophy of the neuromyocardial cells with an increase in the fibrous component in the nodes, His bundle, bundle branches and in the Purkinje fibers (51). In addition connections between the conduction system and the myocardium have been reported to undergo progressive fibrosis (51). Such changes may serve to disrupt the continuity of electrical impulses traveling through the heart.

Dystrophic changes in the myocardium, although not as severe as those observed in skeletal muscle, may also contribute to pathology, including variation in fiber size, myocardial fibers atrophy, fibrosis and fatty infiltration (**Figure 1**). Electron microscopic observation demonstrates an increase in disorganized and degenerating mitochondria, abnormalities of the Z line, and focal dissolution of myofibrils (53,54). These non-specific structural abnormalities can have two consequences to either sever the contact of the myocardium with the conduction system or alternatively localized myocardial atrophy can allow blocks in electrical conduction resulting in reentry and tachyarrhythmias (52-55). Although the distribution and extent of structural abnormalities in the conduction system and myocardium appear to correlate with antemortem ECG conduction block, it is far from absolute. Several studies have reported minor structural changes that do not serve to explain the severity of the cardiac abnormalities manifested in DM (32,34). Thus although progressive structural abnormalities no doubt play a role in the etiology of cardiac disease functional changes may also contribute to pathology.

Functional changes which may lead to pathology in DM
Ion channel dysfunction in DM cardiac muscle is largely unexplored, however given the extensive alterations in skeletal muscle ion channel function, it is highly likely that parallel changes in the heart may contribute to alterations in either the kinetics or magnitude of propagated current. Decreased membrane potential is well documented in skeletal muscle (19,20,21), similar changes are predicted to alter the depolarization and repolarization phases of the cardiac cycle. Thus partial membrane depolarization may inhibit the recovery of rapid sodium channels from inactivation thus reducing the number of available Na^+ channels for depolarization and decreasing the magnitude of the rapid Na^+ current. Such a reduction in Vmax and action potential amplitude could prolong the conduction time of a propagated impulse and result in conduction blocks (56).

Alterations in calcium homeostasis in a manner similar to that observed in skeletal muscle may also serve to prolong conduction times as increased intracellular calcium concentrations may facilitate closure of gap junctions in cardiac tissue (57). In addition, alterations in calcium homeostasis may alter impulse propagation through the AV node, where action potentials are predominantly mediated by slow calcium currents rather than by fast inward sodium currents (58,59). It is also unclear if long term increases in intracellular calcium may lead to cardiac cell inviability and atrophy.

Better understanding of ion channel function in DM cardiac tissue may be key in the development of rational therapy for DM. Development of animal models for DM should greatly facilitate this process.

Drugs
Careful management of DM patients with anesthesia is necessary because of the higher frequency of cardiorespiratory problems during anesthesia and surgery (60).

Antiarrhythmic agents such as quinine, quinidine, and procainamide used in the treatment of myotonia are known to increase the PR interval and depress cardiac conduction and should be avoided. Diphenylhydantoin, which shortens the PR and may be equally effective in the treatment of myotonia, may be a preferential drug (61,62). Slow calcium channel blockers suppress sinus and AV nodal action potentials and may modulate the development of arrhythmias in DM.

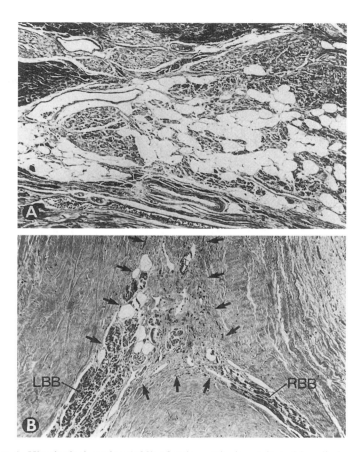

Figure 1. Histological section (x90) of atrioventricular node and bundle branches in humans with myotonic dystrophy. Fibrosis, fatty infiltration, and vacuolization of myocardium are evident. A) There is severe fatty infiltration with interruption of the atrioventricular bundle. B) There is focal replacement fibrosis and atrophy of the right and left bundle branches. Reproduced with permission from (55), ©1988 The American College of Cardiology.

Other Systemic defects in adult onset Myotonic Dystrophy

Smooth muscle

Extensive involvement of smooth muscles in the pharynx and esophagus affect swallowing and peristalsis in DM patients (63). Decreased esophageal pressure and absent or diminished peristaltic waves are documented (64). Abnormal relaxation of smooth muscle can pose a significant problem as it can result in bronchial aspiration, while weakened respiratory muscles can result in pneumonic lung disease which is a cause of death (65).

Eye
Abnormalities of the eye are found in a very high percentage (97%) of adult patients (66). These include cataracts, with lens opacities being found predominantly in the anterior and posterior capsule (67). Degeneration of ciliary muscles results in ocular hypotonia. Visual impairment in DM, unrelated to cataract formation, may be a consequence of retinal degeneration, involving loss of photoreceptors with an increase in pigment cells, cystic changes in the retina and hyalinization and fibrosis of small blood vessels (68).

Endocrine defects
Testicular atrophy is primarily due to hyalinization and fibrosis of the seminiferous tubules (69). Increased basal LH and FSH are reported (70) and fetal loss is frequent in DM patients (2). Elevated fasting insulin, increased insulin response to oral and intravenous glucose and impaired peripheral glucose metabolism are associated with DM (71,72). Frontal balding and benign neoplasm believed to originate from the primitive cells of the hair matrix (calcifying epitheliomas of Malherbe) are associated with DM (2)

Congenital Myotonic Dystrophy
Congenital DM, where newborn infants develop severe symptoms, is a phenotype that is distinctly different from that observed in the adult onset form of the disease. The muscles affected include facial muscles, arthrogrypotic joints, the pharynx and the diaphragm. Severe muscle hypotonia, especially of the diaphragm often results in respiratory failure and death. It is of interest to note that hypotonia and not myotonia predominates in the congenital form of the disease. In fact myotonia is never observed in congenitally affected infants. Skeletal muscle biopsies often demonstrate the presence of decreased muscle fiber size and number, immature fibers which fail to differentiate, the lack of oxidative enzyme activity at the periphery of the fiber and large numbers of satellite cells (2,70,71). Skeletal deformities include thin ribs and talipes. Cardiomyopathy is reported in congenital DM, however neonatal death occurs more as a consequence of respiratory problems rather than cardiac disease (2,72).

Congenitally affected children who survive infancy show marked motor delay and mental retardation. A severe adult onset form of the disease often manifests in the first few decades of life including the development of cardiac dysfunction (1-3). Both atrioventricular and intraventricular conduction defects and echocardiographic abnormalities occur at a much higher frequency (90-100%) in congenital DM compared to the adult onset form (38,39). Echocardiographic abnormalities are primarily impaired however abnormalities of left ventricular systolic function, minor valve defects and mitral valve prolapse are also reported (38).

Prevalence
Because DM shows variable presentation the features in an individual patient may not be typical of DM at the onset and can therefore lead to under diagnosis or even be completely missed as a diagnosis. Thus a conservative estimate of incidence may be 4.5/5.5 per 100,000 (74). However DM prevalence is reported to be as high 75 per 100,000 in certain geographic locales (75).

Genetics
DM is inherited in an autosomal dominant fashion. Both sexes are affected at about the same frequency and approximately 50% of the offspring of DM patients develop the disease (1-3). DM inheritance demonstrates two unique non-Mendelian

features. Both the sex and the position of the parent within a pedigree influences the severity of the disease in the next generation. Thus the adult onset form of the disease appears to be inherited more frequently through the father while congenital DM is almost exclusively maternally inherited (73,76). In addition, DM exhibits genetic anticipation, which refers to the tendency of the disease to increase in severity with successive generations (4). Thus pedigrees often show asymptomatic or mildly affected grandparents who develop minor abnormalities such as cataracts late in life. The second generation often has classic adult onset symptoms. The greater the severity of disease in the second generation the higher is the chance that their offspring will develop serious symptoms early in childhood (1-3).

These confounding features lead to a remarkable hypothesis by Penrose in 1948, who postulated that the pattern of DM inheritance could best be explained to result as a consequence of a gene which showed both marked variability of expression and low correlation between parent and child (77). The accuracy of this statement was realized when the genetic mutation underlying DM was recognized to be an expansion of a CTG repeat sequence located in a gene rich region on chromosome 19q13.3 (78,79,80). Three unique features of CTG tract expansion serve to provide the molecular basis of anticipation in DM pedigrees. First, the probability and amplitude of expansion increases as a function repeat tract length (81,82). Second, the severity of the disease correlates with the length of the repeat sequence (83). Third, the CTG tract expansion results in alterations in the expression of neighboring genes, with the degree of change in gene expression approximately correlating with the size of the expansion (84,85,86).

The probability and amplitude of CTG repeats increase as a function of tract length

DM associated CTG repeat expansions demonstrate two distinct patterns of expansion in human populations. Small ($\pm$ 1-2 repeats) changes in repeat size appear to predominate at tract lengths which are smaller than a 150 bps (35 repeats) in length. Such changes in tract size are reflected in the range (5 to 35 repeats) of repeat tracts observed in the normal populations (78,79,80). However once a threshold of ~50 repeats is reached the pattern of instability appears to change dramatically, such that the frequency of large expansions (> 200 repeats) greatly increases (81). Both the amplitude and frequency of such large expansion events have been shown to increase as a function of tract length (81,82). As the frequency of a large expansion event is critically dependent on the parent tract length (82), a small tract (<35 repeats) is predicted to increase to a size of ~50 repeats, very rarely. Such a rare expansion event would therefore be the origin of a pool of alleles, which having reached a threshold value of ~50 repeats, subsequently mutate at a given frequency per replication event, to result in DM. This prediction is consistent with the fact that alleles between 35 and 49 repeats are very rare in the general population (81) and would explain the linkage disequilibrium observed between the DM mutation and a contiguous 1 kb deletion polymorphism (87).

Studies in model systems suggest that the mechanisms of these two modes of expansion may be distinct, with small changes resulting as a consequence of reiterative synthesis of CTG tracts by the DNA polymerase. Large expansion events may occur as a consequence of large slippage events in Okazaki fragments encoding CTG repeats during replication and/or due to the repair of double strand breaks known to occur in a length dependent fashion in CTG tracts (82, 88,89).

The number of expansion mutations has been shown to increase as function of the number of replication events that the CTG tract undergoes (82). Thus as spermatogenesis involves many more rounds of replication than oogenesis, this observation may explain the higher frequency of mutant DM alleles that are paternally inherited (76). The bias for the maternal inheritance of congenital DM (73), which is associated with enormous expansions reaching sizes of 10 kb or more, is unclear. Several authors suggest that large CTG expansions may either be nonviable with spermatogenesis or alternatively, other factors such as imprinting or intrauterine effects may influence the maternal inheritance of congenital DM (1-3).

The severity of the disease correlates with the length of the repeat sequence
The size of the CTG repeat appears to correlate approximately with both the severity of the DM symptoms and age of disease onset (90,91,92). Thus congenital DM is usually associated with the largest repeat tracts (~1.5->6 kb), while minimally affected patients show the smallest expansions (<0.5 kb) (90,92). There is however a significant overlap in CTG repeat sizes which result in an intermediate adult onset phenotype (90,91,92). This lack of absolute correlation between repeat length and phenotype may be a consequence of somatic mosaicism or age dependent changes in CTG tract size occurring as a consequence of mitotic instability in the affected tissue. Alternatively, the effect of repeat expansion on gene expression within its vicinity, may confirm to a general pattern, but the exact alteration may be stochastic and could therefore give rise to a range of different outcomes as discussed below.

Parent-child comparison of CTG tract lengths confirm that CTG tracts expand in ~90% of the cases and correlates with the earlier and more severe disease onset in succeeding generations (90). In addition, the largest expansions appear to be maternally inherited (93). Thus the correlation of tract length with the severity and age of disease onset provides a molecular explanation for genetic anticipation, variability and the maternal inheritance of congenital DM.

Recent studies also show a significant correlation with CTG tract length with the severity of cardiac disease, suggesting that the number of CTG repeats has value in predicting cardiac risk in DM patients (37,46). Specifically, a good correlation exists between tract length and cardiac conduction defects and wall motion abnormalities. A less significant correlation exists between CTG repeat number and mitral valve prolapse. In addition to CTG tract length, symptom duration and age, are also univariate predictors of cardiac disease in DM (37).

CTG expansion results in length-dependent alterations in gene expression/function
The CTG repeat expansion associated with DM is found in a gene-rich region on chromosome 19q13.3 which contains as many as 6 genes in a 200 Kb region (93,94 pers. comm. D. Brook). The immediate location of the repeat sequence is in the 3' untranslated region of a serine threonine kinase, DMPK (78,79,80) and upstream of a homeodomain-encoding gene, DMAHP (94). Three distinct phenomena have been documented to occur as a consequence of repeat expansion in DM patients (**Figure 2**). These include (i) nuclear retention of the mutant DMPK mRNA (95-97), (ii) abnormal nuclear sequestration of CUG-BP [a putative RNA processing and/or transport protein] by CUG sequences in the mutant DMPK mRNA (98,99) and (iii) decreased transcription of the DMAHP allele linked to the CTG expansion (100,101). The relative contributions of these events in DM etiology are unknown.

Nuclear retention of mutant DMPK mRNA
Three studies have shown nuclear retention of mutant DMPK transcripts in the nuclei of DM fibroblasts (95) and muscle (96,97). The defects underlying abnormal transport of the mutant DMPK mRNA are unknown. Sequestration within the nucleus could occur as consequence of one or more defects. First, the

RNA polymerase may be unable to transcribe through the expanded repeat when it reaches a critical size thus resulting in incomplete 3' end formation and polyadenylation, which in turn may prevent transport of the transcript to the cytoplasm. Second, the mutant transcript could be processed normally but may be trapped in the nucleus because of a conformational change of the expanded CUG repeats or alternatively because the expanded repeats bind proteins which prevent its export from the nucleus. In this regard the presence of high levels of a novel CUG binding protein, CUG-BP (98,99) [believed to play a role in processing and/or transport of CUG encoding RNAs] in DM nuclei is of interest.

One important consequence of nuclear retention of the mutant DMPK mRNA is a decrease in the pool of translatable DMPK mRNA in the cytoplasm. Consistent with this hypothesis several studies have shown decreased DMPK mRNA and protein levels in DM muscle biopsies (84,102-106). Large variations in both DMPK mRNA (102-105) and protein (84,106) have been reported, including some studies showing greater than 50% losses in DMPK levels (103,105). Titration of CUG-BP by the mutant DMPK message could allow DMPK levels to drop below 50% of normal. If CUG-BP is required for processing of wild type DMPK mRNA, specific binding and titration of CUG-BP by the mutant message could hinder the processing of the wild type DMPK mRNAs and result in DMPK protein levels lower than 50% of normal controls.

Abnormal nuclear sequestration of CUG-BP

Abnormally high nuclear levels of CUG-BP, a putative RNA processing/transport protein that specifically binds to CUG repeats, are reported in DM (98,99). The pathological consequences of nuclear sequestration of CUG-BP are unknown. As both RNA splicing and transport are influenced by nuclear levels of splicing/transport proteins [Reviewed in 107], altered nuclear levels of unbound CUG-BP could result in splicing and transport defects of CUG repeat encoding RNAs. Thus nuclear sequestration of CUG-BP could (i) affect processing and transport of the wild type DMPK mRNA resulting in DMPK protein levels which are lower than 50% of normal controls and/or (ii) have a more widespread deleterious effect on one or more messages which require CUG-BP for correct processing and transport. Neurons and germ cells which have high levels of CUG-BP [L.Timchenkov pers. comm.] may be particularly sensitive to such changes. In this regard it is of interest that loss of other RNA binding protein including, hnRNPG [108] and FMR1 [109,110] result in reproductive and brain dysfunction in humans. Thus altered CUG-BP levels may contribute to the DM associated male sterility and behavioral abnormalities.

Decreased transcription of DMAHP

CTG repeat sequences have been shown to adopt hyperflexible, non-B DNA structures [111] which provide one of the strongest known nucleosome positioning elements in nature [112]. Thus expansion of CTG sequences could result in a more condensed chromatin structure and/or alter nucleosome phasing such that gene expression is repressed in its vicinity. Consistent with this hypothesis CTG repeat expansion has been shown eliminate a nuclease hypersensitive site located 3' of the repeat and 5' of a homeodomain-encoding gene, DMAHP [113]. More recent studies have shown that the DMAHP allele linked to the repeat expansion, is expressed at 10-30% of the wild type allele (the extent of transcriptional repression being roughly correlated with the length of the repeat), resulting in lowered steady state levels of DMAHP mRNA [100,101].

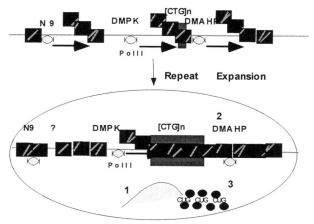

Figure 2: Consequences of CTG repeat expansion in DM
1 Nuclear sequestration of mutant DMPK mRNA
2 Decreased transcription of the DMAHP allele linked to the CTG expansion
3 Abnormal nuclear sequestration of a putative RNA processing and/or transport protein, CUG-BP.

DMAHP loss could contribute to DM pathology as it expressed in several tissues including the cornea, lens capsule, skeletal, smooth and cardiac muscle [114], which show pathological changes in DM. Furthermore, as several DM symptoms could be attributed to defects in ion homeostasis, it is intriguing to note that DMAHP is homologous to mouse transcription factor AREC3/six4, shown to regulate expression of Na^+/K^+-ATPase $\alpha 1$ subunit in developing skeletal muscle [115]. The length-dependent but intrinsically stochastic nature of the changes that repeat expansion cause may explain the phenotypic variability observed in DM. The exact contributions of each mechanism to DM may be resolved using transgenic animals that allow individual mechanisms to be independently tested.

Contribution of partial DMPK loss to DM
To evaluate the contribution of partial DMPK loss in DM, we have previously developed a strain of mice in which DMPK is functionally inactivated (DMPK$^{-/-}$) (116). Our analyses of DMPK$^{-/-}$ mice has shown that loss of DMPK results in a late onset skeletal myopathy characterized by 30-50% loss in muscle twitch and tetanic force development by 11 months of age. Skeletal muscles from mature DMPK$^{-/-}$ mice show variation in fiber size, increased fiber degeneration and fibrosis. Ultra structural changes include Z line loss, mitochondrial and sarcoplasmic reticulum abnormalities. Our data suggests that impaired excitation-contraction and/or abnormalities of the contractile apparatus are likely to underlie the progressive muscle weakness observed in DMPK$^{-/-}$ mice (116).

DMPK and Ion Channel Function
Recent data suggests that the abnormalities in excitation-contraction coupling observed in DMPK$^{+/-}$ and DMPK$^{-/-}$ skeletal may be a consequence of abnormal

calcium and sodium ion channel dysfunction (117; Moorman,R. and S. Reddy unpublished data). Experiments in Xenopus oocytes and other in vitro studies suggest that DMPK regulates sodium and calcium currents by directly phosphorylating the sodium channels and DHPRs (118,119). These observations are of particular interest, as loss of DMPK could result in altered ion homeostasis, which may contribute to several DM symptoms including cardiac dysfunction.

The role of DMPK in DM associated cardiac disease

To test the role of DMPK loss in cardiac arrhythmogenesis in DM, we carried out a series of experiments aimed at evaluating cardiac function in transgenic animals heterozygous and homozygous for DMPK loss (120,121,122). Electrocardiographic and electrophysiological studies developed by us to evaluate cardiac function in transgenic mice are discussed in detail in chapter 3.

Multilead surface ECG and standard pacing protocols were used to determine electrophysiological parameters. Both endocardial and epicardial surgical techniques were utilized. Epicardial studies involved a midline sternotomy for the placement of pacing wires on the outer surface of each chamber. An octapolar mouse EP catheter introduced via the jugular vein allowed pacing electrocardiogram recording. The catheter used was a single-pass octapolar lead, allowing simultaneous stimulation and signal acquisition from the atrium and right ventricle (120,121,122). Pharmacological autonomic manipulations were performed using intravenous isoproterenol (1-3ng/gm) and atropine (1 ng/gm) (120,122). Ambulatory ECG recordings using implantable radiotransmitters were obtained over a period of 5+3 days to study cardiac function at rest and during exertion. A graded exercise swim test was carried out by placing the animals in a warm bath and allowing the animals to swim for incrementally longer intervals each day to a time of nine minutes on the tenth day. Custom software designed for automated acquisition, analysis and computation of heart variability parameters was used. Frequency domain power spectral techniques were used to study sympathetic and parasympathetic influences on heart rate regulation (120).

DMPK$^{+/-}$ and DMPK$^{-/-}$ mice show 1^{O} A-V block

To study cardiac rhythm as a function of DMPK levels the following parameters were studied in wild type animals and DMPK mutant mice. In DMPK$^{-/-}$ mice the resting sinus cycle length was 156.9 ± 40.3 ms (heart rate 404.8 ± 94.6 bpm), in DMPK$^{+/-}$ mice it was 152 ± 34.3 ms (heart rate 413.1 ± 93.7 bpm)], while the mean sinus cycle length in wild-type controls was 148.2 ± 30.8 ms (heart rate 421.7 ± 88.4 bpm). The mean PR intervals [reflecting AV nodal conduction time] were measured to be 48.2 ± 7.4 ms in homozygotes (p-value < 0.001), 48 ± 7.8 ms in heterozygotes (p-value < 0.01) and 34.1 ± 4.8 in controls. On ECG, a prolonged PR interval (mean ± SD = 48 ± 7 msec) was seen in all homozygous DMPK$^{-/-}$ mice and 10 of 11 heterozygous DMPK$^{+/-}$ mice (mean PR interval = 48 ± 8 msec), when compared with wild-type mice (mean PR = 34 ± 5 msec, p < 0.001).

Basal heart rates [reflecting sinus node automaticity] and all other measurements of ECG intervals [QRS (reflecting conduction time in the ventricle), JT, QT (reflecting ventricular action potential duration), QTc, and JTc] in homozygotes and heterozygotes were not statistically significantly different when compared to their littermate controls. Intraventricular conduction abnormalities were present in 22% of mutant mice, but were also apparent in 12% of the wild-type mice (p = 0.07). Thus as DMPK mutant mice showed a prolonged PR interval in conjunction with a normal QRS interval, AV node dysfunction is indicated.

DMPK$^{-/-}$ mice show severe conduction disturbances including 2^0 and 3^0 AV block. In these experiments, mice homozygous for DMPK loss showed more severe disturbances of A-V conduction. Five DMPK$^{-/-}$ mice (5/17) had second-degree AV block [where some P waves are not followed by QRS], and two (2/17) DMPK$^{-/-}$ had third-degree AV block [where no P waves conduct through the A-V node to the ventricles]. No heterozygous or wild-type mice had any form of abnormal atrial or A-V conduction. These results show that DMPK loss results in A-V conduction block which delay or prevent atrial impulses from reaching the ventricles and demonstrate a role for DMPK in AV nodal function (120).

The site of the conduction abnormality was further studied via His bundle recordings in a set of 7 wild-type and 9 age matched (6-13 month) DMPK homozygous mutant mice (121). Both AH and HV components of the AV interval were prolonged in the homozygous mutant mice (39.8 ± 4.5 ms vs. 31± 5.6 ms, p= 0.003 and 15.7 ± 1.7 ms vs. 10.4 ± 1.1 ms, p<0.0001, respectively). Thus AV conduction delay appears to exist both in the AV node per se and in the His-Purkinje system in a manner reminiscent of DM patients (121,31-39).

Ambulation and exercise testing did not lead to an increase in conduction disorders
The implantable telemetry ECG recorder was surgically placed in mice from each group. During the monitoring periods, prolonged PR intervals were evident in the mutant mice. However, there was no further progression of higher-grade A-V block noted during rest, ambulation, or graded exercise testing. None of the animals had any documented ectopy, arrhythmias or sudden death during exercise.

Severity of conduction disturbances increases as a function of age in DMPK$^{-/-}$ mice
We observed a trend towards an increase in PR intervals with age, such that PR intervals greater than 50ms were not observed in 6 month old DMPK$^{-/-}$ mice and manifested only at 16-17 months of age in DMPK$^{-/-}$ mice. However, 2^0 and 3^0 heart block occurred at a higher frequency in adult mice and occurred primarily in mice with PR intervals > 40 ms. This trend was carefully studied using 75 male and 75 female mice, divided into 4 distinct age groups of 1-2 months, 4-6 months, 12-15 months and 18-21 months. The young DMPK$^{-/-}$ and DMPK$^{+/-}$ mice had similar cycle lengths and ECG intervals as their littermate controls. In contrast both DMPK$^{-/-}$ and DMPK$^{+/-}$ adult mice showed prolongation of AV conduction time when compared to their littermates as a function of age. Thus the correlation between the length of the PR interval and the incidence of cardiac arrhythmic events in DMPK mutant mice suggests that A-V conduction is progressively impaired and that prolonged PR intervals precede more serious arrhythmic events. These results suggest that progressive deterioration of the integrity of the conduction system is linked to levels of DMPK and to duration of such alterations in DMPK dosage.

Gross structural differences were not observed in DMPK$^{+/-}$ and DMPK$^{-/-}$ hearts
Histological evaluation of hearts was performed by evaluating serial sections and staining with haemotoxylin-eosin and Gomori trichrome to determine if structural alterations of cardiac muscle and/or increased fibrosis could account for the observed conduction defects. As no significant increase in gross fibrosis and atrophy were detected in the myocardium of mutant mice when compared to wild type controls, our results suggest that functional deficits associated with DMPK loss and/or structural changes of the conduction system per se could underlie the observed conduction defects.

Sympatholytic effects are not responsible for A-V block in DMPK mutant mice

Two likely mechanisms underlying bradycardia and A-V block in humans include calcium channel block in the A-V node and/or sympatholytic effects. To determine if sympatholytic effects are a likely cause for the observed A-V block in DMPK mutant mice, we infused isoproterenol intravenously via the lumen of the mouse EP catheter in a subgroup of 11 mutant mice. On isoproterenol [1-3 ng/gm/min], although the basal heart rates increased on average 25%, no correction of A-V block was observed in DMPK$^{+/-}$ or DMPK$^{-/-}$ mice. These results suggest that sympatholytic effects may not be responsible for the A-V block in DMPK. In this study we show that impulse generation by the sinus node is unaltered by DMPK loss as both heart rate and CSNRT were normal in DMPK mutant mice. A-V node function was however found to be extremely sensitive to DMPK dosage as both DMPK$^{-/-}$ and DMPK$^{+/-}$ mice showed prolonged PR intervals in conjunction with normal QRS intervals on ECG evaluation

The experiments demonstrate that homozygous and heterozygous DMPK mutant mice have distinct cardiac electrophysiological abnormalities specifically affecting atrioventricular conduction. The degree of PR prolongation on surface ECG is similar between mice heterozygous and homozygous for the DMPK mutation. However mice homozygous for DMPK loss show more severe disturbances of A-V conduction. These results demonstrate that cardiac conduction is sensitive to DMPK dosage and link haploinsufficiency of DMPK with atrioventricular conduction disturbances which are the predominant feature of cardiac disease in DM.

Our results contrast with studies performed on transgenic mice which overexpress DMPK and as a consequence develop hypertrophic cardiomyopathy, a phenotype which is not characteristic of DM. Importantly, there were no notable abnormalities in *ex vivo* ventricular hemodynamics or ECG measurements in isolated perfused hearts from DMPK overexpressor mice. Thus our results are consistent with and lend support to the hypothesis that CTG expansion results in decreased DMPK protein levels which in is a critical event leading to subset of key pathological changes observed in DM.

DMPK-deficient mice could provide an excellent model to test the consequence of DMPK loss on ion channel function in cardiac cells. Such studies could lead to the rational development of anti-arrhythmic drugs designed to correct the specific defects associated with DMPK loss in DM patients. It would be of interest to determine if early treatment with corrective drugs will decrease the incidence of more serious conduction disorders later in life. Alternatively DMPK replacement strategies could be developed using DMPK mutant mice in order to prevent the progression of cardiac disease in DM. Such data extrapolated clinically may allow the development of novel therapeutic interventions for cardiac disease in DM patients. Lastly, as the signal transduction processes which govern cardiac rhythm are largely unknown, the biochemical study of DMPK should provide a unique entry point to understand these fundamental processes.

REFERENCES

1. Batten FE, Gibb HP. Myotonia atrophica. *Brain* 1909;32:187-205.

2. Harper, PS. Myotonic Dystrophy. 2nd Ed., Philadelphia, Saunders, 1989.

3. Roses AD, Harper PS, Bossen EH. Myotonic Muscular Dystrophy. *In*: Handbook of Clinical Neurology. 1979;40:485-531.

4. Howeler CJ, Busch HF, Geraedts JP, Niermeijer MF, Staal A. Anticipation in myotonic dystrophy: Fact or fiction? *Brain* 1989;112:779-797.

5. Harper PS, Rudel R. Myotonic Dystrophy. *In*: Myology Basic and Clinical. Engel, AG, Franzini-Armstrong C, eds. Vol 2, 1994;1192-1219.

6. Gold GD. Temporomandibular joint dysfunction in myotonic dystrophy. *Neurology* 1966;16:212-216.

7. Brumlik J, Drechsler B, Vannin TM. The myotonic discharges in various neurological syndromes: a neurophysiological analysis. *Electromyography* 1979;10:369-383.

8. Wohlfart G. Dystrophia myotonica and myotonia congenita: histopathologic studies with special reference to changes in muscles. *J Neuropathol Exp Neurol* 1951;10: 109-124.

9. Dubowitz V, Brooke MH. Muscle Biopsy: A Modern Approach. W.B. Saunders Co., London, 1973.

10. Dubowitz V. Muscle biopsy-technical and diagnostic aspects. Ann Clin Res 1974;6:69-79.

11. Johnson AG. Alteration of the Z lines and I-band myofilaments in human skeletal muscle. *Arch. Neuropathol* 1969;12:218-226.

12. Schotland DL. An electron-microscopic investigation of myotonic dystrophy. *J Neuropathol Exp Neurol* 1970;29:241-253.

13. Horowicz P, Spalding BC. Electrical and Ionic Properties of the Muscle Cell Membrane in Myology Basic and Clinical. Eds, Engel, AG, Franzini-Armstrong C. 1994, 405-422.

14. Rudel R, Lehman-Horn F. *Physiol Rev* 1985;65:310-356.

15. Rudel R, Ruppersberg JP, Spittelmeister W. Abnormalities of the fast sodium current in myotonic dystrophy, recessive generalized myotonia, and adynamia episodica. *Muscle Nerve* 1989;12:281-287.

16. Franke CH, Hatt H, Iaizzo PA, Lehmann-Horn F. Characteristics od Na⁺ channels and Cl⁻ conductance in resealed muscle fiber segments from patients with myotonic dystrophy. *J Physiol Lond* 1990;425:391-405.

17. Desnuelle C, Lombet A, Serratrice G, Lazdunski M. Sodium channel and sodium pump in normal and pathological muscles from patients with myotonic muscular dystrophy and lower motor neuron impairment. *J Clin Invest* 1982;69:358-67.

18. Edstrom L, Wroblewski R. Intracellular elemental composition of single muscle fibers in muscular dystrophy and dystrophia myotonica. *Acta Neurol Scand* 1989;80:419-424.

19. Gruener R, Stern LZ, Markovitz D, Gerdes C. Electrophysiologic properties of intercostal muscle fibers in human neuromuscular diseaes. *Muscle Nerve* 1979;2:165-172.

20. Merickel M, Gray R, Chauvin P, Appel S. Cultured muscle from myotonic muscular dystrophy patients: altered membrane electrical properties. *Proc Natl Acad Sci USA* 1981;78:648-652.

21. Kobayashi T, Askanas V, Saito K, Engel WK, Ishikawa K. Abnormalities of aneural and innervated cultured muscle fibers from patients with myotonic atrophy (dystrophy). *Arch Neurol* 1990;47:893-896.

22. Jacobs AEM, Benders AAGM, Oosterhof A, et al. The calcium homeostasis and the membrane potential of cultured muscle cells from patients with myotonic dystrophy. *Biochem Biophys Acta* 1991;1096:14-19.

23. Benders AAGM, Wevers RA, Veerkamp JH. Ion transport in human skeletal muscle cells: disturbances in myotonic dystrophy and Brody's diseases. *Acta Physiol Scand* 1996;156:355-367.

24. Timchenko L, Nastainczyk W, Schneider T, Patel B, Hofmann F, Caskey CT. Full length myotonin protein kinase (72Kd) displays serine kinase actiity. *Proc Natl Acad Sci USA* 1995;92:5366-5370.

25. Benders AAGM, Timmermans JAH, Oosterhof A, et al. Deficiency of Na⁺/K⁺-ATPase and sarcoplasmic reticulum Ca²⁺-ATPase in skeletal muscle and cultured muscle cells of myotonic dystrophy patients *Biochem J* 1993;293:269-274.

26. Benders AAGM, van Kuppevelt THM, Oosterhof A, Wevers RA, Veerkamp JH. Adenosine triphosphatases during maturation of cultured human skeletal muscle cells and in adult human muscle. *Biochim Biophys Acta* 1992;1112:89-98.

27. Behrens MI, Jalil P, Serani A, Vergara F, Alvarez O. Possible role of apamin-sensitive K⁺ channels in myotonic dystrophy. *Muscle Nerve* 1994;17:1264-1270.

28.Schmid-Antomarchi HJFR, Romey G, Hugues M, Schmid A, Lazdunski M. The all-or-none response of innervation in expression of apamin receptor and apamin-sensitive Ca2+-activated K+ channel in mammalian skeletal muscle. *Proc Natl Acad Sci USA* 1985;82:2188-2191.

29. Behrens MI, Vergara C. Increase of apamin receptors in skeletal muscle induced by colchicine: possible role in myotonia. *Am J Physiol* 1992;263:C794-C802.

30. Vergara C, Ramirez BU. Age-dependent expression of the apamin-sensitive calcium-activated K+ channel in fast and slow rat skeletal muscle. *Exp Neurol* 1997;146:282-285.

31. Appel SH, Roses AD. The muscular dystrophias. In: Stanbury JB, Wyngaarden, JB, Frederickson, DS. eds. The metabolic basis of inherited disease. New York: McGraw Hill, 1978, 1260-1281.

32. Litchfield JA. A-V dissociation in dystrophic myotonica. *Br Heart J* 1953;15:357-359.

33. Petkovich NJ, Dunn M, Reed W. Myotonia distrophica with A-V dissociation and Stokes-Adams attacks. A case report and review of the literature. *Am Heart J* 1964;68:391-396.

34. Perloff JK, Stevenson WG, Roberts NK, Cabeen W, Weiss J. Cardiac involvement in myotonic muscular dystrophy (Steinert's disease): a prospective study of 25 patients. *Am J Cardiol* 1984;54:1074-1081.

35. Fragola PV, Autore C, Magni G, Antonini G, Picelli A, Cannata, D. The natural course of cardiac conduction disturbances in myotonic dystrophy. *Cardiology* 1991;79:93-98.

36. Hawley RJ, Milner MR, Gottdiener JS, Cohen A. Myotonic heart disease: A clinical follow-up. *Neurology* 1991;41:259-262.

37. Tokgozoglu LS, Ashizawa T, Pacifico A, Armstrong RM, Epstein HF, Zoghbi WA. Cardiac involvement in a large kindred with myotonic dystrophy. *JAMA* 1995;274:813-819.

38. Forsberg H, Olofsson B-O, Eriksson A, Andersson S. (1990). Cardiac involvement in congenital myotonic dystrophy . *Br Heart J* 1990;63:119-121.

39. Morgenlander JC, Nohria V, Saba Z. EKG abnormalities in pediatric patients with myotonic dystrophy. *Pediatr Neurol* 1993;9:124-126.

40. Fragola PV, Luzi M, Calo L, et al. Cardiac involvement in myotonic dystrophy.*Am J Cardiol* 1994;74:1070-1072.

41. Fragola PV, Calo L, Antonini G, et al. Signal-averaged electrocardiography in myotonic dystrophy. *Int J Cardiol* 1995;50:61-68.

42. Orndahl G, Thulesius O, Enestrom S, Dehlin O. The heart in myotonic disease.*Acta Med Scand* 1964;176:479-91.

43. Melacini P, Buja G, Fasoli G, et al. The natural history of cardiac involvement in myotonic dystrophy: an eight-year follow-up in 17 patients. *Clin Cardiol* 1988;11:231-238.

44. Olofsson B-O, Forsberg H, Andersson S, Bjerle P, Henriksson A, Wedin I. Electrocardiographic findings in myotonic dystrophy. *Br Heart J* 1988;59:47-52.

45. Winters SJ, Schreiner B, Griggs RC, Rowley P, Nanda NC. Familial mitral valve prolapse and myotonic dystrophy. *Ann Intern Med* 1976;85:19-22.

46. Melacini P, Villanova C, Menegazzo E, et al. Correlation between cardiac involvement and CTG trinucleotide repeat length in myotonic dystrophy. *J Am Coll Cardiol* 1995;25:239-245.

47. Streib EW, Meyers DG, Sun SF. Mitral valve prolapse in myotonic dystrophy. *Muscle Nerve* 1985;8:650-653.

48. Kovick RB, Fogelman AM, Abbasi AS. Echocardiographic evaluation of posterior left ventricular wall motion in muscular dystrophy. *Circulation* 1975;52:447-454.

49. Moorman JR, Coleman RE, Packer DL, et al. Cardiac involvement in myotonic muscular dystrophy. *Medicine* 1985;64:371-387.

50. Badano L, Autore C, Fragola PV, et al. Left ventricular myocardial function in myotonic dystrophy. *Am J Cardiol* 1993;71:987-991.

51. Thompson AMP. Dystrophia cordis myotonia studied by serial histology of the pacemaker and conducting system. *J Path Bact* 1968;96:285-295.

52. Fall LH, Young WW, Power J, Faukner CS, Hettleman BD, Robb JF. Severe congestive heart failure and cardiomyopathy as a complication of myotonic dystrophy in pregnancy*Obstetr Gynecol* 1976;76:481-484.

53. Bulloch RT, Davis JL, Hara M. Dystrophia myotonica with heart block: a light and electron microscopic study. *Arch Pathol* 1967;84:130-140.

54. Tanaka N, Tanaka H, Takada M, Niimura T, Kanehisa T, Terashi S. Cardiomyopathy in myotonic dystrophy. A light and electron microscopic study of the myocardium. *Jpn Heart J* 1973;14:202-212.

55. Nguyen HH, Wolfe JT, Holmes DR Jr, Edwards WD. Pathology of the cardiac conduction system in myotonic dystrophy: a study of 12 cases. *J Am Coll Cardiol* 1988;11:662-671.

56. Zipes DP. Genesis of cardiac arrhythmias: Electrophysiological considerations in "Heart Disease: A textbook of Cardiovascular Medicine". Edited by EugeneBraunwald. W.B. Saunders Company. Philadelphia. 1992;22:588-627.

57. Noma A, Tsuboi N. Dependence of junctional conductance on proton, calcium and magnesium ions in cardiac paired cells of guinea-pig. *J Physiol* 1987;382:193-211.

58. Hess P. Cardiac Calcium Channels in "Cardiac Electrophysiology. From Cell to Bedside". Edited by Zipes DP, Jalife J. WB Saunders: Philadelphia, 1990, 10.

59. Irisawa H, Giles WR. Cardiac Calcium Channels in "Cardiac Electrophysiology. From Cell to Bedside". Edited by Zipes DP, Jalife J. WB Saunders: Philadelphia, 1990, 95.

60. Bourke TD, Zuck D. Thiopentone in dystrophia myotonica. *Br J Anaesth* 1957;29:35-38.

61.Griggs RC, Davies RJ, Anderson DC, Dove JT. Cardiac conduction in myotonic dystrophy*Am J Med* 1975;251:527-529.

62. Munsat TL. Therapy of myotonia. A double-blind evaluation of diphenylhydantoin, procainamide and placebo. *Neurology* 1967;17:359-367.

63. Harvey JC, Sherbourne DH, Siegel,CI. Smooth muscle involvement in myotonic dystrophy.*Am J Med* 1965;39:81-90.

64. Kelley ML. Dysphagia and motor failure of the oesophagus in myotonia dystrophica. *Neurology* 1964;14:955-960.

65. Garrett JM, Dubose TD, Jackson JE, Norman JR. Esophageal and pulmonary disturbances in myotonia dystrophica. *Arch Intern Med* 1969;123:26-32.

66. Harper PS. Pre-symptomatic detection and genetic counselling in myotonic dystrophy.*Clin Genet* 1973;4:134-140.

67. Junge J. Ocular changes in dystrophia myotonica, paramyotonia and myotonia congenita. *Doc Ophthalmol* 1966;21:1-115.

68. Manschot WA. Histological findings in a case of dystrophia myotonica. *Ophthalmologica (Basel)* 1968;155:294-296.

69. Vazquez JA, Pinies JA, Martul P, De los Rios A, Gatzambide S, Busturia MA. Hypothalmic-pituitary-testicular function in 70 patients with myotonic dystrophy*J Endocrinol Invest* 1990;13:375-379.

70. Marinkovic Z, Prelevic G, Wurzburger M, Nogic S. Gonadal dysfunction in patients with myotonic dystrophy. *Exp Clin Endocrinol* 1990;96:37-44.

71. Piccardo MG, Pacini G, Rosa M, Vichi R. Insulin resistance in myotonic dystrophy. *Enzyme* 1991;45:14-22.

72. Krentz AJ, Williams AC, Nattrass M. Insulin resistance in multiple aspects of intermediary metabolism in myotonic dystrophy. *Metabolism* 1991;40:866-872.

73. Harper PS. Congenital myotonic dystrophy in Britain. II. Genetic basis. *Arch Dis Child* 1975;50:514-521.

74. Roig M, Pere-Ramon B, Navarro C, Brugera R, Losada M. Presentation, clinical course and outcome of the congenital form of myotonic dystrophy. *Pediat Neurol* 1994;11:208-213.

75. Mathieu J, De Braekeleer M, Prevost C. Genealogical reconstruction of myotonic dystrophy in the Saguenay-Lac-Saint-Jean area. *Neurology* 1990;40:839-842.

76. Bell J. Dystrophia myotonica and allied diseases. *Treasury Hum Inheritance* 1947;4:342-410.

77. Penrose LS. The problem of anticipation in pedigrees of dystrophia myotonica. *Ann Eugen* 1948;14:125-132.

78. Brook JD, McCurrach ME, Harley HG, et al. Molecular basis of myotonic dystrophy: Expansion of a trinucleotide (CTG) repeat at the 3' end of a transcript encoding a protein kinase family member. *Cell* 1992;68:799-808.

79. Fu Y-H, Pizutti A, Fenwick RG, et al. An unstable triplet repeat in a gene related to myotonic muscular dystrophy. *Science* 1992;255:1256-1258.

80. Mahadevan M, Tsilfidis C, Sabourin L, et al. Myotonic Dystrophy Mutation: An unstable CTG repeat in the 3' untranslated region of the gene. *Science* 1992;255:1253-1255.

81. Barcelo JM, Mahadevan MS, Tsilfidis C, MacKenzie AE, Korneluk RG. Intergenerational stability of the myotonic dystrophy protomutation. *Hum Mol Genet* 1993;2:705-709.

82. Sarkar PS, Chang H-C, Boudi FB, Reddy S. CTG repeats show bimodal amplification in E.coli. *Cell* 1998;95:531-540.

83. Harley HG, Rundle SA, MacMillan JC, et al. Size of the unstable CTGrepeat sequence in relation to phenotype and parental transmission in myotonic dystrophy. *Am J Hum Genet* 1993;52:1164-1174.

84. Fu Y-H, Friedman DL, Richards S, et al. Decreased expression of myotonin-protein kinase messenger RNA and protein in adult form of myotonic dystrophy. *Science* 1993;260:235-237.

85. Klesert TR, Otten AD, Bird T, Tapscott SJ. Trinucleotide repeat expansion at the myotonic dystrophy locus reduces expression of DMAHP. *Nat Genet* 1997;16:402-407.

86. Thornton CA, Wymer JP, Simmons Z, McClain C, Moxley RT. Expansion of the myotonic dystrophy CTG repeat reduces expression of the flanking DMAHP gene. *Nat Genet* 1997;16:407-409.

87. Mahadevan MS, Foitzik MA, Surh LC, Korneluk RG. Characterization and polymerase chain reaction (PCR) detection of an Alu deletion polymorphism in total linkage disequilibrium with myotonic dystrophy. *Genomics* 1993;15:446-448

88. Kang S, Joworaski A, Ohshima K, Wells RD. Expansion and deletion of CTG repeats from human disease genes are determined by the direction of replication in E. coli. *Nat Genet* 1995;10, 213-218.

89. Freudenreich CH, Kantrow SM, Zakian VA. Expansion and length dependent fragility of CTG repeats in yeast. *Science* 1998;279:853-856.

90. Harley HG, Rundle SA, MacMillan JC, et al. Size of the unstable CTG repeat in relation to phenotype and parental transmission in myotonic dystrophy. *Am J Hum Genet* 1993;52:1164-1174.

91. Redman JB, Fenwick RG, Fu Y-H, Pizzuti A, Caskey CT. Relationship between parental trinucleotide GCT repeat length and severity of myotonic dystrophy in offspring. *JAMA* 1993;269,1960-1965.

92. Tsilfidis C, MacKenzie AE, Mettler G, Barcelo J, Korneluk RG. Correlation between CTG trinucleotide repeat length and frequency of severe congenital myotonic dystrophy. *Nat Genet* 1992;1:192-195.

93. Shaw DJ, McCurrach M, Rundle SA, et al. Genomic organization and transcriptional units at the myotonic dystrophy locus. *Genomics* 1993;18:673-679.

94. Boucher CA, King SK, Carey N, et. al. A novel homeodomain-encoding gene is associated with a large CpG island interrupted by the myotonic dystrophy unstable (CTG)n repeat. *Hum Mol Genet* 1995;4:1919-1925.

95. Taneja KL, McCurrach ME, Shalling M, Housman D, Singer R. Foci of trinucleotide repeat transcripts in nuclei of myotonic dystrophy cells and tissues. *J Cell Biol* 1995;128:995-1002.

96. Hamshere MG, Newman EE, Alwazzan M, Athwal BS, Brook JD. Transcriptional abnormality in myotonic dytrophy affects DMPK but not neighbouring genes. *Proc Natl Acad Sci USA* 1997;94:7394-7399.

97. Davis BM, McCurrach ME, Taneja KL, Singer RH, Housman DE. *Proc Natl Acad Sci USA* 1997;94:7388-93.

98. Timchenko LT, Timchenko NA, Caskey CT, Roberts R. Novel proteins with binding specificity for DNA CTG repeats and RNA CUG repeats: implications for myotonic dystrophy. *Hum Mol Genet* 1996;5:115-121.

99. Timchenko LT, Miller JW, Timchenko NA, et al. Identification of a (CUG)n triplet repeat RNA-binding protein and its expression in myotonic dystrophy. *Nuc Acids Res* 1996;24:4407-4414.

100. Klesert TR, Otten AD, Bird TD, Tapscott SJ. Trinucleotide repeat expansion at the myotonic dystrophy locus reduces expression of DMAHP. *Nat Genet* 1997;16:402-407.

101. Thornton CA, Wymer JP, Simmons Z, McClain C, Moxley RT. Expansion of the myotonic dystrophy CTG repeat reduces expression of the flanking DMAHP gene. *Nat Genet* 1997;16:407-409.

102. Carango P, Noble JE, Marks HG, Funanage VL. Absence of myotonic dystrophy protein kinase (DMPK) mRNA as a result of a triplet repeat expansion in myotonic dystrophy.*Genomics* 1993;18:340-348.

103. Hofmann-Radvanyi H, Lavedan C, Rabes JP, et al. Myotonic dystrophy: Absence of CTG enlarged transcript in congenital forms and low expression of the normal allele.*Hum Mol Genet* 1993;2:1263-1267.

104. Krahe R, Ashizawa T, Abbruzzese C, et al. Effect of myotonic dystrophy trinucleotide repeat expansion on DMPK transcription and processing. *Genomics* 1995;28:1-14.

105. Wang J, Pegoraro E, Menegazzo E, et al. Myotonic dystrophy: evidence for a possible dominant-negative RNA mutation. *Hum Mol Genet* 1995;4:599-606.

106. Maeda M, Taft CS, Bush EW, et al. Identification, Tissue-specific expression, and subcellular localization of the 80 and 71 kDa forms of myotonic dystrophy kinase protein. *J Biol Chem* 1995;270:20246-20249.

107. Weighardt F, Biamonti G, Riva S. The roles of heterogenous nuclear ribonucleoproteins (hnRNP) in RNA metabolism. *Bioessays* 1996:18:747-756.

108. Cooke HJ, Elliott DJ. RNA-binding proteins and human male infertility. *Trends Genet* 1997:13;3:87-89.

109. Pieretti M, Zhang F, Fu Y-H, et al. Absence of expression of the FMR-1 gene in fragile X syndrome. *Cell* 1991;66:817-822.

110. Siomi H, Choi M, Siomi MC, Nussbaum RL, Dreyfuss G. Essential role for KH domains in RNA binding: impaired RNA binding by a mutation in the KH domain of FMR1 that causes fragile X syndrome. *Cell* 1994;77:33-39.

111. Gellibolian R, Bacolla A, Wells RD. Triplet repeat instability and DNA topology: An expansion model based on statistical mechanics. *J Biol Chem* 1997;272:167093-167097.

112. Wang Y-H, Griffith J. Expanded CTG triplet blocks from the myotonic dystrophy gene create the strongest known natural nucleosome positioning elements. *Genomics* 1995;25:570-573.

113. Otten AD, Tapscott SJ. Triplet repeat expansion in myotonic dystrophy alters the adjacent chromatin structure. *Proc Natl Acad Sci USA* 1995;92:5465-5469.

114. Heath SK, Carne S, Hoyle C, Johnson JK, Wells DJ. Characterization of expression of mDMAHP, a homeodomain-encoding gene at the murine DM locus. *Hum Mol Genet* 1997;6: 651-657.

115. Kawakami K, Ohto H, Ikeda K, Roeder RG. Structure, function and expression of a murine homeobox protein AREC3, a homologue of Drosophila sineoculis gene product, and implication in development. *Nucl Acids Res* 1996;24:303-310.

116. Reddy S, Smith DBJ, Rich MM, et al. Mice lacking the myotonic dystrophy kinase develop a late onset myopathy. *Nat Genet* 1996;13:423-442.

117. Benders AAGM, Groenen PJTA, Oerlemans FTJJ, Veerkamp JH, Wieringa B. Myotonic dystrophy protein kinase is involved in the modulation of the Ca$^+$ Homeostasis in skeletal muscle cells. *J Clin Invest* 1997;100:1440-1447.

118. Mounsey JP, Xu P, John JE, et al. Modulation of skeletal muscle sodium channels by human myotonin protein kinase. *J Clin Invest* 1995;95:2379-2384.

119. Timchenko L, Nastainczyk W, Schneider T, Patel B, Hofmann F, Caskey CT. Full length myotonin protein kinase (72Kd) displays serine kinase activity. *Proc Natl Acad Sci USA* 1995;92:5366-5370.

120. Berul CI, Maguire CT, Aronovitz MJ, et al. DMPK dosage alterations result in atrioventricular conduction abnormalities in a mouse myotonic dystrophy model. *J Clin Invest* 1999;103:R1-R7.

121. Saba S, VanderBrink BA, Luciano B, et al. Localization of the sites of conduction abnormalities in a mouse model of myotonic dystrophy. *J Cardiovasc Electrophysiol* 1999;10:1214-1220.

122. Berul CI, Maguire CT, Gehrmann J, Reddy S. Progressive atrioventricular conduction block in a mouse myotonic dystrophy model. *J Intervent Card Electrophysiol* 2000;4: (in press).

18

GENETIC CAUSES OF ATRIAL SEPTAL DEFECTS

Kristen Patton, M.D. and Christine E. Seidman, M.D.

Department of Genetics and Medicine, Howard Hughes Medical Institute
Harvard Medical School, Boston, MA 02115

INTRODUCTION

Atrial septal defects (ASDs) are common congenital malformations accounting for over 10% of isolated congenital heart defects (1). Ostium secundum ASDs, located in the region of the fossa ovalis are the most prevalent subtype (Figure 1) and are thought to arise by malformation of the septum primum, resulting in incomplete coverage of the fossa ovalis (2). However little is known about the cellular mechanisms or molecular signals that direct these processes.

Blood flow through the ASD is dependent on several factors: the ratio of left and right ventricular compliance, the size of the defect, and the relative resistance in the pulmonary and systemic circulation systems (3). Uncorrected ASD can therefore result in increased pulmonary circulatory blood, flow, which may lead to the development of pulmonary artery hypertension, right ventricular hypertrophy, subsequent right ventricular volume overload, failure, and death. The electrocardiographic effects of these late complications include ectopic atrial foci, incomplete or complete right bundle branch block, right axis deviation, or right ventricular hypertrophy with strain. Ostium secundum defects can also be associated with variable degrees of atrioventricular block (4). Prolongation of the PR interval has been thought to be due to either the increased size of the atrium or the increased distance for internodal conduction produced by the ASD itself (5).

Although most ASDs occur sporadically, affected individuals sometimes have a family history of septal defects or other congenital heart malformations and heart block (6-9). Given the marked heterogeneity of malformations in relatives and an incidence of ASD in siblings and offspring of affected individuals is less than expected for a single gene defect (10,11), etiologies for septation defects have been thought to be polygenic or multifactorial. Recently however the genetic etiology for two autosomal dominant conditions, Holt Oram syndrome (12,13) and familial ASD with prolonged atrioventricular conduction (14) have been demonstrated to be single gene mutations. These and genetic mapping studies in familial ASDs (15) that occur without other phenotypes indicate the contribution of monogenetic defects to some congenital heart malformations. More broadly, insights derived from these investigations may help to delineate the complex process of human cardiac development.

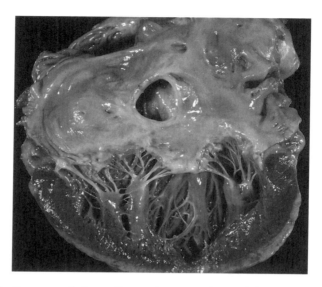

Figure 1. Gross morphology of an ostium secundum atrial septal defect following unsuccessful surgical repair. From Dr. F. Schoen, MD, PhD. Reprinted with permission from *Science* 281:33, ©1998 American Association for the Advancement of Science.

TBX5 Mutations Cause Holt-Oram Syndrome

Holt-Oram syndrome is the prototypic member of a group of poorly understood malformations that affect both the heart and hand (Discussed in further detail in Chapter 19). This unusual disorder occurs in 1 per 100,000 live births and is transmitted as an autosomal dominant trait (16). Upper limb anomalies in Holt-Oram syndrome are fully penetrant but exhibit marked variability in their distribution, symmetry and severity. Abnormalities involve the radial rays, and range from subtle malformations of the carpal bones detectable only by radiography, to extra carpal bones, triphalangism, digitalization or aplasia of the thumbs, absent or hypoplastic radii, upper extremity phocomelia, and syndactyly (16,17). Although skeletal malformations are virtually always bilateral, left sided defects are usually more severe (18).

A wide range of cardiac abnormalities occur in patients with Holt-Oram syndrome (19), but in approximately 15% of affected individuals, heart structure and function is normal. Secundum atrial septal defect is the most common malformation which occur alone, or in combination with other malformations in 60.3% of affected individuals (20). Ventricular muscular septal defects are the second most prevalent malformation and like atrial defects can be singular, multiple ("Swiss cheese" septum), or associated with other malformations. Conduction disease of the sinus and atrioventricular node may be seen with and without associated septal defects and abnormalities such as first degree atrioventricular block, right bundle branch block, or bradycardia occur frequently. Other structural malformations include Tetrology of Fallot, mitral valve prolapse, hypoplastic left heart syndrome, coarctation of the aorta , patent ductus arteriosus , aortic stenosis, anomalous pulmonary venous return, right isomerism, and abnormal ventricular trabeculation (16, 21-23).

Genome-wide linkage analyses defined the map location of the gene responsible for Holt Oram syndrome on chromosome 12p21.3-q22 (19,24) and demonstrated that the wide range of clinical phenotypes found in affected families were accounted for by mutations in a single gene. Subsequent molecular studies (12,13) led to the identification of the Holt-Oram disease gene as TBX5, a member of the T-box family of transcription factor. A diverse range of mutations has subsequently been identified in affected individuals (12,13,25) including insertions, deletions, chromosomal rearrangements, splice site and missense mutations. Most of these mutations result in premature termination signals and thus encode truncated peptides, which may be unstable and rapidly degraded. Even if foreshortened TBX5 peptides are stable they likely have markedly diminished biologic function since residues that comprise the central T-box motif are critical for binding target DNA sequences. Since affected Holt-Oram patients are heterozygous and also have one normal TBX5 gene, haploinsufficiency or a 50% reduction of this transcription factor during development accounts for the pleiotropic manifestations of disease. The phenotype resulting from different degrees of TBX5 truncation is similar; all cause severe malformation of the upper limbs and congenital heart defects. Missense mutations are defects that alter only one amino acid in TBX5. These are a rare cause of Holt-Oram syndrome and effect distinct domains of the T-box motif. Surprisingly, these mutations have unique clinical consequences (25). Mutations in residues at the carboxyl region of the T-box motif cause more severe skeletal than cardiac malformations, whereas a missense mutation at the amino region of the motif cause a predominance of cardiac malformations.

Nkx.2-5 Mutations Cause Familial ASD with Conduction Defects
Several kindred have been reported (6-9) that have congenital cardiac malformations with associated conduction system defects (Figure 2). Pedigree analyses indicate autosomal dominant disorder with age-related penetrance. Secundum atrial septal defects occurred commonly but other cardiac malformations were often found in family members including ventricular septal defects, tetralogy of Fallot, subvalvular aortic stenosis, pulmonary atresia and redundant mitral valve leaflets with fenestrations (26). Abnormalities in conduction included variable degrees of atrioventricular block (6,7,26). Serial electrocardiographic studies in some families indicated post-natal onset of conduction disease with long-term progression (14). Electrophysiologic studies localized defects to the atrioventricular node. Notably, sudden death occurred in six individuals from three of the families in asymptomatic adults, years after the surgical correction of an ASD. None of these individuals had undergone a pacemaker implantation.

Genome-wide linkage analysis in one large affected family defined a disease locus on chromosome 5q35 (14), where the gene encoding the transcription factor Nkx2.5 is located (27). Given the recognized role of this molecule in cardiac development of lower species (see below), Nkx2.5 sequences were screened for mutation and unique defects were identified in affected individuals from different families (14).

A

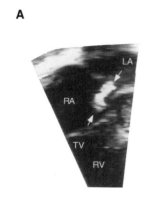

B

Age (years)	PR interval (s)	ECG
0.75	0.19	
2	0.19	
Surgical closure of ASD		
5	0.23	
6	0.28	
7	0.29 (2:1)	
14	0.42	

1 s

Figure 2. Clinical manifestations of ASD with conduction system disease. (A) ASD detected by two-dimensional echocardiography. Doppler pulse signal detects blood flow between the left and right atria. (B) ECGs show progressive atrioventricular nodal delay in an individual with a familial ASD. Reprinted with permission from *Science* 281:108, ©1998 American Association for the Advancement of Science.

Two mutations were identified that encode premature termination signals, and therefore are predicted to truncate the Nkx2-5 peptide. Another defect is a missense that alters one highly conserved amino acid residue in the homeodomain, a motif that binds target DNA.

Nkx2-5 mutations that encode foreshortened peptides are potentially unstable; alternatively these truncated peptides may disrupt the molecule's ability to target DNA binding. Hence like most TBX5 mutations, Nkx2-5 defects appear to cause haploinsufficiency of a transcription factor that is critical for normal cardiac morphogenesis. In addition to defining a role for this transcription factor in atrial septation, the associated electrical abnormalities in affected individuals indicates an important role for Nkx2-5 in the development or maintenance of the human atrioventricular node. The electrophysiology of nodal tissue is recognized to be distinct from that of surrounding myocardium: nodal cells express few gap junctions and propagate impulses slowly and are physiologically comparable to embryonic myocardium (28). Such observations raise the possibility that atrioventricular nodal cells are the vestigial remnants of primordial myocardial cells. Since Nkx2.5 expression is required for development of cardiac progenitor tissues, continued expression may necessary throughout postnatal life in primitive myocardial cells such as those found in nodal tissues.

Mutations on Chromosome 5p Cause Familial ASD
Genetic analyses of two families with secundum ASD, transmitted as a dominant trait with reduced penetrance and variable expressivity led to the identification of another ASD locus on chromosome 5p (15). The disease gene encoded here remains unknown. Clinical manifestations of this mutation were variable and included atrial septal aneurysms, vascular anomalies (left superior vena cava) and aortic valve disease. Notably ASDs were not demonstrable in several individuals whose DNA samples exhibited the affected genotype. Nonpenetrance, or the absence of a disease phenotype in an individual with a disease-causing mutation may be due to unknown molecular events, or can be caused by inadequate diagnostic studies or spontaneously closure of the defect. Regardless of the mechanism, nonpenetrance is likely to result in an underestimation of the incidence of heritable gene mutations that cause ASDs.

The cardiac phenotypes of individuals with a mutation of a locus on chromosome 5p also provide insights into the relationship of atrial septal aneurysm and secundum ASD. These aneurysms have been considered congenital malformation of the septum (29), which may play a role in postnatal ASD closure (30). Genetic studies in a study family support this cause and effect relationship in that an affected genotype was found in individuals with secundum ASD and individuals with atrial septal aneurysm. Serial evaluation of these individuals and ultimately gene identification should help to define postnatal changes in the atrial septal formation and maturation.

INSIGHTS FROM CARDIAC DEVELOPMENT OF LOWER ORGANISMS

The complex processes of heart tube formation, looping, and septation has been greatly illuminated in recent years by analyses of these events in lower organisms (31). Prior to gastrulation, precursors of cardiac cells located lateral to the primitive streak ingress and migrate into anterior-lateral plate mesoderm (32-33) to form the cardiac crescent. (34). Bone morphogenetic protein plays a central role in selecting cells destined for a myocyte lineage (35) and expression of Nkx 2-5 marks these earliest cardiac progenitor cells (36,37).

While heterozygous Nkx 2.5 mutations in humans cause ASDs, homozygous null mutations in the related Drosophila Nkx gene, tinman, results in absence of heart and other muscle groups (37). Targeted homozygous knockout of Nkx2.5 in mice (38, 39) results in normal formation of the heart tube, but severely deranged looping and mal-development of trabeculation and formation of the endocardial cushions, and early embryonic death. In situ hybridization studies of Nkx2.5 null mice show disturbed expression of a wide array of cardiac transcripts including atrial and brain natriuretic peptides, myosin light chain (MCL2V) and transcription factors, N-myc, MEF2C, HAND1, and Msx2 (39,40). Collectively these data provide compelling evidence that the level of Nkx2.5 in mammalian cardiac development is critical. With moderate deficiency, ASDs and other structural anomalies are evident; greater deficiency results in abolition of a ordered genetic cascade for myogenic lineages, cardiac looping and morphogenesis.

The role of *Tbx5* in cardiac development is less fully understood. Expression is evident throughout the cardiac crescent, but as these bilateral fields further coalesce and fuse to form the segmented primitive heart tube regional expression becomes evident (41). At this stage *Tbx5* transcripts are detected in posterior poles that ultimately become cardiac atria. With subsequent looping, asymmetric expression continues and *Tbx5* transcripts become localized to the trabeculated left ventricle. Notably these are absent from the distal right ventricle or developing outflow tract. This strong transmural atrial wall and septa expression and preponderant left ventricular expression pattern is maintained throughout subsequent maturation (Figure 3A). The patterns of *Tbx5* expression provide an embryological basis for the prevalence of atrial septal defects (ostium primum and secundum) and other cardiac malformations observed in patients with Holt-Oram syndrome (Figure 3B).

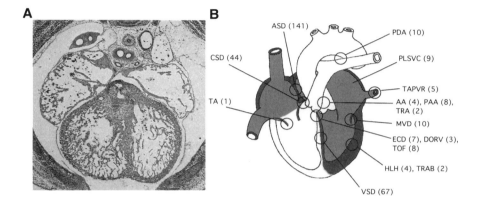

Figure 3. (A) In situ hybridization of *Tbx5* to transverse sections of an E13.5 mouse embryo produces a red signal in both atria and left ventricle. (B) Schematic representation of the mature heart indicating regions of Tbx5 expression (shaded areas) and the location of Holt-Oram cardiac defects in 240 patients. Atrial septal defect (ASD), atrioventricular block (AVB), conduction system defects (CSD), double outlet right ventricle (DORV), endocardial cushion defect (ECD), hypoplastic left heart (HLH), mitral atresia (MA), mitral valve prolapse (MVP), right isomerism (RI), total anomalous pulmonary venous return (TAPVR), tetralogy of Fallot (TF), trabecular anomalies (Trab), tricuspid atresia (TA), ventricular septal defects (VSD). The number of defects described in the literature. Reprinted with permission from Bruneau et al. *Develop Biol* 1999; 211:100-108.

CONCLUSIONS

Human genetic studies of inherited ASDs clearly indicate heterogeneity in both the clinical manifestations of these malformations and their molecular etiologies. These defects occur in isolation, or have associated conduction system disease or other structural malformations of the heart and other organs. Further identification and characterization of mutations in known disease genes and those yet to be defined should therefore provide a better understanding of human cardiac morphogenesis and help to define a molecular basis for the co-appearance of a spectrum of cardiac malformations. The wide phenotypic variation seen in affected individuals who share a common gene remains an intriguing finding. Development and characterization of animal models with these mutations may elucidate the mechanisms for variable expression of these mutations. Ultimately these studies may also improve our understanding of nonfamilial ASDs.

REFERENCES

1. Hoffman JE. Congenital heart disease: Incidence and inheritance. *Pediatr Clin N Am.* 1990:37:25-43.

2. Van Mierop LHS. Embryology of the atrioventricular canal region and pathogenesis of endocardial cushion defects. *In* Feldt RH, McGoon DC, Ongley PA, Rastelli GC, Titus JL, Van Mierop LHS (eds). Atrioventricular canal defects. Philadelphia: WB Saunders, 1976:1-3.

3. Moore KL, Persaud TVN. The Developing Human: Clinically Oriented Embryology.W.B. Saunders, Co. 1998, pp.349-404.

4. Ellison RC, Sloss, LJ. Electrocardiographic features of congenital heart disease in the adult. *In* Roberts, WC: Congenital Heart Disease in Adults. Philadelphia, FA Davis Co., 1979, p. 267

5. Takahashi H, Sakamoto T, Hada Y, Amano K , Hasegawa I , Takahashi T, Suzuki J. Left ventricular function in atrial septal defect by two-dimensional echocardiography.*J Cardiovasc Ultrasonography.* 1985;4:283.

6. Emanuel R, O'Brien K, Somerville J, Jefferson K, Hegde M. Association of secundum atrial septal defect with atrioventricular conduction abnormalities or left axis deviation. *Br Heart J* 1975;7:1085-92.

7. Pease WE, Nordenberg A , Ladda RL. Familial atrial septal defect with prolonged atrioventricular conduction. *Circulation* 1976; 53:759-762.

8. Kahler RL, Braunwald E, Plauth Jr WH, Morrow AG. Familial congenital heart disease: Familial occurrence of atrial septal defects with A-V conduction abnormalities;supravalvular aortic and pulmonic stenosis; and ventricular septal defect. *Am J Med.* 1966; 40: 384.

9. Bharati S, Lev M. Conduction system in sudden unexpected death a considerable time after repair of atrial septal defect. *Chest* 1988; 94:142-8

10. Boughman JA, Berg KA, Astemberski JA, Clark EB, McCarter RJ, Rubin JD, Ferencz C. Familial risks of congenital heart defects assessed in a population basedepidemiologic study. *Am J Med Genet.* 1987; 26:839-849.

11. Whittemore R, Wells, JA, Castellsague X. A second-generation study of 427 probands with congenital heart defects and their 837 children. *J Am Coll Cardiol.* 1994; 23:1459-1467.

12. Basson CT, Bachinsky DR, Lin RC, Levi T, Elkins JA, Soults J, Grayzel D, Kroumpouzou E, Traill TA, Leblanc-Straceski J, Renault B, Kucherlapati R, Seidman JG, Seidman CE. Mutations in human *Tbx 5* cause limb and cardiac malformation in Holt-Oram syndrome. *Nature Genet.* 1997; 15:30-35.

13. Li, QY, Newbury-Ecob RA, Terrett JA, Wilson DI, Curtis ARJ, Yi CH, Gebuhr T, Bullen PJ, Robson SC, Strachan T, Bonnet D, Lyonnet S, Young ID, Raeburn JA, Buckler AJ, Law DJ, Brook JD. Holt-Oram syndrome is caused by mutations in *TBX5*, a member of the *Brachyury (T)* gene family. *Nature Genet.* 1997; 15:21-29.

14. Schott J-J, Benson DW, Basson CT, Pease W, Siberbach GM, Moak JP, Maron BJ, Seidman CE, Seidman JG. Congenital heart disease caused by mutations in the transcription factor *NKX2-5*. *Science* 1998; 281:108-111.

15. Benson DW, Sharkey A, Fatkin D, Lang P, Basson CT, McDonough B, Strauss AW, Seidman JG, Seidman CE. Reduced penetrance, variable expressivity, and genetic heterogeneity of familial atrial septal defects. *Circulation* 1998; 97:2043-2048.

16. OMIM: Online Mendelian inheritance in Man, OMIM. Johns Hopkins University, Baltimore, MD. WWW url: hhtp://www3.ncbi;mlm.nih.gov/omim/.

17. Poznanski AK, Gall JC Jr., Stern AM. Skeletal manifestations of the Holt-Oram syndrome. *Radiol.* 1970; 94:45-53.

18. Smith AT, Sach GH Jr, Taylor GJ. Holt-Oram syndrome. *J Pediatrics* 1979; 95:538-543.

19. Basson CT, Cowley GS, Solomon SD, Weissman B, Poznanski AK, Traill TA, Seidman JG, Seidman CE. The clinical and genetic spectrum of the Holt-Oram syndrome (heart-hand syndrome). *N Engl J Med* 1994; 330: 885-891.

20. Sletten LJ, Pierpont ME. Variation in severity of cardiac disease in Holt-Oram syndrome. *Am J Med Genet* 1966; 65:128-32.

21. Holt M, Oram S. Familial heart disease with skeletal malformations. *Br Heart J* 1960; 22:236-242.

22. Newbury-Ecob R, Leanage R, Raeburn JA, Young ID. The Holt-Oram syndrome: a clinical genetic study. *J Med Genet* 1996; 33:300-307

23. Gall JC Jr, Stern AM, Cohen MM, Adams MS, Davidson RT. Holt-Oram syndrome: clinical and genetic study of a large family. *Am J Hum Genet.* 1966; 18:187-200.

24. Terrett JA, Newbury-Ecob R, Cross GS, Fenton I, Raeburn JA, Young ID, Brook JD. Holt-Oram syndrome is a genetically heterogeneous disease with one locus mapping to human chromosome 12q. *Nature Genet.* 1994; 6:401-404.

25. Basson CT, Huang T, Lin RC, Bachinsky DR, Weremowicz S, Vaglio A, Bruzzone R, Quadrelli R, Lerone M, Romeo G, Silengo M, Pereira A, Krieger J, Mesquita SF, Kamisago M, Morton CC, Pierpont MEM, Muller CW, Seidman JG, Seidman CE. Different *TBX5* interactions in heart and limb defined by Holt-Oram syndrome mutations. *Proc Natl Acad Sci USA* 1999; 96:2919-2924.

26. Bjornstad PG. Secundum-type atrial septal defect with prolonged PR interval and autosomal dominant mode of inheritance. *Br. Heart J.* 1974; 36:1149.

27. Turby D, Wechsler SB, Blanchard KM, Izumo S. Molecular cloning, chromosomal mapping, and characterization of the human cardiac-specific homeobox gene *hCsx*. *Molec Med.* 1996; 2:86-96.

28. Moorman AFM, Lamer WH. Molecular anatomy of the developing heart. *Trends Cardiovasc Med.* 1994; 4:257-64.

29. Hanley PC, Tajik AJ, Hynes JK, Edwards WD, Reeder GS, Hagler DJ, Seward JB.. Diagnosis and classification of atrial septal aneurysm by two-dimensional echocardiography: report of 80 consecutive cases. *J Am Coll Cardiol.* 1985; 6:1370-82.

30. Brand A, Keren A, Branski D, Abrahamov A, Stern S. Natural course of atrial septal aneurysm in children and the potential for spontaneous closure of associated septal defect. *Am J Cardiol* 1989; 64:996-1001

31. Olson EN, Srivastava D. Molecular pathways controlling heart development. *Science* 1996;272:671-676.

32. Lawson KA, Meneses JJ, Pederson RA. Clonal analysis of epiblast during germ layer formation in the mouse embryo. *Development* 1991; 113:891-911.

33. Tam PP, Parameswaran M, Kinder SJ, Weinberger RP. The allocation of epiblast cells to the embryonic heart and other mesodermal lineages: the role of ingression and tissue movement during gastrulation. *Development* 1997; 124:1631-1642.

34. Schultheiss TM, Xydas S, Lassar AB, Induction of avian cardiac myogenesis by anterior endoderm. *Development* 1995; 121:4203-4214.

35. Schultheiss TM, Burch JB, Lassar AL. A role for bone morphogenetic proteins in the induction of cardiac myogenesis. *Genes Devel* 1997; 11:451-462.

36. Lints TJ, Parsons LM, Hartley L, Lyons I, Harvey RP. Nkx2.5: a novel murine homeobox gene expressed in early heart progenitor cells and their myogenic descendants. *Development* 1993; 119:419-431.

37. Bodmer R. The gene tinman is required for specification of the heart and visceral muscles in Drosophila. *Development* 1993; 118:719-729.

38. Lyons M, Parsons LM, Hartley L, Li R, Andrews JE, Robb L, Harvey RP. Myogenic and morphogenetic defects in the heart tubes of murine embryos lacking the homeobox gene Nkx2-5*Genes Devel* 1995; 9:1654-1666.

39. Tanaka M, Chen Z, Bartunkova S, Yamasaki N, Izumo S. The cardiac homeobox gene Csx/Nkx2.5 lies genetically upstream of multiple genes essential for heart development. *Development* 1999; 126:1269-80.

40. Durocher D, Chen CY, Ardati A, Schwartz RJ, Nemer M. The atrial natriuretic factor promoter is a downstream target for Nkx2.5 in the myocardium. *Mol Cell Biol* 1996; 16:4648-4655.

41. Bruneau BG, Logan M, Davis N, Levi T, Tabin CJ, Seidman JG, Seidman CE. Chamber-specific cardiac expression of Tbx5 and heart defects in Holt-Oram syndrome. *Develop Bio* 1999; 211:100-108.

19

HOLT-ORAM SYNDROME AND THE TBX5 TRANSCRIPTION FACTOR IN CARDIOGENESIS

Cathy J. Hatcher, Ph.D. and Craig T. Basson, M.D., Ph.D.
Cardiology Division, Department of Medicine and Department of Cell Biology
Weill Medical College of Cornell University, New York, NY 10021

INTRODUCTION

The lives of 3% of newborn infants are threatened by serious birth defects, and of these, congenital cardiac malformations are the most common and affect between 0.5 and 1% of all live births (1). Congenital cardiac structural anomalies that are not immediately life-threatening, including bicuspid aortic valve, mitral valve prolapse, and self-resolving ventricular septal defects, occur in more than 5% of live births (2-4). Despite a reported 92% sensitivity for fetal echocardiography of high risk patients in the hands of experienced investigators, congenital structural heart disease remains among the most frequently undiagnosed anomalies by current prenatal evaluations. The recognition of an association between macroscopic karyotypic abnormalities such as trisomies of chromosomes 13, 18, and 21 and complex cardiac syndromes including malformation of the ventricular and atrial septa has permitted improved sensitivity of prenatal detection for congenital heart disease by cytogenetic studies. In some cases, such as deletions and rearrangements of chromosome 22 in individuals with velocardiofacial syndrome, cytogenetic analyses have also provided important clinical information about microscopic karyotypic abnormalities. However, definitive diagnosis of congenital heart disease remains elusive and awaits determination of molecular genetic etiologies. The advent of genome mapping and improved techniques of linkage analysis and positional cloning have been applied to simple congenital heart disease in humans. Chromosomal loci and genes (3) have been assigned to familial hypertrophic cardiomyopathy, long QT syndrome, supravalvular aortic stenosis and Marfan syndrome. However, given a 25-45% risk of extracardiac defects in the setting of cardiac malformation, molecular genetic analysis of complex congenital heart disease remains an issue with significant clinical consequences. Over the past year, we and other investigators have employed such experimental tools to identify the gene defects in Holt-Oram syndrome (5), Alagille syndrome (6), situs inversus / visceral heterotaxy (7), and atrial septal defects with progressive atrioventricular block (8). In this chapter, we will focus on the identification of the TBX5 transcription factor as the mutated gene in Holt-Oram syndrome and the contribution of TBX5 to human cardiac septation and isomerism.

DaVinci first recognized in 1513 that communication between right and left cardiac chambers was a result of defects in the atrial and ventricular septum. As early as 1664, Stenon (9) observed an association between congenital cardiac malformation and upper limb deformity. In 1960, Holt and Oram (10) described a family affected by the heart-hand syndrome now known as Holt-Oram syndrome, [Online Mendelian Inheritance of Man #142900; (11)]; individuals exhibited malformed thumbs in the setting of atrial septal defects. Subsequent study of multiple families affected by Holt-Oram syndrome (12-27) revealed an autosomal dominant pattern of inheritance. Penetrance of the disorder appeared complete but the expression of the syndrome was highly variable in the presence, severity, and location of limb and cardiac malformations. Despite the presence of multisystem anomalies, intellectual function was always intact, and craniofacial abnormalities were invariably absent.

SKELETAL AND CARDIAC PHENOTYPES

All individuals with Holt-Oram syndrome exhibit some upper limb skeletal abnormality in the developmental distribution of the preaxial radial ray (11, 28-30). Such deformity may be bilateral and asymmetric or unilateral, and, in either limb, may be mild and subclinical or severe and overt. For instance, despite initial descriptions of the typical Holt-Oram syndrome patient being characterized by thumb deformity (either triphalangism or hypoplasia / absence), the most common skeletal manifestation of Holt-Oram syndrome is malformation of one or more of the carpal bones. (Figure 1) These wrist bones may be absent, misshapen or fused, and diagnosis may only be possible by x-rays. However, with adequate testing every Holt-Oram syndrome patient will be demonstrated to have such carpal bone malformation (30). These subtle aberrations of the thumb and/or wrist may be the only manifestation of this disorder. By contrast, some individuals have severe foreshortening of the radius bone that extends proximally in a preaxial distribution to include the humerus bone and shoulder girdle. Such severe limb deformity may present as phocomelia similar to the familiar effects of thalidomide, and thus when Holt-Oram syndrome was first described, it was dubbed a "pseudo-thalidomide" syndrome (11).

Unlike Holt-Oram skeletal malformation, not all individuals affected by Holt-Oram syndrome have congenital heart disease, but approximately three quarters of individuals with Holt-Oram syndrome have cardiac manifestations (30). As with Holt-Oram skeletal manifestations, these may be severe or clinically insignificant, and the severity of cardiac disease is not necessarily proportional to the severity of skeletal disease. Holt-Oram syndrome cardiac disease may manifest in the anatomical structure and/or the electrical conduction properties of the heart (Figure 2). Most commonly, individuals present with ostium secundum defects of the atrial septum; ostium primum atrial septum defects are seen only rarely. Many affected individuals will, however, present with ventricular septal defects, most often in the membranous portion of the ventricular septum.

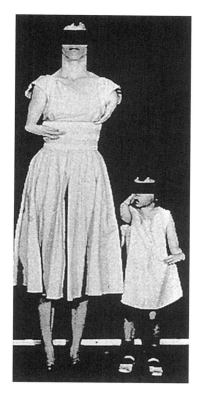

Figure 1. Skeletal manifestations of Holt-Oram syndrome. A mother and daughter from Family B affected by Holt-Oram syndrome exhibit typical severe skeletal deformity (phocomelia and ectromelia). [Photograph courtesy of Haig H. Kazazian, Jr., M.D., University of Pennsylvania School of Medicine, Philadelphia, PA.]

The consequences of these anatomic cardiac defects and associated intracardiac shunts are not unique to Holt-Oram syndrome, and as with any severe septal defect, such disorder may ultimately lead to right-to-left shunting, cyanotic heart disease, and pulmonary hypertension. This aggregation of findings, Eisenmenger's syndrome, results in high morbidity and mortality in patients with septal defects. Rarely, more complex congenital heart disease (e.g. anomalous pulmonary venous drainage, Tetralogy of Fallot, truncus arteriosus, atrioventricular defects, isomerism, abnormal right ventricular trabeculation, and hypoplastic left heart syndrome) are noted in Holt-Oram syndrome (9-33).

Holt-Oram syndrome cardiac conduction disease is not a simple consequence of an anatomic septal defect interrupting intracardiac conduction pathways. In fact, Holt-Oram syndrome patients may exhibit progressive conduction disease in the absence of any observable septal defect (29). Conversely, septation defects may occur without conduction disease. Conduction disease often initially manifests as sinus bradycardia with mild first-degree atrioventricular block (Figure 2). However, over time the function of the sinus node and block at the atrioventricular node can deteriorate further to produce atrial fibrillation and higher grade Mobitz II and complete heart block. Worsening intraventricular (particularly right) conduction delay may be seen as well. These conditions may cause significant morbidity and require medical and/or pacemaker therapy.

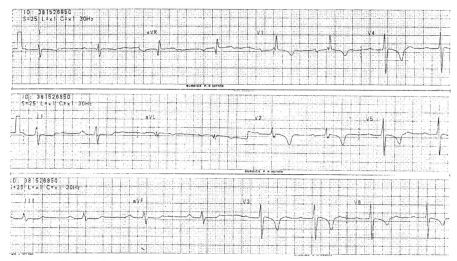

Figure 2. Conduction abnormalities in Holt-Oram syndrome. Typical 12 lead electrocardiogram of a Holt-Oram syndrome patient shows sinus bradycardia, first degree atrioventricular block, right bundle branch block, and a right superior axis.

EPIDEMIOLOGY AND GENETICS

Incidence of Holt-Oram syndrome has been difficult to estimate because of a lack of large population studies, but disease has been noted throughout the world including North America, South America, Europe, Asia, Australia, and Africa and in individuals of all major ethnic groups (9-34). Elek et al. (34) surveyed the Hungarian Congenital Malformation Registry and noted a birth prevalence of 0.95 per 100,000 total births. 85% of these were consequences of new mutations giving a calculated mutation rate on the order of 1 in a million. In the many familial Holt-Oram cases reported, the syndrome has always been inherited as an autosomal dominant trait with complete penetrance despite its highly variable expression.

No consistent familial cytogenetic abnormalities have been associated with Holt-Oram syndrome, although a variety of karyotypic abnormalities were identified in sporadic cases (23-27) prior to modern molecular genetic analyses. Thus, cytogenetic studies had not been helpful in localizing and identifying the gene defect that caused the limb and heart defects of Holt-Oram syndrome. Nevertheless, it seemed clear that identification of the Holt-Oram syndrome gene defect would yield important information about regulatory pathways in both cardiac and skeletal development. Moreover, the elucidation of the Holt-Oram syndrome defect might allow analogization of heart development with limb development, and the large body of information on molecular mechanisms underlying limb morphogenesis (reviewed in 35) might provide a critical scaffolding to understand cardiac morphogenesis.

CHROMOSOMAL MAPPING STUDIES

Our initial investigations of Holt-Oram syndrome (29) focused on two large affected families. Family A includes 49 family members in five generations at risk for inheriting the disorder, and of these individuals 26 (11 male and 15 female) were affected by Holt-Oram syndrome. Family B includes 31 members in 3 generations at risk for inheriting Holt-Oram syndrome with 19 (10 male and 9 female) affected individuals. While most families affected by Holt-Oram syndrome exhibit a range of mild to severe skeletal and cardiac deformity, Families A and B represent opposite poles of the phenotypic spectrum. Individuals in Family A only have mild skeletal deformity which largely manifests as thumb or wrist bone abnormalities; no individual has severe ectromelia or phocomelia. All Family A affected individuals, however, have some form of congenital heart disease, and in many cases these defects, including multiple concomitant septation defects and a complete atrioventricular canal defect, are severe and life threatening. We refer to these multiple septal defects or severe complex congenital heart disease as "composite" cardiac defects. By contrast, Family B affected individuals often have severe skeletal malformations including ectromelia and phocomelia (Figure 1), but most affected individuals have no structural cardiac disease. Congenital heart disease in Family B, when it does occur, is limited to hemodynamically insignificant atrial septal defects.

We used linkage analysis to determine whether defects at a single genetic locus might cause the disparate Holt-Oram syndrome phenotypes in Families A and B. Highly polymorphic short tandem repeats (STRs) randomly distributed throughout the genome were analyzed to test for linkage to the Holt-Oram syndrome locus first in Family A. After approximately 60% of the human genome was excluded, linkage was identified to microsatellites located on the long arm of chromosome 12 (29). Further linkage analyses confirmed that the Holt-Oram syndrome gene defect in Family B resides at this chromosome 12q2 locus. Subsequent analyses by us (36) and others (37,38) have demonstrated that mutations at this chromosome 12q24.1 locus produce Holt-Oram syndrome in more than thirty families.

Although there is no doubt that chromosome 12q2 is the major genetic locus for Holt-Oram syndrome, there remains some controversy as to whether genetic heterogeneity exists in Holt-Oram syndrome. We and others (29,30,36,37) have found no evidence for such heterogeneity. However, Terrett et al. (38) were unable to establish linkage to chromosome 12q2 in two families. In one case, this appeared to the result of the uninformativeness of the microsatellites tested, and nonlinkage could not be definitively established. In the case of the other family reported, LOD scores were significantly less than -2.0, and nonlinkage was clear. However, the diagnostic criteria used for Holt-Oram syndrome by Terrett et al. (38) differed from standard criteria (11,13,28) and thus may have obfuscated the linkage analysis. For instance, Terrett et al. (38) required individuals to have bilateral limb deformity whereas we (5,29,30) and others (11,13,28) generally include individuals who have unilateral limb deformity only. Moreover, x-ray studies were not included in all individuals' clinical evaluations, and therefore subtle subclinical evidence of carpal bone malformation may not have been detected. Thus, it remains difficult to interpret discordance of chromosome 12q2 microsatellites with the Holt-Oram syndrome trait in this family.

An alternative explanation for the "nonlinkage" observed by Terrett et al. (38) may be that this family was not, in fact, affected by Holt-Oram syndrome but by a related phenocopy heart-hand syndrome. Several such syndromes have been described (11,36), and all include upper limb and congenital cardiac disease like that observed in Holt-Oram syndrome. To address whether such similar syndromes are associated with the same genetic locus, we examined (36) a family affected by Heart-Hand Syndrome Type III. Like Holt-Oram syndrome, Heart-Hand Syndrome Type III is an autosomal dominant syndrome. All individuals have some upper limb abnormality including carpal bone malformations, and digital manifestations often include hyperphalangism of the index finger as well as radial ray defects. In addition, abnormalities may be seen in the lower limb (unlike Holt-Oram syndrome) and particularly involve the first and second toes. Cardiac abnormalities primarily include sinus and atrioventricular node disease and intraventricular conduction delays, and conduction disease appears to be fixed in the few patients followed serially unlike the progressive disease seen in Holt-Oram syndrome. However, the limited number of individuals affected by this rare syndrome available for study precludes establishing statistically significant differences in structural cardiac defects when compared with Holt-Oram syndrome patients. When chromosome 12q2 STRs linked to Holt-Oram syndrome were employed for linkage analysis of a Heart-Hand Syndrome Type III family, LOD scores <-2.0 were obtained. Similar results were also achieved when we analyzed a family with autosomal dominantly inherited atrial septal defects and conduction disease but without any limb deformity (8,36). Thus, these phenocopy syndromes appear clinically related to Holt-Oram syndrome but are genetically distinct. These findings may, in fact, suggest that in families with Holt-Oram-like syndromes, genetic linkage analysis may often be sufficient to distinguish Holt-Oram syndrome from its phenocopies. Such distinctions may provide important bases for diagnosis and prognostication in families affected by heart-hand syndromes.

IDENTIFICATION OF THE *TBX5* GENE AND MUTATIONS

Ultimately, such clinical differentiation as well as basic delineation of developmental mechanisms underlying congenital deformity are best facilitated by defining the specific gene mutated at the chromosomal locus identified for a heritable condition. Although a number of known genes had been mapped to the general cytogenetic location of the Holt-Oram syndrome locus (12q24.1), all such candidates were excluded from the interval by refined genetic and physical mapping studies. Faced with identifying novel genes at chromosome 12q24.1, we first set out (5) to limit the size of the Holt-Oram locus by refining the genetic and physical maps of the locus. Haplotype analyses along with these mapping studies first demonstrated that the Holt-Oram syndrome disease gene was located within a 1 cM interval between anonymous STRs D12S129 and D12S354 that was encoded on a single 880 kb yeast artificial chromosome (887b9) from the CEPH MegaYAC library. Further studies refined this to a minimal interval between STRs D12S1646 and D12S2185 which was cloned into a contig of four P1 bacteriophage clones.

Because random sequence analysis of these clones failed to reveal any known genes, strategies were designed to identify novel gene segments. All four P1 clones encompassing the Holt-Oram syndrome locus were subjected to exon trapping (5), and more than 20 trapped sequences were subcloned into plasmid vectors for subsequent sequence analysis. When these sequences were compared to the Genbank database, homology was observed to the *Drosophila optomotor blind* (*omb*) gene, a member of the T-box gene family of transcription factors. T-box transcription factors are defined by their high degree homology between their DNA binding domains, so called T-boxes (39-42). Prototypical members of this family such as the *brachyury* or *T* gene are important for epithelial-mesenchymal interactions during vertebrate development of a wide variety of tissues including notochord, kidney, limb and heart (42). T-box gene family members are highly evolutionarily conserved and are present from lower order organisms such as worms to higher order mammals including rodents and man. In *Drosophila*, the *omb* gene has been shown to be both necessary and sufficient for wing formation (43). Both hypomorphic and null alleles in *omb* yield disorganization of wings, and ectopic expression of *omb* is sufficient to produce abnormal supernumerary wings.

Reverse transcriptase PCR demonstrated that Holt-Oram locus "trapped" exon sequences were expressed in both adult and embryonic (13 week of gestation) human total cardiac RNA. Trapped exons were then used as probes to screen a 26 week human embryonic heart cDNA library, and five corresponding cDNA clones were identified. Sequence analysis of the cardiac cDNA clones demonstrated that all five contained overlapping sequence. A single open reading frame was initially identified (5) amongst these clones that is predicted to encode a 349 amino acid polypeptide. Comparison of the cDNA nucleotide sequence and the predicted amino acid sequence of this polypeptide demonstrated high homology to the T-box domain of other T-box gene family members. This region of homology extended from amino acid residues 56 to 238. This newly identified human T-box exhibited 65% identity with human TBX2 T-box, 53% identity with human TBR1 T-box, 52% identity with human T (Brachyury) T-box, and 62% identity with the *Drosophila omb* T-box that was originally detected by the homology search with trapped exon sequences. However, the highest degree of homology was observed with the mouse Tbx5 T-box, described by Papaioannou and colleagues (40,41). These two T-boxes were 97% identical, and therefore we designated (5) the human chromosome 12q24.1 T-box gene as human TBX5.

Subsequent analysis (30) of additional genomic and cDNA clones for TBX5 identified alternatively spliced isoforms. Alternative splicing occurs at the 3' end of the molecule and alters the open reading frame. In this isoform, alternative splicing occurs after the nucleotides encoding amino acid residue 327, and additional coding sequence predicts a 517 amino acid polypeptide. Recently, we have performed western blot and immunohistochemical studies of human tissues with antiserum to

TBX5 which demonstrate that polypeptides corresponding to both the predicted alternatively spliced TBX5 isoforms are expressed in mammalian cells (Hatcher, Mah, Basson, unpublished data). cDNA analyses also demonstrated alternative splicing at the 5' end of TBX5. However, all such splicing occurs 5' to the coding sequence and only modifies untranslated sequence.

In situ hybridization studies (44,45) with mouse Tbx5 to localize its expression during embryonic development further supported the hypothesis that mutations in the human TBX5 gene might cause limb and cardiac defects typical of Holt-Oram syndrome. Robust expression of *Tbx5* was observed in the developing mouse forelimb with a striking intense staining of the precartilaginous zones of the developing carpal bones. No significant expression was observed in the hindlimbs. Thus, murine *Tbx5* is expressed during development in skeletal regions that correspond to human anatomical locations affected by Holt-Oram syndrome. *Tbx5* expression in the murine thoracic body wall might correlate with pectoral muscle abnormalities occasionally seen in Holt-Oram syndrome patients. Moreover, murine *Tbx5* is expressed throughout the atria during development. Bruneau et al. (46) have recently described asymmetry (left > right) of *Tbx5* mRNA in the developing and neonatal mouse and chicken ventricles. Such asymmetry is less obvious in Li et al.'s (47) *in situ* hybridization studies of human cardiac tissue. Additionally, our recent immunohistochemical studies have now analyzed the expression of human TBX5 protein. TBX5 protein persists in both human ventricles during fetal and adult life (Figure 3; Hatcher, Goldstein, and Basson, unpublished data). Thus, the regulated expression of human TBX5 during cardiogenesis remains to be completely detailed. Nonetheless, it was clear even from early data on *Tbx5* cardiac expression that TBX5 mutations might cause cardiac defects. *Tbx5* expression in murine embryonic genital papilla, trachea, lung and pharynx do not have obvious correlates with the Holt-Oram syndrome phenotype.

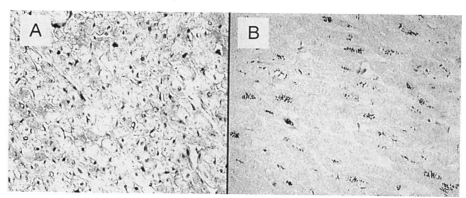

Figure 3. Immunolocalization of TBX5 protein in the human heart. Paraffin sections of normal adult human left and right ventricles treated with antibody to human TBX5, and bound antibody visualized with secondary antibody coupled to horseradish peroxidase. Myofibrils cut (A) transversely in the left ventricular myocardium and (B) longitudinally in the right ventricular myocardium. Dark staining of myocyte nuclei in myocardium from both ventricles demonstrates continued presence of TBX5 transcription factor during adulthood.

Given these correlative findings, we set out to examine the TBX5 gene in individuals with Holt-Oram syndrome to identify mutations. We chose to analyze genomic DNA as the source of TBX5 for mutational analysis. To do so, we established the genomic structure of the TBX5 gene by comparison of TBX5 cDNA clone sequences with the genomic clone sequences. Nine exons were identified (5,30) with the translation start site beginning in exon 2. As described above, alternative splicing at the 3' end created the variable presence of exon 9. 5' untranslated region alternative splicing generated three possible exon 1's, referred to as exon 1a, 1b, and 1c. In all, the TBX5 gene is greater than 50 kb in size. To perform mutational analysis, oligonucleotide primers were designed from intron sequences flanking each exon containing coding sequence (exons 2-9). Each exon was then PCR amplified for unafffected and affected probands and subjected to cycle sequencing to look for sequence variants. Sequence variants were considered mutations if they met three criteria: 1) Variants were not present in the chromosomes of more than 100 unaffected unrelated individuals as well as unaffected individuals related to the proband, 2) Variants were present in all affected individuals related to the proband, and 3) Variants would alter the predicted protein encoded by the TBX5 gene. All mutations were confirmed by another technique besides sequence analysis, usually restriction fragment length polymorphism analysis or allele specific oligonucleotide hybridization. We have to date identified (5,30) 12 mutations in individuals affected by Holt-Oram syndrome. In each case, the mutations satisfy the criteria described above. Three additional mutations have also been identified by Li et al. (47). Most of these mutations are predicted to modify sequence within the T-box DNA binding domain (Table 1).

Table 1. TBX5 Mutations in Individuals Affected by Holt-Oram Syndrome

Family	Mutation*	Class of Mutation
A	Gly80Arg	Missense
B	Arg237Gln	Missense
IIg	Arg237Gln	Missense
V	Arg237Trp	Missense
E	ΔGlu243FSter	Frameshift; truncated at codon 263
F	Glu69ter	Nonsense; truncated at codon 69
IIa	t(5;12)(q15;q24)	Intron 1A disruption; translocation
IIb	Ser196ter	Nonsense; truncated at codon 196
IId	ΔAsp140FSter	Frameshift; truncated at codon 145
IIj	Int2ASC-2A	Intron 2 splice acceptor site; truncation
III	Int2ASG+1C	Intron 2 splice acceptor site; truncation
IIq	insMet83Fster	Frameshift; truncated at codon 94
GG	-4,+der(4),t(4;12)(p16;q24.1)	Gene duplication
8,12,22	Arg279ter	Nonsense; truncated at codon 287
16	insSer387FSter	Frameshift; truncated at codon 393

* Amino acid residues are numbered as previously described (5,30). IIj and III are splice acceptor site (AS) mutations; the nucleotides are numbered as described (30). Identification of mutations in families with letter codes is described in references 5 and 30, and with number codes in reference 47.

Analysis of Family IIb provides typical evidence that mutations in TBX5 cause Holt-Oram syndrome (30). The *TBX5* sequence of affected individuals from Family IIb contained a C→A transversion at nucleotide residue 587 (Figure 4). Substitution of an adenosine residue for the normal cytosine produces a nonsense codon, designated Ser196ter, that would be predicted to encode a prematurely truncated protein even in the unlikely case that the aberrant message RNA was stable and translated. The Ser196ter mutation was independently confirmed by oligonucleotide specific hybridization and heteroduplex analysis and was present in all clinically affected individuals. Of note, the eldest affected individual in Family IIb represents a sporadic case of Holt-Oram syndrome; both this individual's mother and father are clearly unaffected by the syndrome. Therefore, assuming that the syndrome is completely penetrant, one would predict that no mutation would be found in the unaffected parents' TBX5 gene. This hypothesis proved to be true, and the Ser196ter mutation in the eldest affected individual represents a *de novo* event. Moreover, the mutation apparently also occurred in the eldest affected individual's germ cells, since the mutation was then passed on to subsequent descendants and showed complete cosegregation with Holt-Oram syndrome. Thus, this family provides a natural set of genetic experiments which fulfill Koch's postulates of disease causation in that an etiologic factor (a TBX5 mutation) was correlated with a disorder (Holt-Oram syndrome), the factor was isolated, and then reintroduced (i.e. in subsequent offspring) and shown to reproduce the disease phenotype.

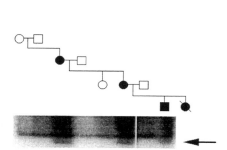

Figure 4. Detection of *TBX5* Truncation Mutations in Family IIb. Products of a dideoxyadenine cycle sequencing reaction demonstrate a Ser196ter nonsense mutation in Family IIb. Family IIb pedigree is shown above sequencing gel. Affected individuals have an adenine residue (arrow), while unaffected exhibit a cytosine residue at nucleotide position 587. Samples from the youngest affected child (deceased) were not available for genetic analyses.

HOW DO *TBX5* MUTATIONS CAUSE HOLT-ORAM SYNDROME?

Of the 15 *TBX5* gene mutations identified, 11, as a result of nonsense / frameshift mutations, splice site mutations, or chromosomal rearrangements, are predicted to produce markedly truncated forms of TBX5 protein or no TBX5 protein at all. For instance, we have identified (30) one individual with severe limb and cardiac manifestations of Holt-Oram syndrome: left arm phocomelia and right arm severe ectromelia in the setting of a complete atrioventricular canal defect and abnormal atrial isomerism. Karyotype studies of this individual demonstrated that a translocation had occurred between chromosomes 5 and 12 [46,XX,t(5;12)(q15;q24)]. No sequence variants were seen in the *TBX5* coding sequence, exons 2-9. However, when fluorescence *in situ* hybridization studies were done using either TBX5 cDNA clones or genomic clones containing only 5' untranslated exon 1a, it became clear that the translocation breakpoint had occurred in the 5' untranslated region of the TBX5 gene. Thus, it is likely that this chromosomal abnormality separated the as yet unidentified TBX5 regulatory regions from the TBX5 coding sequence, and thus the mutated allele would be null. Such findings suggest that *TBX5* haploinsufficiency is at least one mechanism by which perturbed TBX5 expression might produce Holt-Oram syndrome.

Other truncation mutations identified (Glu69ter, insMet83Fster, ΔAsp140FSter, Ser196ter, insAsn198Fster, ΔGlu243Fster, Int2ASC$_{-2}$A, and Int2ASG$_{+1}$C) are all consistent with the hypothesis of haploinsufficiency. All of these mutations would truncate the T-box DNA binding domain of TBX5, and investigation of the *T (Brachyury)* gene has shown that deletion of even a single base at either end of the T-box can inhibit DNA binding (48). Therefore, even if the shortened transcripts were stable (and it is likely that they are not) and were translated, the truncated protein would be expected to be unable to bind DNA, and therefore a "functional" haploinsufficiency would exist. An additional truncation mutation (ΔGlu243FSter) may produce a functional haploinsufficiency by inhibiting DNA binding as well since recent crystallography studies (49) of the T(Brachyury) T-box (described below) suggest that these residues immediately flanking the T-box may be important for stabilization of T-box binding to DNA.

Two additional truncating mutations (Arg279ter and insSer387FSter) described by Li et al. (47) clearly could not function in this manner since they occur well 3' to the T-box domain. It remains unclear what their mode of action is (i.e. haploinsufficiency vs. dominant negative effect). Li et al. (47) have suggested that they may truncate activating / repressing domains in the 3' half of the TBX5 molecule. Such domains have been shown to be present in T (Brachyury) and are therefore hypothesized to be present in TBX5. However, no significant homology exists between these genes outside of the T-box DNA binding domain, and therefore it is difficult to predict how structure/function analysis of the T (Brachyury) gene might correlate with TBX5 in this region of the molecule.

If TBX5 haploinsufficiency is one mechanism by which Holt-Oram syndrome is produced, is there a generalized gene dose effect? Can overexpression of TBX5 produce a similar phenotype? To date, there is no definitive evidence that this is true. However, that there may be substance to such a hypothesis is suggested by the several patients reported with chromosome 12q2 duplication syndromes that share similar elements with Holt-Oram syndrome. For instance, we have studied one individual (GG) with the karyotype 46, XY, -4, +der(4), t(4;12)(p16;q24.1) which indicates a duplication of the chromosome 12q24.1 region. Thus, this duplication should produce an increased gene dose of the *TBX5* gene, albeit along with nearby genes, including the *TBX3* gene within 500 kb of *TBX5*. GG exhibits a variety of features consistent with Holt-Oram syndrome including upper limb brachydactyly and a cardiac ventricular septal defect which in sum may be related to *TBX5* overexpression. Notably the patient also exhibits a variety of genitourinary abnormalities including left renal agenesis and hypospadias which are similar to some features of ulnar-mammary syndrome (11) caused by mutations in *TBX3*.

Experimental data from animal models support the hypothesis that normal *TBX5* gene dose is essential for cardiac development. Several investigators have shown that gene dose of other T-box transcription factors is critical for appropriate *Xenopus laevis* axial patterning (42,50-53). Horb and Thomsen (54) specifically studied the contribution of *Xenopus laevis TBX5* gene dose to cardiac development. As in chick, mouse, and human (44-47,55-57), their *in situ* hybridization studies showed that XTbx5 mRNA is distributed throughout the posterior structures of the developing heart. Expression of a dominant negative *XTbx5* repressor construct resulted in a lethal gastrulation defect that prevented analysis of its effect on the heart. Therefore, Horb and Thomsen (54) placed the *XTbx5* repressor construct under the control of a steroid inducible promoter, injected this switchable construct into *Xenopus* embryo hearts and then treated embryos expressing this repressor with dexamethasone at stage 15 (after gastrulation has been completed but prior to the onset of cardiac expression of *XTbx5* at stage 17). Depending on the level of XTbx5 repression achieved, the hearts of these embryos were either absent or severely malformed. Injection of low levels of *XTbx5* along with the repressor either partially or completely rescued the cardiac defects. Interestingly, coinjection of higher concentrations of *XTbx5* were less effective at rescuing the cardiac defect and suggested that XTbx5 overexpression might produce malformation through a gain of function mechanism. Thus, Horb and Thomsen (54) concluded that as in human Holt-Oram syndrome, precise regulation of Tbx5 levels were essential for normal cardiogenesis in *Xenopus*.

Does, then, abnormal gene dose explain all individuals with Holt-Oram syndrome? The answer is almost certainly no. Although the vast majority of TBX5 mutations identified thus far are mutations predicted to truncate the TBX5 protein, we have now identified three families which inherit TBX5 missense mutations (Gly80Arg - Family A, Arg237Gln - Family B, and Arg237Trp - Family V) at the 5' and 3' ends of the T-box DNA binding domain, and since these should only produce single amino acid substitutions in the TBX5 protein, there is no reason to suspect that they alter gene dose. How then might these mutations have their effects? We hypothesize that such missense mutations have a dominant negative effect by stoichiometric inhibition of TBX5 binding to DNA. For this hypothesis to be true, TBX5 protein altered by one of these missense mutations ought be less efficient at DNA binding than the wild type TBX5. Recent evidence supports this speculation. Muller and Herrmann (49) have now successfully resolved the crystallographic structure of the *Xenopus* T (Brachyury) [*Xbra*] gene T-box which is highly homologous to the TBX5 T-box. These studies modeled the T-box in its bound state to DNA and document a novel binding mechanism in which the T-boxes bind as dimers to DNA with the 5' end of the T-box binding in the minor groove of DNA and the 3' end of the T-box binding in the major groove. Strikingly, the amino acid residues in *Xbra* which correspond to the TBX5 Gly80 and Arg237 that are involved in the human missense mutations described above immediately flank the residues which form the T-box DNA recognition surfaces that permit T-box hydrophobic interactions with DNA in the minor groove and polar hydrophilic interactions with DNA in the major groove (30). Therefore, it seems likely that the significant charge alterations produced by these missense mutations adjacent to DNA binding sites would alter and abrogate these interactions. Thus, it follows that such missense mutations might produce their phenotypic consequences through a dominant negative effect rather than through haploinsufficiency as postulated for "truncation" mutations.

GENOTYPE - PHENOTYPE CORRELATIONS

If different genetic mechanisms underlie the phenotypic effects of missense and truncation mutations, can one detect different phenotypic consequences of these mechanisms? To assess this hypothesis, we have compared (30) the phenotypes of individuals affected by Holt-Oram syndrome with characterized TBX5 mutations (Figure 5). 59 individuals were included in analyses - 17 with truncation mutations, 19 with the Gly80Arg missense mutation, 18 with the Arg237Gln missense mutation, and 5 with the Arg237Trp missense mutation. As would be expected for a completely penetrant disorder, all individuals with TBX5 mutations, regardless of specific mutation, exhibited some form of skeletal disorder, and 75% of such individuals exhibited some form of cardiovascular disorder. However, when comparing the effects of different mutation classes, statistically significant differences in the kinds of skeletal or cardiac disorders comprising Holt-Oram syndrome phenotypic expression were observed.

Strikingly, two of the missense mutations described above occur in Families A and B, the two families with which genetic analysis of Holt-Oram syndrome were initiated (29) and which were observed from the beginning to have unusual Holt-Oram phenotypes: either severe cardiac (Family A) or severe skeletal (Family B) disease. Family V (affected by the third missense mutation) also resided in this unusual category of Holt-Oram syndrome phenotypes; Holt-Oram syndrome phenotypic expression in this family was similar to Family B, i.e. with severe skeletal disease without severe cardiac disease. Therefore, we correlated (30) mutation class with incidence of severe skeletal disease (defined as malformation involving bones outside of the proximal radial ray, i.e. more than thumb, carpal bones, and radius bone) and incidence of composite cardiac disease (defined as either more than one septation defect or complex congenital heart disease). Individuals with truncation mutations exhibited high incidences of severe disease of both the skeletal (53%) and the cardiac (41%) systems. By contrast, individuals with missense mutations exhibited high incidences either of severe skeletal disease or of composite cardiac disease but not both. 21% of individuals with the Gly80Arg mutation had composite cardiac disease with no individual with this mutation exhibiting severe skeletal disease. Individuals with the Arg237Gln or Arg237Trp mutations exhibited high incidence of severe skeletal disease, 33% and 40% respectively, while no individual with these mutations exhibited composite cardiac disease. Thus, TBX5 truncation mutations appear to affect severely both limb and heart, while TBX5 missense mutations appear to affect severely only one organ system or the other (Figure 5), and these phenotypic distinctions seem likely to reflect different genetic mechanisms, such as haploinsufficiency or dominant negative effects.

Phenotypic distinctions amongst individuals with different missense mutations are more difficult to statistically validate given the limited number of such mutations identified and the limited number of individuals with such mutations. However, it is striking that two TBX5 missense mutations (Arg237Gln and Arg237Trp) at the 3' end of the T-box (which binds to target DNA minor groove) have severe effects on the skeletal system without severely affecting the heart. On the other hand, a TBX5 missense mutation (Gly80Arg) at the 5' end of the T-box (which binds target DNA major groove) conversely severely affects the heart but not the limb. We have, therefore, hypothesized that differential DNA binding (i.e. major vs. minor groove) may imply unique consequences in different tissues. Ongoing investigation seeks to identify more such missense mutations to further evaluate this hypothesis and to identify modifying genes that might interact with TBX5 and produce the intrafamilial variations seen in Holt-Oram syndrome phenotypes even in the face of a single TBX5 mutation, missense or truncation.

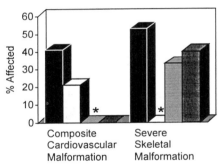

Figure 5. Incidence of composite congenital cardiovascular and severe skeletal malformation in individuals with *TBX5* mutations causing Holt-Oram syndrome. Clinical phenotypes were analyzed in 17 individuals (Families E, F, IIa, IIb, and IId).

affected by *TBX5* truncation mutations, 19 individuals (Family A) affected by the Gly80Arg *TBX5* missense mutation, 18 individuals (Family B) affected by the Arg237Gln *TBX5* missense mutation, and 5 individuals (Family V) affected by the Arg237Trp *TBX5* missense mutation. Within each class of *TBX5* mutation [truncation (black), Gly80Arg (stippled), Arg237Gln (striped), and Arg237Trp (cross-hatched)], the percent of affected individuals with either severe cardiovascular or severe skeletal malformation was determined. Asterisks indicate $p<0.005$ when compared with malformation caused by *TBX5* truncation mutations.

It should be noted that the genotype-phenotype correlations and TBX5 structural studies alone do not definitively exclude other mechanisms of action of TBX5 mutations. In fact, the finding that T-box domains may bind DNA as dimers certainly allows for such possibilities as truncated TBX5 proteins disrupting DNA binding through a dominant negative effect. Moreover, the observation of T-box dimerization suggests possible explanations as to why morphologic consequences are not seen in all tissues in which mutant TBX5 is expressed, for instance lung and genital papilla. While such reduced tissue penetrance may reflect a relative differential sensitivity to gene dose, particularly if haploinsufficiency is invoked as the underlying genetic mechanism of disease, it is also possible that other homologous non-TBX5 T-box genes expressed in lung and genital papilla (e.g. TBX2 and TBX3) may be able to dimerize with TBX5 and function in a redundant fashion in these tissues. In fact, it remains to seen if TBX4 (also reportedly expressed in the murine heart [44]) can interact with TBX5 and modify mutant TBX5 effects. These questions will be addressed in the future by the identification of the TBX5 domains critical for dimerization and the TBX5 binding sequences in target DNA (42,49,58).

TBX5 CONTRIBUTION TO CARDIOGENESIS

An increasing number of important transcription factors, cytokines, and extracellular matrix components are now being identified that regulate cardiac morphogenesis. The challenge ahead is to determine how these many molecular agents interact, and the ability to compare and to contrast TBX5 contribution to limb and heart development may assist us to generate hypotheses to be tested in the future. As discussed earlier, the *Drosophila* T-box gene, *omb* has been directly demonstrated (45) to be involved in wing formation. *Drosophila* wing formation requires establishment of an anterior (A) - posterior (P) axis, created by a decapentaplegic (*dpp*) morphogen gradient which activates TBX genes such as *omb* and leads to the development of distal limb structures (35,59,60). Our investigations demonstrate that TBX5 mutations cause distal limb hypomorphism (thumb and wrist bone abnormalities) as well as proximal defects (such as phocomelia) that are analogous to the developmental wing defects in *Drosophila omb*. These findings imply that TBX5, like other T-box genes, may be expressed in response to a *dpp*-like morphogen gradient in limb. Based on the paradigm of vertebrate and invertebrate limb development, we have, then, hypothesized that TBX5 is expressed in response to a morphogen gradient in heart development in a fashion analogous to limb development. Our preliminary immunohistochemical findings suggest that such TBX5 protein gradients do in fact exist within the ventricular myocardium (Hatcher, Goldstein, and Basson, unpublished data).

What might be the relationships between such putative morphogen gradients, TBX5 gene expression and axis formation in the developing human heart? Genes (11,61) such as Tinman, MEF2, and GATA transcription factors regulate initial myocyte differentiation along the AP axis of the developing straight heart tube into atrial and ventricular myocytes. Normal rightward bending of the heart tube may involve the asymmetric expression of ZIC3, sonic hedgehog, activin, nodal, *iv*, and *inv* (7,61). With the establishment of an asymmetric left (L) - right (R) axis, the heart loops under the influence of genes such as Csx and HAND transcription factors. Establishment of a dorsal (D) - ventral (V) axis results in neural crest cell migration and differentiation of the conotruncal regions. Expression of TGFß, BMP isoforms and transcription factors MSX1 and MOX1 in endocardial cushions result in division of atria from ventricles and form atrioventricular valves. Further development requires septation of both the atria and the ventricles as well as chamber specification. Therefore, we speculate that during development of a four chambered heart, morphogen gradients (perhaps human homologues of *Drosophila dpp*) direct expression of the TBX5 transcription factor to produce the atrial and ventricular septal anlages.

However, we also suspect that TBX5 mediated pathways participate in cardiac chamber isomerization, the morphologic definition of each chamber which occurs independently of anatomical location (situs). Each atria and ventricle has unique anatomic features. For example, atrial appendage morphology and pulmonary venous return, are different in the right and left atria, while ventricular trabeculation and conduction system development are different in left and right ventricles. Because these morphologic features can be abnormal in Holt-Oram syndrome patients (9-34) such as the individual described with a chromosome 12q24 translocation and a presumed *TBX5* null allele (30), we suggest that TBX5 and/or its as yet unidentified downstream target genes participate in isomerization during cardiac morphogenesis in addition to physical septation of the heart. It is of note that TBX5 is not expressed only in the interatrial septum but throughout the walls of both atria during human development (Hatcher, Goldstein, Basson, unpublished data). Presumably other genes, such as neuregulin, TEF1, RXRα, and N-myc already known to participate in this process, are either activated by the same morphogen gradient as TBX5 or are activated by TBX5 and its downstream target genes, and all contribute to the establishment of cardiac chamber identity.

In other organ systems, animals studies have demonstrated that TBX5 contributes to the establishment of tissue identity. Correlation between Tbx5 and Tbx4 expression patterns and developmental regions that give rise to forelimb and hindlimb respectively have been observed in the mouse (45), chicken (54-57), and newt (62). Several investigators have studied the contribution of the T-box transcription factors Tbx5 and Tbx4 to specification of limb identity (wing vs. leg) in the developing chick. Induction of supernumerary limbs that, based on positioning of fibroblast growth factor - 8 releasing beads, are either wing-like or leg-like has demonstrated that as with normal chick limbs, wing vs. leg identity correlates with Tbx5 or Tbx4 expression respectively (54-57). Recently, Takeuchi et al. (63) and Rodriguez-Esteban et al. (64) have used electroporation and viral vectors to ectopically express Tbx5 in the developing chick leg and Tbx4 in the developing chick wing. Ectopic Tbx5 induces an at least partial conversion of leg morphology to wing morphology, and similarly ectopic Tbx4 induces an at least partial conversion of wing to leg morphology. Thus, these T-box transcription factors contribute to establishment of limb identity in the chick, and we expect that they similarly contribute to establishment of cardiac chamber identity.

SUMMARY

Demonstration, then, that TBX5 mutations are responsible for the autosomal dominant condition Holt-Oram syndrome provides significant information and suggests many new hypotheses about the molecular mechanisms that lead to limb development, cardiac septation and cardiac isomerization. These studies have broad implications for understanding both developmental biology and human pathology. We predict that the human homologues of components identified in other species will be operant in the TBX5 signaling pathway of man. Furthermore, we suspect that these other components are likely candidate genes for mutations that cause other congenital limb and heart disorders. Thus, definition of all components of this pathway may improve diagnosis of additional congenital hand and heart disorders and may also provide clinical approaches to these complex human conditions.

Although gene based therapy for Holt-Oram syndrome and related cardiac anomalies may be some years away, the current knowledge on hand now permits DNA-based diagnosis for Holt-Oram syndrome. We have already used such information, for instance, to demonstrate by both linkage/haplotype analysis and mutational analysis that one individual originally classified as having an indeterminate diagnosis, based on the findings of a muscular ventricular septal defect with no limb anomalies, is, in fact, unaffected by Holt-Oram syndrome. Such findings have significant impact on patients and their families, but as with all DNA-based diagnoses, the application of genetic testing may also carry a variety of financial, psychological, social, and ethical burdens. In the future, a full appreciation of the TBX5 dependent pathways in the development of the cardiac structure and conduction system will suggest appropriate diagnostic and therapeutic modalities for individuals with congenital heart disease.

REFERENCES

1. D'Alton ME, DeCherney AH. Prenatal diagnosis. *N Engl J Med* 328:114-120,1993.
2. Roguin N, Du ZD, Barak M. High prevalence of muscular ventricular septal defect in neonates. *J Am Coll Cardiol* 26:1545-1548,1995.
3. Mah CS, Vaughan CJ, Basson CT. Advances in the molecular genetics of congenital structural heart disease. *Genet Testing* 3:157-172,1999.
4. Freed L et al. Prevalence and clinical outcome of mitral valve prolapse.*N Engl J Med* 341:1-7,1999.
5. Basson CT et al. Mutations in human *TBX5* cause limb and cardiac malformation in Holt-Oram syndrome. *Nat Genet* 15:30-35,1997.
6. Li L et al. Alagille syndrome is caused by mutations in human Jagged1, which encodes a ligand for Notch1. *Nat Genet* 16:243-251,1997.
7. Gebbia M et al. X-linked situs abnormalities result from mutations in ZIC3. *Nat Genet* 17:305-308,1997.
8. Schott JJ et al. Congenital heart disease caused by mutations in the transcription factor NKX2-5. *Science* 281:108-111,1998.
9. Pruznanski W. Familial congenital malformations of the heart and upper limb.A syndrome of Holt-Oram. Cardiologia 45:21-38,1964.
10. Holt M, Oram S. Familial heart disease with skeletal malformations. *Br Heart J* 22:236-242,1960.
11. Online Mendelian Inheritance in Man, OMIM (TM), Johns Hopkins University, Baltimore, MD. World Wide Web URL:http://ww3.ncbi.nlm.nih.gov/omim/.

12. Smith AT, Sack GH, Taylor GT. Holt-Oram syndrome. *J Pediatr* 95:538-543,1979.
13. Hurst JA, Hall CM, Baraitser M. The Holt-Oram syndrome. *J Med Genet* 28:406-10,1991.
14. Letts RM, Chudley AE, Cumming G, Shokier MH. The upper limb - cardiovascular syndrome (Holt-Oram syndrome). *Clin Orthop Rel Res* 116:149-154,1976.
15. Kullman F, Grimm,T. Holt-Oram-Syndrom. *Dtsch Med Wochenschr* 118:1455-62,1993.
16. Sahn DJ, Goldberg SJ, Allen HD, Canale JM. Cross-sectional echocardiographic imaging of supracardiac total anomalous pulmonary venous drainage to a vertical vein in a patient with Holt-Oram syndrome. *Chest* 79:113-115,1981.
17. Starke H, Schimke RN, Dunn M. Upper-limb cardiovascular syndrome.*Am J Cardiol* 19:588-592,1967.
18. Newbury-Ecob RA, Leanage R, Raeburn JA, Young ID. Holt-Oram syndrome: a clinical genetic study. *J Med Genet* 33:300-307,1996.
19. Sletten LJ, Pierpont, ME. Variation in severity of cardiac disease in Holt-Oram syndrome.*Am J Med Genet* 65:128-132,1996.
20. Marcus RH, Marcus BD, Levin SE. The upper limb-cardiovascular syndrome (Holt-Oram syndrome) in a South African family. *S Afr Med J* 67:1013-1014,1985.
21. Gall JC, Stern AM, Cohen MM, Adams MS, Davidson RT. Holt-Oram syndrome: clinical and genetic study of a large family. *Am J Hum Genet* 18:187-200,1966.
22. Zhang K, Sun Q, Cheng TO. Holt-Oram syndrome in China: A collective review of 18 cases. *Am Heart J* 111:572-577,1986.
23. Rybak M, et al. Holt-Oram syndrome associated with ectromelia and chromosomal aberrations. *Am J Dis Child* 121:490-495,1971.
24. Turleau C, et al. Two patients with interstitial del (14q), one with features of Holt-Oram syndrome. Exclusion mapping of PI (alpha-1-antitrypsin). *Ann Genet* 27:237-240,1984.
25. Ockey CH, Feldman GV, MacAulay ME, Delaney MJ. A large deletion of the long arm of chromosome no. 4 in a child with limb abnormalities. *Arch Dis Child* 42:428-434,1967.
26. Yang SP, Sherman S, Derstine JB, Schonberg SA. Holt-Oram syndrome gene may be on chromosome 20. (Abst) *Pediat Res* 127:137A,1990.
27. Kristoffersson U, Mineur A, Heim S, Mandahl N, Mitelman F. Normal high-resolution Karyotypes in 3 patients with the Holt-Oram syndrome. *Am J Med Genet* 28:229-231,1987.
28. Poznanski AK, Gall JC, Stern AM. Skeletal manifestations of the Holt-Oram syndrome. *Radiology* 94:45-53,1970.
29. Basson CT, et al. The clinical and genetic spectrum of the Holt-Oram syndrome (Heart-Hand syndrome). *N Engl J Med* 330:885-891,1994.
30. Basson CT, et al. Different *TBX5* interactions in the heart and limb defined by Holt-Oram syndrome mutations. *Proc NatlAcad Sci* USA 96:2919-2924,199.
31. Najjar H, Mardini M, Tabbaa R, Nyhan W. Variability of the Holt-Oram syndrome in Saudi individuals.*Am J Med Genet* 29:851-855,1988.
32. Glauser TA, Sakai E, Weinberg P, Clancy R. Holt-Oram syndrome associated with hypoplastic left heart syndrome. *Clin Genet* 36:69-72,1989.
33. Ruzic B, Bosnar B, Beleznay O. Ein seltener herzfehler als symptom des Holt-Oram syndroms. *Radiologe* 21:296-299,1981.
34. Elek C, Marta V, Czeizel E. Holt-Oram syndroma. *Orvosi Heitlap* 132:72-78,1991.
35. Cohn MJ, Tickle C. Limbs: a model for pattern formation within the vertebrate body plan. *Trends Genet* 12:253-257,1996.
36. Basson CT et al. Genetic heterogeneity of heart-hand syndromes. *Circulation* 91:1326-1329,1995.
37. Bonnet D, et al. A gene for Holt-Oram syndrome maps to the distal long arm of chromosome 12. *Nat Genet* 6:405-408,1994.
38. Terrett JA, et al. Holt-Oram syndrome is a genetically heterogeneous disease with one locus mapping to human chromosome 12q. *Nat Genet* 6:401-404,1994.
39. Bollag RJ, et al. An ancient family of embryonically expressed genes sharing a conserved protein motif with the T locus. *Nat Genet* 7:383-389,1994.
40. Agulnik SI, et al. Evolution of mouse T-box genes by tandem duplication and cluster dispersion. *Genetics* 144:249-254,1996.
41. Herrmann BG, Kispert A. The T genes in embryogenesis. *Trends Genet* 10:280-286,1994.
42. Smith J. T-box genes: what they do and how they do it. *Trends Gen* 15:154-158,1999.
43. Grimm S, Pflugfelder GO. Control of the gene optomotor-blind in Drosophila wing development by decapentaplegic and wingless. *Science* 271:1601-1604,1996.

44. Chapman DL, et al. Expression of the T-box family genes, Tbx1-Tbx5, during early mouse development. *Develop Dyn* 206:379-390,1996.
45. Gibson-Brown JJ, et al. Evidence of a role for T-box genes in the evolution of limb morphogenesis and specification of forelimb/hindlimb identity. *Mech Devel* 56:93-101,1996.
46. Bruneau B, et al. Chamber specific cardiac expression of *TBX5* and heart defects in Holt-Oram syndrome. *Devel Biol* 211:100-108,1999.
47. Li Q, et al. Holt-Oram syndrome is caused by mutations in TBX5, a member of theBrachyury (T) gene family. *Nat Genet* 15:21-29,1997.
48. Kispert A, Herrmann BG. The *Brachyury* gene encodes a novel DNA binding protein.*EMBO J* 12:3211-3220,1993.
49. Muller CW, Herrmann BG. Crystallographic structure of the T domain - DNA complex of the Brachyury transcription factor. *Nature* 389:884-888,1997.
50. Zhang J, et al. The role of maternal VegT in establishing the primary germ layers in Xenopus embryos. *Cell* 94:515-524,1998.
51. Papaioannou VE, Silver LM. The T-box gene family. *BioEssays* 20:9-19,1998.
52. Isaacs HV, et al. eFGF regulates Xbra expression during Xenopus gastrulation. *EMBO J* 13:4469-4481,1994.
53. Schulte-Merker S, Smith JC. Mesoderm formation in response to *Brachyury* requires FGF signaling. *Curr Biol* 5:62-67,1995.
54. Horb ME, Thomsen GH. *Tbx5* is essential for heart development. *Development* 125:1739-1751,1999.
55. Isaac A, et al. Tbx genes and limb identity in chick embryo development. *Development* 125:1867-1875,1999.
56. Ohuchi H, et al. Correlation of wing-leg identity in ectopic FGF-inducedchimeric limbs with the differential expression of chick *Tbx5* and *Tbx4*. *Development* 125:51-60,1998.
57. Logan M, Simon H-G, Tabin C. Differential regulation of T-box and homeobox transcription factors suggests roles in controlling chick limb-type identity. *Development* 125:2825-2835,1998.
58. Carreira S, Dexter TJ, Yavuzer U, Easty DJ, Goding CR. Brachyury-related transcription factor Tbx2 and repression of the melanocyte-specific TRP-1 promoter. *Mol Cell Biol* 18:5099-5108,1998.
59. Lawrence PA, Struhl G. Morphogens, compartments and pattern: lessons from *Drosophila*. *Cell* 85:951-961,1996.
60. Nellen D, Burke R, Struhl G, Basler K. Direct and long-range action of a *dpp* morphogen gradient. *Cell* 85:357-368,1996.
61. Olson EN, Srivastava D. Molecular pathways controlling heart development. *Science* 272:671-676,1996.
62. Simon H-G, Kittappa R, Khan PA, Tsilfidis C, Liversage RA, Oppenhiemer S. A novel family of T-box genes in urodele amphibian limb development and regeneration: candidate genes involved in vertebrate forelimb/hindlimb patterning. Development 124:1355-366, 1997.
63. Takeuchi JK, et al. *Tbx5* and *Tbx4* genes determine the wing/leg identity of limb buds.Nature 398:810-814, 199.
64. Rodriguez-Esteban C, Tsukui T, Yonei S, Magallon J, Tamura K, Belmont JCI. The T-box genes *Tbx4* and *Tbx5* regulate limb outgrowth and identity. Nature 398:814-818, 1999.

20

INHERITED STRUCTURAL HEART DISEASES ASSOCIATED WITH ARRHYTHMIAS: DEFECTS IN LATERALITY

Baruch S. Ticho, M.D., Ph.D.
Massachusetts General Hospital, Boston, MA 02114

Richard Van Praagh, M.D.
Children's Hospital, Boston, MA 02115

INTRODUCTION

The clinical presentation of patients with defects in the determination of laterality is extremely varied. Abnormalities can occur in 1) establishment of visceral and atrial situs resulting in situs inversus or heterotaxy, 2) looping of the cardiac tube resulting in ventricular inversion, and 3) positioning of the heart in the chest resulting in dextrocardia. These disorders are usually easily recognized, and can be associated with complex cardiac anomalies. Affected individuals may be completely asymptomatic or may present at any age with a broad range of severity of symptoms. Conduction defects occur most frequently in patients with heterotaxy or with "corrected" transposition of the great arteries. The clinical and conduction system manifestations of these diseases will be presented, followed by a discussion of the molecular and genetic bases for these disorders.

Conduction Disturbances In Heterotaxy Syndromes
The fundamental characteristics of heterotaxy are an abnormal symmetry of certain viscera and veins (lungs, liver, venae cavae) and situs discordance between various organ systems, as well as between the various segments of the heart.

The usual orientation of the heart and visceral organs is known as situs solitus. Situs inversus refers to a mirror-image reversal of organs such that the heart and stomach are on the right side, the liver on the left and the lobation and bronchial patterns of the lungs are reversed. The incidence of cardiac disease among affected individuals is similar to the general population, and no association with conduction defects is known.

Any arrangement other than situs solitus or inversus, that is, any random orientation of different organs, is known as heterotaxy, heterotaxia, or situs ambiguus (1). These patients have asplenia or polysplenia syndromes and can have the appearance of isomerism, which is a loss of pulmonary and cardiac asymmetry at some levels resulting in apparent bilaterally right- or left–sidedness, respectively.

Asplenia

In asplenia syndrome, frequently both lungs are trilobed, both bronchi are eparterial and the spleen is hypoplastic or absent. In addition, the liver commonly overrides the midline. Previous terminology for asplenia included use of the term right atrial isomerism, however bilateral right atria have never been observed. The appearance of bilateral right atrial appendages has been described (2,3). Right atrial appendage isomerism occurs exclusively with asplenia, and not with polysplenia, but only in 20 percent of cases (4). Eighty percent of asplenia patients have either normal or inverted atrial appendage situs. The other cardiac anomalies in asplenia syndrome are often characteristic and include common atrium, complete AV canal, double-outlet right ventricle, pulmonic stenosis, transposition of the great arteries and anomalous pulmonary venous connections (5).

Although complete AV canal defects are common in asplenia, AV block rarely occurs. One series of 58 asplenia patients found sinus rhythm in all (5). In another series, 98 percent of patients with the diagnosis of right atrial isomerism had sinus rhythm and in 34 percent of these the axis was rightward (+90° to +179 °) (6). Complete AV block was documented in a newborn with asplenia syndrome and bilateral superior vena cavae (7). The histologic findings in this case revealed a discontinuity between the atria and the AV conduction tissue. Two AV nodes, of which only the posterior was continuous with a penetrating and bifurcating bundle, were also demonstrated.

Several reports of bilateral sinus nodes in asplenia patients have been used to support the notion of bilateral right-sidedness of the atria. In four cases characterized as having isomerism of the right atrial appendages and bilateral superior vena cavae it was reported that two sinus nodes were found (8). A sling of conduction tissue was thought to link the two nodes. Dual AV nodes were also noted. A separate report of two cases of asplenia syndrome with common AV canal demonstrated 2 discrete AV conduction systems, one posterior and the other anterior (9). In these 2 cases the posterior AV conduction system was well developed, whereas the anterior one was hypoplastic.

The dual AV nodes may predispose patients to supraventricular tachycardia (SVT). One series of 101 patients with right atrial isomerism documented SVT in 25 percent of cases (10). Patients with two ventricles were more likely to develop SVT than those with a univentricular heart. The type of ventricular loop and the position of the apex were not correlated with SVT. Seven patients underwent electrophysiologic studies which demonstrated that sinus node function, and atrial and ventricular refractory periods were all normal. The mechanism for SVT was postulated to be "AV nodal to AV nodal" reentry. The retrograde accessory pathway for SVT was mapped to an anterior AV node in two cases and a left lateral pathway in one case. Radiofrequency ablation was successfully attempted in two patients (10). In another study three patients with asplenia and SVT underwent radiofrequency ablation successfully (11). The accessory pathways were associated with the tricuspid valve in all three hearts.

Polysplenia

The designation polysplenia syndrome is used for a complex association of abnormalities of the spleen and of visceral lateralization with congenital heart malformations (12,13). The phenotype of polysplenia suggests bilateral 'left-sidedness' (12) and mirror imaging of the lungs is frequent such that both lungs have the appearance of the left lung, with 2 lobes and hyparterial bronchi. Anomalous pulmonary venous return is frequent. The renal to hepatic segment of the inferior vena cava is often missing. Return of blood from the lower part of the body is by the azygos or hemiazygos system, a venous defect that occurs almost exclusively in this syndrome. Left atrial isomerism has never been documented. Although bilateral left atrial appendages have been described in polysplenia, are not a consistent feature, appearing at most in 31 percent of cases (4). Cardiac defects found in polysplenia include atrial and ventricular septal defects, pulmonic stenosis, AV canal defects, and others (5). The cardiac anomalies are distinct from, and less severe than, asplenia.

Conduction disturbances are common in polysplenia. It has been noted that the P wave axis in polysplenia is difficult to determine (5). The atrial pacemaker appears to vary from one examination to the next in some patients. One series of 67 patients with reported left atrial isomerism revealed sinus rhythm in 73 percent, nodal rhythm in 12 percent and AV block in 15 percent; of these 30 percent had first degree block, 20 percent second degree and 50 percent complete block (6). The P wave axis was normal in 37 percent and superior in 49 percent, and in one third of cases the P wave axis shifted more than 90 ° on subsequent electrocardiograms. There was no relation found between the P wave axis and the nature of the systemic or pulmonary venous connection. Another study of 50 left isomerism patients observed a P wave axis of -30 ° to -90 ° in 70% of the individuals, with frequent variability in axis (14). They also noted an increasing incidence of slow junctional escape rate with age.

Histologic findings in nine cases of polysplenia could not identify a sinus node in two instances. In the other cases the sinus nodes were single, hypoplastic and abnormally located either in the lateral wall of the right atrium in five cases, or in the left atrium in two cases (8). Dual AV nodes were identified in six of these hearts which appeared to be connected by conduction tissue. In two of these connections there was a discontinuity of the tissue. Two AV nodes and a connecting sling were found in two other polysplenia patients (15).

Congenital complete atrioventricular block can accompany polysplenia. One survey found a 20 percent incidence of complete AV block among 30 children with polysplenia (16). All of these cases of complete AV block had interrupted IVC, two thirds had complete AV canal defect, and one third had two intact AV valves. A 20% incidence of complete heart block was also noted in another report (17).

The third degree heart block in polysplenia has been postulated to be due to discontinuity between the AV node and the ventricular conduction pathway. An analysis of 10 cases of polysplenia and complete heart block revealed that the AV conduction axis was interrupted at the level of the penetrating bundle in all cases (18). A single AV node in contact with atrial tissue was present in all cases. Eight of these hearts had common AV canal and two had ventricular septal defects.

Conduction Disturbances In Ventricular Inversion
Left-right asymmetry is first evident during the fourth week of human gestation when the primitive heart tube loops to the right (D-looping). As a result the right ventricle lies to the right of the left ventricle. Occasionally the heart tube bends to the left and the morphologic right ventricle is positioned to the left of the left ventricle.

Isolated ventricular inversion is a relatively rare lesion, accounting for only 0.5% of clinically apparent congenital heart disease (19). In 99% of the cases of inverted ventricles, transposition of the great arteries also occurs, resulting in physiologically corrected transposition, also called transposition {S,L,L}, or L-transposition of the great arteries (L-TGA)) by its segmental diagnosis. There are atrioventricular and ventriculoarterial discordances, thus fully saturated pulmonary venous return is correctly directed to the aorta.

In addition to transposition of the great arteries, other cardiac lesions also occur with ventricular inversion. A detailed study of the pathologic anatomy of 77 postmortem cases found that in classical corrected TGA {S,L,L} with two ventricles, anomalies of the left-sided systemic tricuspid valve were present in 97%, and malformations of the left-sided systemic right ventricle in 91% (20). Ventricular septal defects (VSD), pulmonary stenosis and dextrocardia are also common.

Rhythm disturbance in corrected TGA occurs frequently, in up to 69 percent of patients (21). Usually there is a QS or qR pattern in V_1 and an rS or RS pattern in V_6 on standard ECG. Preexcitation can be present as well.

Atrial tachyarrhythmias are a common occurrence in L-TGA. In one survey of 52 patients under 54 years of age who had survived with VSD, pulmonic stenosis and/or systemic AV valve deformity, 36 percent had documented atrial fibrillation or flutter or SVT (21). The presence of associated cardiac defects may predispose patients to early arrhythmias. A long term follow up of 18 patients without associated cardiac anomalies found that SVT did not appear until the fifth decade but was present in all patients after the age of 60 (22).

In some cases arrhythmias may be due to AV valve regurgitation or ventricular dysfunction. Other cases are due to accessory pathways which have been documented histologically (23) and electrophysiologically (24,25). The association of L-TGA, Wolff-Parkinson-White syndrome and Ebstein anomaly occurred in several of these cases.

Heart block in L-TGA is common, even in patients without associated cardiac defects. In 17 patients with L-TGA and no coexisting lesions, 12 percent had first degree AV block and 29 percent had complete AV block (25). First- and second-degree AV block preceded complete AV block in 2 patients. Electrophysiologic studies confirmed that the site of AV block was supra-Hisian in 2 patients and intra-Hisian in 1 patient. Another survey of 107 patients with L-TGA, most of whom had cardiac defects, revealed that 22 percent had complete AV block (26). Only 4 percent of the patients had congenital block; the remainder developed complete block (in the absence of surgery) over an average of 18 years. The risk for block was higher in patients who did not have a VSD. Complete AV block could occur spontaneously even in the absence of pre-existing lesser degrees of block (26).

The site of the block has clinical implications on patient outcome. This was confirmed in a series of electrophysiologic studies on 40 patients with L-TGA which showed normal conduction in 38 percent, first degree block in 35 percent, and complete AV block in 27 percent (27). The site of complete block was above the His potential in four, below in two and within the bundle in one. The two patients with block below the bundle of His were the only ones who had symptoms.

Dissection of the conduction pathways in 11 patients with L-TGA revealed that the AV node in all cases was located anteriorly in the right atrium connecting with a His bundle which encircled the anterolateral region of the pulmonary valve (28). In most cases a hypoplastic posterior AV node was also present. It was proposed that complete AV block resulted from fibrous degeneration of the of the AV bundle due to its increased length.

Conduction Disturbances in Dextrocardia
A wide variety of definitions and descriptions of dextrocardia exist. In primary (congenital) dextrocardia, the cardiac mass lies in the right chest in the absence of mechanical effects, and the apex points to the right. The majority of cases (50-80%) of primary dextrocardia are associated with L-loop ventricles. Corrected transposition of the great arteries occurs frequently. Dextrocardia is also common in both heterotaxy syndromes. The conduction disturbances seen in dextrocardia reflect the underlying heart defects. Thus heart block occurring with L-TGA or polysplenia is often seen with dextrocardia.

CHILDREN'S HOSPITAL EXPERIENCE - CONGENITAL HEART BLOCK

Since complete heart block is a common complication of laterality defects, we undertook to examine the causes of congenital AV block among autopsy patients at Children's Hospital, Boston. We reviewed the medical records at the Cardiac Registry at Children's Hospital to identify patients with the diagnosis of congenital complete heart block for the period from 1927 to 1997. All cases of complete heart block listed in the Cardiac Registry had a cardiac lesion. There were 15 Cardiac

Registry cases from patients who died at Children's Hospital, and 8 consult cases of patients who had died elsewhere. In the consult cases, the autopsies were done at another institution and the autopsy report was provided, and only the heart (and attached organs, if any) were examined at Children's Hospital. Patients were included in this review if they had documented 3° heart block based on surface ECG or electrophysiologic study. Cases in which heart block occurred post-operatively were excluded. For each of the 23 patients, the medical record was reviewed for clinical and autopsy diagnoses. Data were collected for cardiac malformations and segmental diagnosis (Table 1). The largest group, 9 cases (40%), was comprised of patients with polysplenia, 6 individuals (26%) had L-TGA and the remainder had other diagnoses.

Table I. Cardiac Diagnoses in 23 Autopsy Cases of Congenital Complete Heart Block

Number	Malformation†	Segmental diagnosis*
1	ASD I	SDS
2	ASD II	SDS
3	PFO	SDS
4	ASD II, VSD	SDS
5	VSD	SDS
6	TOF	SDS
7	MVP	SDS
8	PS	SDS
9	L-TGA	SLL
10	L-TGA	SLL
11	L-TGA	SLL
12	L-TGA	SLL
13	L-TGA	SLL
14	L-TGA	SLL
15	Polysplenia	SDS
16	Polysplenia	ADS
17	Polysplenia	ILL
18	Polysplenia	ILL
19	Polysplenia	ILS
20	Polysplenia	ILS
21	Polysplenia	IDL
22	Polysplenia	IDD
23	Polysplenia	IDS

*Nomenclature for the segmental diagnosis is as follows: atrial situs (S = solitus, I = inversus, A = ambiguous), right ventricular situs (D = right sided right ventricle, L = left-sided right ventricle), aorta situs (S = normal aortic situs, L = aorta to the left of the pulmonary artery, D = aorta to the right and anterior of the pulmonary artery). Abbreviations: ASD I = primum atrial septal defect, ASD II = secundum atrial septal defect, PFO = patent foramen ovale, VSD = ventricular septal defect, TOF = tetralogy of Fallot, MVP = mitral valve prolapse, PS = pulmonary stenosis, L-TGA = "corrected" transposition of the great arteries.

In the general population the majority (67-75%) of congenital heart block is not associated with structural heart disease. Most often these cases are due to maternal generalized autoimmune diseases (29). The patients reported here all had cardiac lesions. It is possible that the patients with congenital heart block in our sample who did not have L-TGA or polysplenia may have been born to mothers with autoimmune disorders, but unfortunately, maternal histories were unavailable.

In our necropsy cases, atrioventricular concordance was present in 13 of 23 patients (57%), with AV discordance being found in 9 cases (39%) (Table I). In one patient with polysplenia (4%) (case 16, Table I) AV concordance or discordance was not determined since the atrial situs could not be diagnosed with confidence. Atrioventricular discordance alone clearly does not account for the complete heart block since block occurred in cases of atrioventricular concordance as well as discordance, as above.

GENETIC MECHANISMS FOR LATERALITY DEFECTS

Evidence for the genetic basis of disorders of left-right (LR) asymmetry derives from work done on 1) the molecular basis of LR orientation, 2) animal models, and 3) clinical genetic studies.

The Molecular Basis Of Left-Right Asymmetry
There have recently been tremendous advances in our knowledge of the molecules which contribute to the establishment of LR asymmetries (30). Many of these molecules, including nodal, activin (31), lefty (32), and Vg1 (33) are members of the transforming growth factor β (TGFβ) superfamily and are implicated in guiding LR decisions in the heart (31,34).

Mouse Models Of Aberrant Left-Right Asymmetry
Mouse models of aberrant left-right asymmetry offer a powerful opportunity for dissecting the genetic and embryological basis of laterality (35). The first such model is the iv (inversus viscerum) mouse, which has heterotaxy in 50% of homozygous progeny, with the remainder developing normal visceral situs. The iv gene is left-right dynein (lrd), an axonemal dynein heavy chain gene, which is expressed in the embryonic midline, along the node and rostral floorplate (36). In the *inv* mouse, whose genetic cause has been recently shown to be due to a defect in an ankyrin-repeat protein (37,38), situs inversus and heterotaxy occur in 85% and 15%, respectively, of homozygous offspring (39).

The lefty protein is a ligand in the TGFβ pathway that is important for left-right determination. When the lefty gene was selectively disrupted in mice the most common feature was thoracic left isomerism, including bilateral left lungs and left atria (32). The overall phenotype is strikingly similar to human polysplenia syndrome.

Mice with mutations in the activin receptor type IIB (ActR IIB) gene have abnormal spleens, and randomization of the positioning and apical orientation of the heart, in addition to bilateral right-sidedness of the pulmonary and atrial anatomy (40). These findings resemble the asplenia syndrome in humans. Mice that had selective disruption of the ActR IIB gene also manifest abnormalities of the axial skeleton, with additional thoracic vertebrae, anterior transformation of multiple vertebrae, and altered expression of HOX genes along the cranio-caudal axis. This is compatible with a role for the midline in directing LR asymmetry. Several members of the TGF-β family may act via ActR IIB, including BMP-4 (41), Vg1 (42) and nodal (43). Thus, the effect of the mutation may be to interfere with signaling by several ligands.

Clinical Genetics Of Heterotaxy Syndromes

Asplenia   The estimated incidence of all heterotaxy is in the range of 1 per 10,000 births (44). Although many cases of asplenia appear to be sporadic, there are numerous documented familial occurrences. Instances of parental consanguinity in 3 families and multiple affected sibs in other families support autosomal recessive inheritance as a mechanism (45,46). Inheritance in an X-linked pattern has also been documented (see below). In one reported family 3 siblings had asplenia with cyanotic heart disease while another family had 2 affected boys (47,48). Overall empiric recurrence risk after birth of a single case of asplenia is probably on the order of 5% or less.

Polysplenia Families of 2 sisters with polysplenia syndrome or 2 affected brothers have been reported (12,49,50). Other families with affected sibs were also reported (49,51,52,53). In an Amish family, 5 persons in 2 generations showed congenital cardiac and visceral defects consistent with the polysplenia syndrome (53). The parents of 4 affected sibs were fourth cousins; a deceased sister of the father was affected. Families in which 1 person had polysplenia and another person asplenia suggest that in some cases asplenia and polysplenia syndromes may be caused by disruption of the same gene (52,54,55).

Mutations in the gene for human activin type IIB are associated with left-right axis malformations. Kosaki et al. (56) reported two missense mutations that were identified in three individuals with heterotaxy. These individuals had polysplenia and "corrected transposition". Neither nucleotide substitution was identified in over 100 normal controls. The patients were heterozygous for the mutations indicating that the mutations may be acting as dominant-negatives. In our unpublished results from DNA obtained from autopsy samples of Cardiac Registry patients with asplenia syndrome we have found two nonsense mutations in the activin receptor IIB gene that have not been identified in normal controls.

Other genes are associated with heterotaxy syndromes. Casey et al. (57) performed linkage studies in a large family with X-linked heterotaxy, affecting 11 males in 2 generations. All but perhaps one of the affected males suffered from congenital heart disease, and all but one of the affected males manifested alterations of visceral situs, including asplenia or polysplenia, symmetric liver, intestinal malrotation, and abnormal lung lobation. Other midline malformations identified were sacral agenesis, posteriorly placed anus, rectal stenosis, meningomyelocele, cerebellar hypoplasia and arhinencephaly. Gebbia et al. (58) positionally cloned a gene from a region where the X-linked phenotype had been mapped. The gene encodes a putative zinc-finger transcription factor that they designated ZIC3. One frameshift, 2 missense, and 2 nonsense mutations were identified in familial and sporadic situs ambiguus. The frameshift allele was also associated with situs inversus among some heterozygous females, suggesting that ZIC3 functions in the earliest stages of left-right (LR) body axis formation. ZIC3 was the first gene unequivocally associated with human situs abnormalities.

Gebbia et al. (58) found a normal male who had fathered a daughter with situs ambiguus. Neither she nor the father carried any mutation in ZIC3 and both parents were anatomically normal. The daughter and her unaffected mother who was unrelated to the father were found to be heterozygous for an arg182-to-gln mutation in the prodomain of the NODAL gene. Mutations in NODAL, LEFTY and HNF-3β have been identified in subjects with situs malformations (59,60,61).

Genetic Mechanisms Of Transposition Of The Great Arteries Or Dextrocardia
Limited data are available on the genetic transmission of L-TGA or dextrocardia. Few reports of familial cases are published. A review of the frequency of cardiovascular malformations in first-degree relatives of 19 patients with L-TGA found that 1 of 50 sibs had a cardiovascular malformation while all parents were normal (63). They report that the overall recurrence risk in sibs of patients with any form of transposition of the great arteries was 5 in 612 (0.82%). The incidence of congenital heart disease in the children whose parents had one of four selected defects (dextrocardia, atrial septal defect, coarctation of the aorta or aortic valve stenosis) was 8.8% (64). This is a much higher incidence than that reported in most comparable studies.

SUMMARY

There is clearly a genetic basis to some diseases with disrupted left-right asymmetry. Despite the disparity in clinical appearance of syndromes associated with laterality defects, the human and animal data seem to imply that these entities may be interrelated etiologically and embryologically. Targeted mutation of a single gene in mice can cause phenotypes representative of situs inversus or heterotaxy and also result in disruptions in cardiac laterality. This would imply that differing anomalies of left-right asymmetry in humans may result from perturbations of a single gene. Components of the TGFβ pathway are crucial for establishing normal left-right asymmetry. The data presented above confirms that disruption of this pathway can cause laterality defects in humans. Further evidence on the role of dyneins and extra-cellular flow at the embryonic midline in human laterality defects should be forthcoming (62).

REFERENCES

1.   Splitt MR, Burn J, Goodship J. Defects in the determination of left-right asymmetry. *J Med Genet* 1996;33:498-503.
2.   Sapire DW, Ho SY, Anderson RH, Rigby ML. Diagnosis and significance of atrial isomerism. *Am J Cardiol* 1986;58:342-6.
3.   Uemura H, Ho SY, Devine WA, Anderson RH. Analysis of visceral heterotaxy according to splenic status, appendage morphology, or both. *Am J Cardiol* 1995;76:846-9.
4.   Van Praagh R. The anatomy of the heterotaxy syndromes: anomalies of right-left asymmetry with asplenia, polysplenia and a right-sided spleen. Gold, J ed., Montefiore Medical Center and the New York Society of Thoracic Surgery: State of the Art Review. 1999 (Course syllabus in press).
5.   Van Praagh S, Santini F, Sanders SP. Cardiac malpositions with special emphasis on visceral heterotaxy (asplenia and polysplenia syndromes). In Fyler DC (ed): "Nadas' Pediatric Cardiology." Philadelphia: Hanley & Belfus, Inc., 1992, 589-608.
6.   Wren C, Macartney FJ, Deanfield JE. Cardiac rhythm in atrial isomerism. *Am J Cardiol* 1987;59:1156-8.
7.   Rossi L, Montella S, Frescura C, Thiene G. Congenital atrioventricular block in right atrial isomerism (asplenia). A case due to atrionodal discontinuity. *Chest* 1984;85:578-80.
8.   Dickinson DF, Wilkinson JL, Anderson KR, Smith A, Ho SY, Anderson RH. The cardiac conduction system in situs ambiguus. *Circulation* 1979;59:879-85.
9.   Ih S, Fukuda K, Okada R, Saitoh S. The location and course of the atrioventricular conduction system in common atrioventricular orifice and in its related anomalies with transposition of the great arteries. *Jpn Circ J* 1983;47:1262-73.
10. Wu MH, Wang JK, Lin JL, Lai LP, Lue HC, Young ML, Hsieh FJ. Supraventricular tachycardia in patients with right atrial isomerism. *J Am Coll Cardiol* 1998;32:773-9.
11. Levine JC, Walsh EP, Saul JP. Radiofrequency ablation of accessory pathways associated with congenital heart disease including heterotaxy syndrome. *Am J Cardiol* 1993;72:689-93.
12. Moller JH, Nakib A, Anderson RC, Edwards JE. Congenital cardiac disease associated with polysplenia, a developmental complex of bilateral 'left-sidedness.'. *Circulation* 1967;36: 789-799.
13. Rose V, Izukawa T, Moes CAF. Syndromes of asplenia and polysplenia: a review of cardiac and non-cardiac malformation in 60 cases with special reference to diagnosis and prognosis. *Brit Heart J* 1975;37:840-852.
14. Momma K, Takao A, Shibata T. Characteristics and natural history of abnormal atrial rhythms in left isomerism. *Am J Cardiol* 1990;65:231-6.
15. Bharati S, Lev M. The course of the conduction system in dextrocardia. *Circulation* 1990;57:163-71.
16. Garcia OL, Metha AV, Pickoff AS, Tamer DF, Ferrer PL, Wolff GS, Gelband H. Left isomerism and complete atrioventricular block: a report of six cases. *Am J Cardiol* 1981;48:1103-7.
17. Roguin N, Pelled B, Freundlich E, Yahalom M, Riss E. Atrioventricular block in situs ambiguus and left isomerism (polysplenia syndrome). *PACE* 1984;7:18-22.
18. Ho SY, Fagg N, Anderson RH, Cook A, Allan L. Disposition of the atrioventricular conduction tissues in the heart with isomerism of the atrial appendages: its relation to congenital complete heart block. *J Am Coll Cardiol* 1992;20:904-10.
19. Bjarke BB, Kidd BS. Proceedings: Congenitally corrected transposition of the great arteries: a clinical study of 101 cases. *Br Heart J* 1976;38:535.
20. Van Praagh R, Papagiannis J, Grunenfelder J, Bartram U, Martanovic P. Pathologic anatomy of corrected transposition of the great arteries: medical and surgical implications. *Am Heart J* 1998;135:772-85.
21. Connelly MS, Liu PP, Williams WG, Webb GD, Robertson P, McLaughlin PR. Congenitally corrected transposition of the great arteries in the adult: functional status and complications. *J Am Coll Cardiol* 1996;27:1238-43.
22. Presbitero P, Somerville J, Rabajoli F, Stone S, Conte MR. Corrected transposition of the great arteries without associated defects in adult patients: clinical profile and follow up. *Br Heart J* 1995;74:57-9.
23. Bharati S, Rosen K, Steinfield L, Miller RA, Lev M. The anatomic substrate for preexcitation in corrected transposition. *Circulation* 1980;62:831-42.

24. Benson DW Jr, Gallagher JJ, Oldham HN, Sealy WC, Sterba R, Spach MS. Corrected transposition with severe intracardiac deformities with Wolff-Parkinson-White syndrome in a child. Electrophysiologic investigation and surgical correction. *Circulation* 1980;61:1256-61.
25. Daliento L, Corrado D, Buja G, John N, Nava A, Thiene G. Rhythm and conduction disturbances in isolated, congenitally corrected transposition of the great arteries. *Am J Cardiol* 1986;58:314-8.
26. Huhta JC, Maloney JD, Ritter DG, Ilstrup DM, Feldt RH. Complete atrioventricular block in patients with atrioventricular discordance. *Circulation* 1983;67:1374-7.
27. Gillette PC, Busch U, Mullins CE, McNamara DG. Electrophysiologic studies in patients with ventricular inversion and "corrected transposition". *Circulation* 1979;60:939-45.
28. Anderson RH, Becker AE, Arnold R, Wilkinson JL. The conducting tissues in congenitally corrected transposition. *Circulation* 50:911-23.
29. Smeenk RJ. Immunological aspects of congenital atrioventricular block. 1997. *PACE* 1974;20:2093-7.
30. Yost HJ. Left-right development in Xenopus and zebrafish. *Semin Cell Dev* 1998;9:61-66.
31. Levin M, Johnson RL, Stern CD, Kuehn M, Tabin C. A molecular pathway determining left-right asymmetry in chick embyogenesis. *Cell* 1995;82:803-814.
32. Meno C, Shimono A, Saijoh Y, et al. Lefty-1 is required for left-right determination as a regulator of lefty-2 and nodal. *Cell* 1998;94:287-97.
33. Hyatt BA, Lohr JL, Yost H.J. Initiation of verebrate left-right axis formation by maternal Vg1. *Nature* 1996;384:62-65.
34. Isaac A, Sargent MG, Cooke J. Control of vertebrate left-right asymmetry by a Snail-related zinc finger gene. *Science* 1997;275:1301-1304.
35. Supp DM, Brueckner M, Potter SS. Handed asymmetry in the mouse: understanding how things go right (or left) by studying how they go wrong. *Semin Cell Dev Biol* 1998;9:77-87.
36. Supp DM, Witte DP, Potter SS, Brueckner M. Mutation of an axonemal dynein in the left-right asymmetry mouse mutant inversus viscerum. *Nature* 1997;389:963-966.
37. Mochizuki T, Saijoh Y, Tsuchiya K, et al. Cloning of inv, a gene that controls left/right asymmetry and kidney development. *Nature* 1998;395:177-81.
38. Morgan D, Turnpenny L, Goodship J, et al. Inversin, a novel gene in the vertebrate left-right axis pathway, is partially deleted in the inv mouse. *Nat Genet* 1998;20:149-56.
39. Yokoyama T, Copeland NG, Jenkins NA, Montgomery CA, Elder FFB, Overbeek PA. Reversal of left-right asymetry: a situs inversus mutation. *Science* 1993;260:679-682.
40. Oh SP, Li E. The signaling pathway mediated by the type IIB activin receptor controls axial patterning and lateral asymmetry in the mouse. *Genes Dev.* 1997;11:1812-1826.
41. Chang C, Wilson PA, Mathews LS, Hemmati-Brivanlou A. A Xenopus type I activin receptor mediates mesodermal but not neural specification during embryogenesis. *Development* 1997;124:827-837.
42. Schulte-Merker S, Smith JC, Dale L. Effects of truncated activin and FGF receptors and of follistatin on the inducing activities of Bvg1 and activin: does activin play a role in mesoderm induction? *EMBO J* 1994;13:3533-3541.
43. Nomura M, Li E. Roles for Smad2 in mesoderm formation, left-right patterning and craniofacial development in mice. *Nature* 1998;393:786-90.
44. Lin AE ,Ticho BS, Houde KK, Westgate MN, Holmes LB. Heterotaxy: Etiology and prevalence in a newborn population. *Am J Human Gene*t 1998;63:A112.
45. Simpson J, Zellweger H. Familial occurrence of Ivemark syndrome with splenic hypoplasia and asplenia in sibs. *J Med Genet* 1973;10:303-304.
46. Hurwitz RC, Caskey, CT. Ivemark syndrome in siblings. *Clin Genet* 1982;22:7-11.
47. Ruttenberg HD, Neufeld HN, Lucas RV, Carey LS, Adams P, Anderson RC, Edwards JE. Syndrome of congenital cardiac disease with asplenia. *Am J Cardiol* 1964;13:387-406.
48. Chen SC, Monteleone PL. Familial splenic anomaly syndrome. *J Pediat* 1977;91:160-161.
49. Hallett JJ, Gang DL, Holmes LB. Familial polysplenia and cardiovascular defects. *Pediatr Res* 1979;13:344,
50. de la Monte SM, Hutchins GM. Sisters with polysplenia. *Am J Med Genet* 1985;21:171-173.
51. Kawagoe K, Hara K, Jimbo T, Mizuno M, Sakamoto S. Occurrence of Ivemark syndrome with polysplenia in sibs of a family. *Proc Jpn Acad* 1980;56 633-637.
52. Niikawa N, Kohsaka S, Mizumoto M, Hamada I, Kajii T. Familial clustering of situs inversus totalis, and asplenia and polysplenia syndromes. *Am J Med Genet* 1983;16:43-47.

53.   Arnold GL, Bixler D, Girod D. Probable autosomal recessive inheritance of polysplenia, situs inversus and cardiac defects in an Amish family. *Am J Med Genet* 1983;16:35-42.

54.   Polhemus DW, Schafer WB. Congenital absence of spleen; syndrome with atrioventricularis and situs inversus. *Pediatrics* 1952;9:696-708.

55.   Zlotogora J, Elian E. Asplenia and polysplenia syndromes with abnormalities of lateralization in a sibship. *J Med Genet* 1981;18:301-302.

56.   Kosaki R, Gebbia M, Kosaki K, Lewin M, Bowers P, Towbin JA, Casey B. Left-Right axis malformations associated with mutations in ACVR2B, the gene for human activin receptor type IIB. *Am J Med Genet* 1999;82:70-76.

57.   Casey B, Devoto M, Jones KL, Ballabio A. Mapping a gene for familial situs abnormalities to human chromosome Xq24-q27.1. *Nat Genet* 1993;5:403-407.

58.   Gebbia M, Ferrero GB, Pilia G, et al B. X-linked situs abnormalities result from mutations in ZIC3. *Nat Genet* 1997;17:305-308.

59.   Bassi MT, Kosaki K, Belmont J, Casey B. NODAL, LEFTY and HNF-3b nucleotide changes associated with complex heart defects and other features of left-right axis malformations.*Am J Hum Genet* 1997;61:A4.

60.   Kosaki K, Casey B. Genetics of human left-right axis malformations. *Semin Cell Dev Biol* 1998;9:89-99.

61.   Kosaki K, Bassi MT, Kosaki R, Lewin M, Belmont J, Schauer G, Casey B. Characterization and mutation analysis of human LEFTY A and LEFTY B, homologues of murine genes implicated in left-right axis development. *Am J Hum Genet* 1999;64:712-21.

62.   Vogel G. Developmental biology. How to get a heart in the right place. *Science* 1999;285:23.

63.   Becker TA, Van Amber R, Moller JH, Pierpont ME. Occurrence of cardiac malformations in relatives of children with transposition of the great arteries. *Am J Med Genet* 1996;66:28-32.

64.   Rose V, Gold RJ, Lindsay G, Allen M. A possible increase in the incidence of congenital heart defects among the offspring of affected parents. *J Am Coll Cardiol* 1985;6:376-82.

21
MARFAN SYNDROME AND RELATED DISORDERS OF FIBRILLIN

Ronald V. Lacro, M.D.

Department of Cardiology, Children's Hospital • Boston
Department of Pediatrics, Harvard Medical School, Boston, MA 02115

INTRODUCTION

Marfan syndrome is a heritable disorder of connective tissue affecting approximately one in every 5 - 10,000 individuals. If all related disorders of fibrillin are included, the incidence of fibrillin abnormalities may be as high as one in every 3 – 5,000 (1). The cardinal clinical manifestations of the syndrome involve the skeletal, cardiovascular, and ocular systems (2,3). A characteristic body habitus, aneurysmal dilatation of the aorta (Figure 1), and ectopia lentis (subluxation or dislocation of the ocular lens) are the hallmarks of this condition. In addition, the skin, fascia, central nervous system, and lung may show characteristic involvement. Marfan syndrome is inherited in an autosomal dominant fashion, although an estimated 15 to 30 percent of cases are sporadic, representing new mutations in otherwise unaffected families. Males and females are equally affected, and there is no preference for race or ethnic group.

The first known reference to what is now called Marfan syndrome is in the fifth century in the Babylonian Talmud (4). It has been suggested that Abraham Lincoln had Marfan syndrome (5,6), and the world-renowned violin virtuoso, Nicolo Paganini, had long fingers and hyperextensible joints that were said to be attributable to Marfan syndrome (7). In 1986, the U.S. Olympic volleyball star, Flo Hyman, died from a ruptured aortic aneurysm associated with Marfan syndrome. Unfortunately, the diagnosis was only made posthumously; however, this tragic event focused widespread public attention on the syndrome for the first time (2).

Aortic dilatation and aortic dissection are the major causes of morbidity and mortality (8-10). Before the advent of surgical repair of aortic aneurysms, the median expected survival for individuals with Marfan syndrome was 47 years (11). Recent studies have revealed that life expectancy in persons with Marfan syndrome has increased significantly overall since 1972. The increase in longevity seems partially attributable to advances in clinical care such as improvements in medical management and aortic surgery (12-15).

There is considerable intrafamilial and interfamilial variability in the clinical phenotype (16). The mutant gene exerts a pleiotropic effect; that is, multiple, apparently unrelated phenotypic features stem from a single genetic change. Many features are age-dependent and progressive. Recently, the gene (*FBN1*) encoding for

Marfan Syndrome and Related Disorders of Fibrillin

fibrillin-1, a major connective tissue protein, has been identified and extensively studied (1,17-18). Fibrillin-1 is expressed in many tissues affected in Marfan syndrome (19). Genetic studies have shown that mutations in the *FBN1* gene, located on the long arm of chromosome 15 (15q21.1), are responsible for the Marfan syndrome phenotype (6,20-22). More than 70 different mutations of *FBN1* causing Marfan syndrome have been identified to date (1,17-18,22-24). Furthermore, additional mutations in *FBN1,* account for a number of related phenotypes which overlap with the classical Marfan phenotype (see discussion below) (1,17,25-42). Finally, mutations in a related gene (*FBN2*) encoding the protein, fibrillin-2, have been documented in individuals with congenital contractural arachnodactyly, a connective tissue disorder clinically distinct from Marfan syndrome (20,29,43-45).

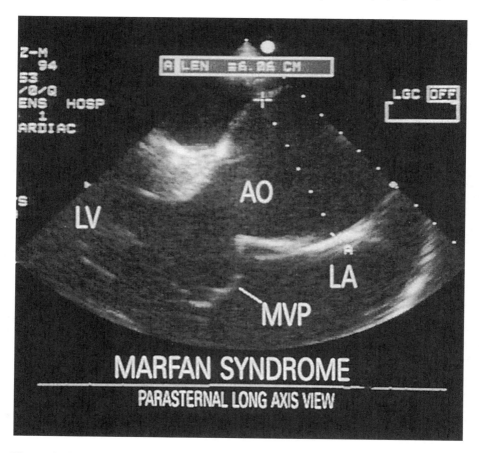

Figure 1: Mitral valve prolapse and severe aortic root dilatation in a 17-year-old boy with classical Marfan syndrome (parasternal long-axis view). The aortic root measured 6.06 cm, z-score = + 10.9 standard deviations > mean for BSA.

History of Marfan Syndrome

In 1896, Marfan, the first professor of pediatrics in Paris, described a 5-year-old girl named Gabrielle who had long, thin fingers and limbs, which he termed dolichostenomelia (dolicho=long, steno=thin or narrow, melia=limbs) (46). Gabrielle also had multiple joint contractures and developed scoliosis. Achard reported on a similar patient with loose-jointedness of the hands, long digits, and dolichostenomelia, and called the condition arachnodactyly (47). Purists now argue that Achard's patient had the condition which is now regarded as Marfan syndrome, while Marfan's original patient more likely had congenital contractural arachnodactyly (Beals syndrome) rather than Marfan syndrome (43). Over the next 40 years, other clinical manifestations of Marfan syndrome were associated with those affecting the skeletal system. In 1914, Börger (48) associated subluxation of the lens (ectopia lentis) with the dolichostenomelic body habitus, although two tall, loose-jointed siblings with ectopia lentis had been described many years previously (49). In 1931, Weve noted the heritable nature of the condition and primary involvement of tissue derived from embryonic mesoderm, and associated Marfan's name with the phenotype for the first time, calling the syndrome dystrophia mesodermalis congenita, typus Marfanis (50). The cardiovascular system was first implicated when severe mitral regurgitation was noted in affected patients in 1912 (51-52). The aortic complications of dilatation and dissection were clearly associated with the skeletal findings in 1943 (8-9). It was McKusick, in 1955, who recognized that disease of the aorta accounts for most deaths in affected individuals (53). In the 1950's, studies of large pedigrees of affected families delineated a great part of the natural history of Marfan syndrome, defined the range of pleiotropism and variability, and established its autosomal dominant inheritance (53-54). Characteristic abnormalities have been identified not only in the three major systems, but also in the skin and integument, the central nervous system, and the pulmonary system (Tables 1 and 2).

By the late 1950's, McKusick codified heritable disorders of connective tissue as a nosological grouping of human phenotypes. In the first edition of his monograph, *Heritable Disorders of Connective Tissue*, eight disorders, including Marfan syndrome, were included (currently there are over 150). In 1956, McKusick wrote: "What the suspensory ligament of the lens has in common with the media of the aorta is obscure. If (this were) known, the basic defect of the syndrome might be understood (54)."

Molecular Genetics: The Fibrillin Gene (*FBN1*)

Although McKusick predicted in 1956 that a biochemical defect in connective tissue would be responsible for Marfan syndrome, few at that time could have guessed that it would take over 35 years to track down the underlying defect. Because of the large size of connective tissue proteins and their peculiar physico-chemical properties, methods were required to study the fibrillin gene rather than the protein itself. Thus, it was largely through molecular genetics that the biochemical defect underlying Marfan syndrome has been identified.

In 1986, Sakai and colleagues isolated a *"new"* connective tissue protein of the extracellular matrix and called it fibrillin (19). Fibrillin, a high molecular weight glycoprotein (350 kDa), is a major constituent of the microfibril, which is an important constituent of extracellular matrices in most tissues and organs of humans and virtually all lower species. Microfibrils provide the framework upon which tropoelastin is deposited to form the elastic fiber (55-57). As elastic fibers are an abundant element in tissues affected in the Marfan syndrome (the aortic media, the suspensory ligament of the lens, and the periosteum), fibrillin was strongly suspected to be the site of the abnormality in Marfan syndrome. Proof of the genetic defect in Marfan syndrome was established by a series of elegant studies by several groups of investigators. First, immunohistologic studies of skin and cultured fibroblasts obtained from patients with Marfan syndrome showed qualitative and quantitative abnormalities of the microfibrillar fibers (58). Second, the mapping of Marfan syndrome to the long arm of chromosome 15 (15q) was achieved through family linkage studies utilizing polymorphic markers of the human genome (59-60). Third, a probe from the partially cloned fibrillin gene (*FBN1*) was mapped by *in situ* hybridization to the same region on the long arm of chromosome 15 (15q21.1) (61). Fourth, Lee et al. (20) and Dietz et al. (22) demonstrated a tight linkage of an intragenic DNA polymorphism to the Marfan phenotype (no recombinants identified). Finally, Dietz et al. (22), using clones of the fibrillin gene isolated by Maslen et al. (21), identified *de novo* point mutations in the fibrillin gene in individuals with sporadic Marfan syndrome.

FBN1 is a large gene at 15q21 with 65 exons, spanning 110 kb. There are 47 tandemly repeated domains with homology to epidermal growth factor (EGF), of which 43 satisfy the consensus for calcium binding (20,22,62-64). To date more than 70 different *FBN1* mutations that cause Marfan syndrome have been identified. Only four mutations have been found in unrelated individuals. Hence, there is extensive intragenic heterogeneity at *FBN1*, and a "common" mutation is unlikely (1,17-18). There have been no large deletions. The most common mutation is missense and most affect calcium-binding EGF-like domains. Nearly all mutations substitute one of the six predictably spaced cysteine residues of the EGF-like motifs that interact via intradomain disulfide linkage, one of the highly conserved residues within the calcium-binding sequence, or residues important for interdomain hydrophobic packing interactions (1,17-18).

In addition to classical Marfan syndrome, mutations in *FBN1* account for a number of related phenotypes which overlap with the classical Marfan phenotype (reviewed in references 1,17), including familial aortic aneurysm and dissection (25-28), familial isolated ectopia lentis (29-32), familial tall stature with Marfan-like habitus (33), Shprintzen-Goldberg syndrome (34-35), familial mitral valve prolapse syndrome (36-40), MASS phenotype (23-24,41), and atypical skeletal phenotype without cardiovascular manifestations (42). Some of the factors that modulate phenotypic severity, both between and within families include 1) intragenic heterogeneity, 2) clinically similar but etiologically distinct disorders cosegregating independently in the same family, and 2) somatic mosaicism (1,17,40,64). Finally, mutations in a related gene encoding the protein, fibrillin-2 (*FBN2*), have been documented in individuals with congenital contractural arachnodactyly, a connective tissue disorder clinically distinct from Marfan syndrome (20,29,43-45).

Pathogenesis: Molecular pathogenesis of fibrillinopathies (Figure 2)

The molecular pathogenesis of Marfan syndrome and related disorders of fibrillin have been reviewed recently in great detail (1,17). Microfibrils are aggregates of multiple structural proteins. The most important of these proteins are the fibrillins, which are organized in multimeric fibers composed of dozens and perhaps hundreds of monomers. The impact of *FBN1* mutations has been characterized, primarily in cultured dermal fibroblasts, by (1) the amount of mutant mRNA expressed; (2) the size of the mutant monomer; (3) the amount of mutant monomer synthesized; (4) the amount secreted; (5) the amount of fibrillin deposited in the extracellular matrix; and (6) the ultrastructure of microfibrils. Most mutations in *FBN1* are of the missense variety and therefore do not reduce the size of the fibrillin monomer. Furthmayr and colleagues (65-66) identified five classes of defects based on the amount of fibrillin synthesized and the amount of fibrillin deposited in the extracellular matrix. Most mutations result in deposition of less than 35% of the expected amount of fibrillin in the extracelllular matrix.

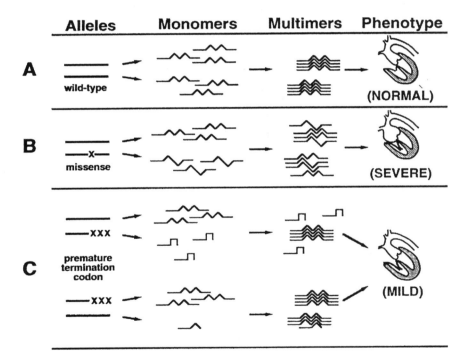

Figure 2. Molecular pathogenesis of the fibrillinopathies: The dominant-negative model. (A) Normal synthesis, secretion, and processing of fibrillin-1 monomers leads to normal microfibrillar aggregates and a normal phenotype. (B) A mutation that alters primary structure but does not interfere with synthesis and secretion produces a pool of abnormal fibrillin-1 monomers that interfere with microfibril assembly, resulting in a severe phenotype. (C) Mutations that result in either a marked reduction of transcript (mRNA) or a mutant peptide incapable of aggregating with the normal monomers lead to a reduced number of relatively normal microfibrils, and a mild phenotype. (From Reference 67, 1994, with permission)

In most instances, the results of fibrillin studies are consistent with a dominant-negative model to explain molecular pathogenesis (Figure 2). According to the dominant-negative model (67), the mutant fibrillin-1 monomer must interact with nonmutant fibrillin-1 monomers; this potentially delays or prevents secretion of both, but certainly interferes with formation of microfibrillar aggregates and deposition of fibrillin in the extracelllular matrix. A dominant-negative effect explains why heterozygosity for a fibrillin mutation should be so severe when 50% of the normal complement of monomers is being synthesized (from the normal allele). Mutations that result in either a marked reduction of transcript (mRNA) or a mutant peptide incapable of aggregating with the normal monomers, lead to a reduced number of relatively normal microfibrils, and a mild phenotype.

Although much has been learned about the role of *FBN1* mutations in the pathogenesis of Marfan syndrome and related connective tissue disorders, the precise mechanisms by which genotype determines phenotype remain largely unknown. Until we further understand how *FBN1* mutations produce a particular phenotype, we cannot determine with certainty which individuals with *FBN1* gene mutations will have the life-threatening cardiovascular complications associated with Marfan syndrome. The prospects for specific gene therapy depend on improved delineation of the mechanisms which modulate genotype-phenotype correlation.

Diagnosis: Berlin Criteria (1986) and Revised Criteria (1996)

The diagnosis of Marfan syndrome is made clinically based on characteristic phenotypic abnormalities and a positive family history for the syndrome. Up to 15 to 30 percent of cases are sporadic (new mutations) without a positive family history. Because of the unfavorable prognosis if untreated, an early diagnosis of Marfan syndrome is of great practical importance. The primary care physician plays a key role in identifying patients with features suggestive of Marfan syndrome, a task which is more difficult in younger patients. The family practitioner or pediatrician must be familiar with the major manifestations of Marfan syndrome and must make the initial referrals, usually to a geneticist or, if available, to a Marfan syndrome clinic (Table 1).

Two specialized studies are required of any person in whom the Marfan diagnosis is suspected: slit-lamp examination of the eyes and echocardiography. The former is needed to establish whether ectopia lentis is present. Echocardiography is necessary to determine whether mitral valve prolapse and aortic root dilatation are present. Conditions that must be excluded routinely when considering the diagnosis of Marfan syndrome include homocystinuria, contractural arachnodactyly, a number of the Ehlers-Danlos variants, Stickler syndrome, and familial mitral valve prolapse syndrome or MASS phenotype. The "marfanoid hypermobility syndrome" (68) and the "neonatal or infantile Marfan syndrome" (69-71) are not separate entities; rather they represent phenotypic extremes of the classic phenotype.

The phenotypic spectrum of connective tissue disorders is a continuum. At one end of this continuum one can find the so-called "classical" cases--more severely affected individuals with characteristic manifestations allowing easy diagnosis. At the other end, however, mild cases merge with the normal population. At some point along the continuum, a somewhat arbitrary line must be drawn between individuals affected with Marfan syndrome and individuals with a phenotype falling within the admissible range of deviation for the normal population. To this end, and to aid physicians in making uniform diagnoses, diagnostic criteria were codified in the International Nosology of Inherited Connective Tissue Disorders (72), the so-called Berlin Nosology of 1986. These **"Berlin criteria"** allow systematic diagnosis of Marfan syndrome based on phenotype and a positive family history for the syndrome (Table 1). A system is said to be "involved" when one or more manifestations is present. The Berlin Nosology differentiates major manifestations from minor manifestations. Major manifestations (dilatation of the ascending aorta, ectopia lentis, and dural ectasia) are uncommon in the general population and therefore carry high specificity for the syndrome. According to the Berlin Nosology, requirements for diagnosis in the absence of an unequivocally affected first-degree relative include involvement of the skeleton and at least two other systems, and at least one major manifestation. Requirements for diagnosis in the presence of an unequivocally affected first-degree relative include involvement of at least 2 systems; a major manifestation is preferred but not required, depending on the family's phenotype.

Since 1986, the Berlin criteria have been applied more or less successfully throughout the world, and because affected status can be assigned within a family pedigree, they have assisted in finding the Marfan gene through linkage analysis studies. On the other hand, the identification of the Marfan gene and the emerging possibility of molecular testing that accompanied its discovery emphasized an important shortcoming of the Berlin criteria--the purely clinical (and therefore subjective) character of the criteria on which the diagnosis is based. Molecular testing has the potential of reducing this subjectivity. Furthermore, the Berlin criteria allowed frequent overdiagnosis of first degree relatives of the unequivocally affected proband, as evidence by molecular testing (40,73). To counter these shortcomings, a group of Marfan experts recently proposed the **"Revised Diagnostic Criteria,"** hereafter referred to as the **"Revised criteria"** (Table 2) (74).

As the diagnosis of Marfan syndrome cannot rely solely on molecular testing, the Revised Nosology uses the same matrix system as the Berlin Nosology, involving major clinical criteria with a high specificity and minor clinical criteria which are more common in the general population. The major differences in the new Revised criteria include the following: (1) more stringent requirements for the diagnosis of Marfan syndrome for the index case as well as for relatives of an unequivocally affected individual; (2) skeletal involvement as a major criterion if at least 4 of 8 typical skeletal manifestations are present; (3) potential contribution of molecular analysis to the diagnosis of Marfan syndrome; and (4) delineation of initial criteria for diagnosis of other heritable conditions with partially overlapping phenotypes (74).

Requirements for diagnosis for the index case include 2 major manifestations (as compared to 1 for Berlin) and involvement of a third system. Requirements for diagnosis for a relative of an index case include 1 major manifestation (preferred but not required for Berlin) and involvement of a second system. The Revised Nosology introduces a new system, the "Family/Genetic History" specifying 3 major criteria, including having a first-degree relative who meets the Revised criteria independently; presence of a mutation in *FBN1* known to cause the Marfan syndrome; and presence of a haplotype around *FBN1*, inherited by descent, known to be associated with unequivocally diagnosed Marfan syndrome in the family. Specific criteria for the individual systems are more stringent. Criteria in the skeletal system are more specific or more quantifiable than in the Berlin nosology (e.g., instead of the subjective term, "dolichostenomelia," the criterion is quantitatively formulated as reduced upper to lower segment ratio or arm span to height ratio greater than 1.05 (75); pes planus must be associated with medial displacement of the medial malleolus). For the ocular system, the use of keratometry (76) and ocular ultrasound (77) is required to meet minor clinical criteria, and at least two minor criteria are necessary for ocular system involvement. A clinical diagnosis of myopia without documentation by ultrasound of an increased axial length of the globe is no longer sufficient. Retinal detachment has also been excluded from the list of minor criteria. For the cardiovascular system, aortic regurgitation, endocarditis, and dysrhythmias are excluded from the list of minor criteria, while dilatation of the main pulmonary artery below the age of 40 years is added as a minor criterion. In addition, age restrictions are stipulated for calcification of the mitral annulus (below the age of 40 years) and dilatation or dissection of the descending thoracic or abdominal aorta (below the age of 50 years). For skin and integument, only striae atrophicae and recurrent or incisional herniae are included in the minor criteria. For the central nervous system, only dural ectasia, a major manifestation, is included. Hyperactivity with or without attention deficit disorder, learning disability (verbal-performance discrepancy), and dilated cisterna magna have been excluded. Finally, De Paepe et al. (74) delineate the initial criteria for diagnosis of other heritable disorders partially overlapping with Marfan syndrome including congenital contractural arachnodactyly, familial thoracic aortic aneurysm, familial aortic dissection, familial ectopia lentis, familial Marfan-like habitus, MASS phenotype, and mitral valve prolapse syndrome. It is emphasized that these conditions constitute diagnostic entities completely separate from Marfan syndrome. Mutations in *FBN2* have been documented in congenital contractural arachnodactyly, while mutations in *FBN1* have been documented in all of the others.

The Berlin criteria (Table 1) are useful as a screening tool for primary care practitioners and other physicians deciding whether a particular patient should be referred for further diagnostic evaluation and testing, whereas the Revised criteria (Table 2) are most useful to clinical and molecular geneticists and other Marfan syndrome specialists. The Berlin criteria allow some overdiagnosis. In our experience, the Revised criteria allow fewer false positive diagnoses, but allow frequent false negative diagnoses, particularly in young children. In our Marfan syndrome clinic, we use both sets of criteria to determine where on the spectrum of connective tissue disorders a given individual sits. It is sometimes difficult to differentiate clinically an individual with very mild manifestations of Marfan syndrome in one family from another individual with the MASS phenotype in a different family. From a purely clinical standpoint, deciding whether an individual meets diagnostic criteria for Marfan syndrome is less important than appropriately identifying, treating, and following specific clinical manifestations, such as aortic root dilatation or lens subluxation. For example, it is possible to have severe aortic dilatation and dissection without satisfying diagnostic criteria for Marfan syndrome. Individuals with clinical manifestations consistent with Marfan syndrome who do not fulfill the Revised criteria should be monitored and managed with the same principles used for patients who meet the Revised criteria. Furthermore, family members who are at risk for these clinical manifestations should undergo clinical evaluation and possible echocardiography and slit-lamp examination.

Use of Molecular Diagnostics in Marfan syndrome

Although the gene responsible for Marfan syndrome has been identified, there is no readily available laboratory test which, in isolation, allows the assignment of affected status for Marfan syndrome. Although biochemical and genetic studies of fibrillin have greatly aided diagnosis in specific instances, it is not appropriate at present to seek routinely to determine whether a person with equivocal signs has a mutation in *FBN1* for at least two reasons. First, discovering mutations is neither simple nor widely attempted. Mutation detection is time-consuming and costly. Second, both fibrillin protein abnormalities and *FBN1* mutations have been identified in individuals who have conditions other than Marfan syndrome (1). Hence, Marfan syndrome is, and shall remain, a clinical diagnosis.

When a *FBN1* mutation has been identified in a particular family, prenatal and presymptomatic diagnosis is possible by direct mutation detection or by DNA linkage studies. When the *FBN1* mutation is unknown, but an affected individual is heterozygous for at least one of the *FBN1* polymorphisms, phase can be established, and relatives are cooperative, prenatal and presymptomatic diagnosis is possible by DNA linkage analysis. When linkage analysis is not possible, the *FBN1* mutation must be determined in an affected person (1). Prenatal diagnosis is possible by either linkage or mutation analysis using DNA from amniocytes or chorionic villi (73,78-79). Mutation analysis using DNA from single cells removed from preimplantation blastocysts is also feasible (80), but successful clinical application has not yet been reported.

Natural History and Management

Given involvement of multiple systems, persons affected by Marfan syndrome are best served by a coordinated multidisciplinary team experienced in all issues relevant to this condition. Because of the variability in phenotypic expression, the clinical approach should be customized to the individual patient. The age-dependency of some features, and the potential for preventive treatment mandate careful follow-up examinations (81-82).

Major and minor manifestations of Marfan syndrome are listed by system in Tables 1 and 2, and recommended management of patients with Marfan syndrome is outlined in Table 3. All patients should undergo a comprehensive medical evaluation at least annually, with more frequent examinations depending on the severity of clinical manifestations. Complete care for the Marfan syndrome patient should include regular counseling for the patient, parents, spouse or significant other, and siblings. New advances in treatment and research, psychosocial concerns, and genetic counseling should be addressed periodically.

Cardiovascular Manifestations

The advent of 2-dimensional echocardiography has had important consequences for the diagnosis, management, and follow-up of patients with Marfan syndrome and related connective tissue disorders (10,83-84). The widespread availability of echocardiography has greatly contributed to earlier diagnosis and more intensive follow-up of patients affected by this syndrome. Echocardiograms usually provide the information needed to decide whether medical or surgical intervention is indicated. Cases with milder cardiovascular expression are now more likely to be identified than in previous decades (13).

Up to a third of affected individuals have normal findings on clinical examination, yet almost all show abnormal echocardiograms (2-3,69,84-85). The most frequent echocardiographic findings are mitral valve prolapse and aortic root dilatation (Figure 1). While the absence of aortic dilatation does not exclude the diagnosis of Marfan syndrome, it does rule out the life-threatening complications of the syndrome.

Aortic dimensions obtained by two-dimensional echocardiography are compared to published standards obtained in normal children and adults, normalized for age and body surface area. In our pediatric echocardiography laboratory, aortic dimensions are compared to our normal pediatric population, normalizing for body surface area. The degree of aortic dilatation is expressed as a z-score, which indicates the number of standard deviations above or below the expected mean value for body surface area. For example, an aortic root z-score of +3 indicates an aortic root dimension 3 standard deviations above the mean for body surface area. If the z-score is > +2 but < +4, the dilatation is considered to be mild, without significant risk for aortic complications. In contrast, we know of two unrepaired children who died of acute aortic dissection with aortic root z-scores of approximately 10. The risk for aortic complications is considered high if the aortic root z-score is > +8.

The risk for aortic complications including regurgitation, dissection, and rupture, increases in proportion to the size of the aortic root. The stongest predictors of dissection of the ascending aorta, aside from the actual caliber of the root, are generalized dilatation of the ascending aorta extending beyond the sinotubular junction and a family history of dissection (84). Clinical and echocardiographic predictors of adverse outcome in childhood Marfan syndrome include the neonatal phenotype, a family history of dissection, and generalized dilatation of the ascending aorta (86).

Although the entire aortic wall is susceptible to enlargement, aortic dilatation usually occurs at the sinuses of Valsalva (Figure 1), presumably because this part of the aorta is most subject to pulsatile expansion and stress during contraction of the left ventricle. As the weakened aortic root progressively dilates, the leaflets of the aortic valve fail to coapt completely resulting in regurgitation. Significant aortic dilatation can occur without symptoms. Against this background of dilatation, an intimal tear may develop resulting in subacute or acute aortic dissection. Aortic dissection usually begins immediately above the aortic valve and can either extend retrograde into the coronary arteries or extend antegrade through the aortic arch to the descending aorta. The aortic root aneurysm may rupture into the pericardium or mediastinum and cause sudden death.

Mitral valve prolapse may be accompanied by mitral regurgitation which may be progressive, necessitating mitral valve repair or replacement (39,52,87). Other cardiovascular manifestations observed in Marfan syndrome include calcification of the mitral valve annulus (unusual in the general population before the age of 40 years), dilatation of the main pulmonary artery, and aneurysm of the descending thoracic or abdominal aorta.

Electrophysiologic Manifestations

No typical electrocardiographic (ECG) abnormalities occur. Resting 12-lead electrocardiograms have shown abnormalities of conduction and repolarization, but mainly in association with aortic or mitral valve dysfunction (88-90). Axis deviations occur because of rotation of the heart by severe pectus excavatum or thoracic lordosis (1).

Most premature deaths associated with Marfan syndrome relate to aortic dissection but sudden presumably arrhythmic deaths have also been reported (13,15). Patients with severely regurgitant valve lesions, as well as those who have undergone surgery, understandably are prone to disorders of cardiac rhythm, both supraventricular and ventricular (91-92). Mitral regurgitation promotes left atrial enlargement, which in turn predisposes to atrial fibrillation and atrial flutter. Uncontrolled studies using 24-hour ambulatory electrocardiograms have revealed ventricular premature beats and short runs of ventricular tachycardia in occasional patients (92-93).

Savolainen and colleagues studied the prevalence of cardiac dysrhythmias and abnormalities of conduction and repolarization in Marfan syndrome (94). Forty-five adult Marfan syndrome patients (25 men) and healthy age and sex matched controls underwent 24-hour ambulatory electrocardiograms. Patients with Marfan syndrome had a higher prevalence of cardiac dysrhythmias than healthy persons. Two Marfan syndrome patients had atrial fibrillation. The median number of atrial premature beats and ventricular premature beats was significantly higher among Marfan patients. Five patients but no controls had runs of $>= 3$ premature ventricular complexes, and nine patients but no controls had ventricular premature beats with R on T configuration. The Marfan patients had prolonged atrioventricular conduction time and disturbed depolarization as suggested by longer QT intervals and more common ST segment depression. The findings at ambulatory electrocardiography showed no association with echocardiographically determined aortic root dimension, left atrial size, or left ventricular dimension, wall thickness and systolic function; nor did the electrocardiographic findings correlate with the presence of mitral or tricuspid valve prolapse.

Patients with Marfan syndrome should always be questioned about palpitations and lightheadedness or near-syncope, at rest and with exercise. Any symptoms of more than trivial nature should prompt further evaluation.

CARDIOVASCULAR MANAGEMENT

Beta-Adrenergic Blockade

Beta-blockers have been effective in slowing the rate of aortic root dilatation, as well as in decreasing the incidence of aortic regurgitation and dissection (12). In 1971, Halpern et al. first suggested that beta-adrenergic-blockade might reduce the risk of dissection (95). This proposal was based on a few lines of evidence, including animal studies which showed a much improved survival in turkeys prone to aortic rupture when propranolol was added to their feed (96,97). In 1994, Shores et al. published the results of a prospective randomized trial of propranolol in adolescents and adult patients with classic Marfan syndrome. They demonstrated that prophylactic beta-adrenergic-blockade is effective in slowing the rate of aortic dilatation and reducing the risk of aortic complications such as regurgitation and dissection (12). In the same year, Salim et al. reported on another study which showed the effectiveness of beta-blockers in slowing the rate of aortic root dilatation. They compared the effect of atenolol and propranolol on the rate of aortic root enlargement in patients under the age of 21, most of whom were adolescent, concluded that atenolol and propranolol did not differ in efficacy, and recommended that prophylactic beta-blockade be started at the earliest possible age (98). To date, no randomized, prospective study has been reported documenting the efficacy of beta-blockade in very young patients with aortic dilatation. Furthermore, there has not been a report of a study evaluating the efficacy of other classes of medications, such as angiotensin converting enzyme inhibitors or calcium channel blockers, in retarding aortic root growth in Marfan syndrome individuals at any age. Nor has there been a study of the impact of these other medications on an animal model of aortic aneurysms.

The exact mechanism by which beta-blockers slow the rate of aortic enlargement in Marfan syndrome has not been proven. Beta-blockers (99) exhibit negative inotropy and negative chronotropy, two mechanisms thought to be the main contributors to the retardation of aortic dilatation. Through their negative inotropic effect, beta blockers reduce the abruptness of ventricular ejection, thereby diminishing the physiological impact on the weakened aortic wall. Through their negative chronotropic effect, the heart rate is slowed, and the ratio of pre-ejection period to ejection time is reported to increase.

A number of different beta-blockers have been used to slow aortic root growth in Marfan syndrome. Atenolol has the advantages of increased cardiac selectivity and once or twice daily dosing, but propranolol and other beta-blockers are also effective. Due to its low lipid solubility, atenolol has a lower incidence of central nervous system side effects than propranolol. A lower first-pass metabolism and considerably longer plasma half-life allow once or twice daily dosing. Controversy still exists as to whether the absorption pharmacokinetics of atenolol in Marfan patients differ from those in unaffected individuals (100).

Although beta-blockers are the only class of medications that have been shown to slow the rate of aortic dilatation in Marfan syndrome, the timing of its use, particularly in young patients, remains somewhat controversial. Any adult patient with classic Marfan syndrome should be considered for prophylactic therapy, particularly if there is more than mild aortic dilatation. In our pediatric patients, we generally recommend beta-blocker therapy and exercise modification when there is moderate aortic root dilatation, defined as an aortic root dimension with a z-score > +4 (> 4 standard deviations above the mean for body surface area).

Due to the marked variation in individual responsiveness to all beta-adrenergic blocking agents, the dose must be titrated for patients of all ages. Counting a patient's heart rate after several minutes of moderate exercise is an easy way to monitor drug compliance and efficacy. In older children, adolescents, and adults, the resting heart rate should be less than 60 beats per minute and the heart rate during exercise should not exceed 100. Patients should be counseled and monitored closely for possible side effects including lethargy or fatigue, depression, bronchospasm and other respiratory problems, and hypoglycemia. Some young children develop irritability and hyperactivity, which usually subside after a week or two of treatment.

Exercise Modification

Exercise modification is prescribed for individuals with Marfan syndrome and other connective tissue disorders associated with aortic dilatation. These individuals should avoid contact and competitive sports, isometric exercises, weight-lifting, and participation in physical activity at maximal exertion or to the point of exhaustion. We generally implement these exercise recommendations when the aortic root z-score is > +4. For pediatric patients, we recommend that their interests and activities be channeled away from competitive sports. The exercise prescription should also be tailored to the severity of ocular and skeletal manifestations.

Bacterial Endocarditis Prophylaxis

All patients with Marfan syndrome should receive prophylaxis for bacterial endocarditis, regardless of evident valve pathology. For those individuals who have undergone composite graft repair, more aggressive prophylaxis (i.e., with parenteral antibiotics) should be considered.

Aortic Root Replacement

For adults and older adolescents, prophylactic aortic root replacement is recommended when the aortic root diameter is greater than 5.5 cm (14-15,101-102). This recommendation is based on the fact that the relative risk for aortic dissection is significantly higher when the aortic root is greater than 5.5 cm. If there is a family history of aortic dissection, aortic root replacement is recommended when the aortic root diameter is greater than 5.0 cm. Morbidity and mortality are significantly higher if root replacement is performed after a dissection has already occurred. Additional indications for aortic root replacement include severe aortic regurgitation with left ventricular strain and in an acute emergency due to rupture, dissection, or severe left ventricular decompensation.

There are no strict criteria for timing of aortic root replacement in younger patients. Recommended guidelines include when the aortic root dimension exceeds twice the predicted for the age and body surface area (83) or twice the diameter of the distal ascending aorta or proximal descending aorta (1). At our pediatric center, indications for surgical repair include an aortic root z-score > +8, rapid change in aortic root z-score, and severe aortic regurgitation (86).

The composite graft operation (the Bentall procedure) (103) which was first performed in 1966 but not widely used until the mid-1970's, has proven to have low operative as well as long-term mortality, and has greatly increased the life-expectancy of Marfan patients (14-15,101-102). In this operation, the ascending aorta and valve are replaced by a synthetic tube that has a prosthetic valve sewn into the proximal end. A prosthetic valve requires lifetime anticoagulation therapy.

More recently, aortic root replacement with an aortic homograft rather than a prosthetic valve has obviated the need for long-term anti-coagulant therapy. However, there is a risk of developing homograft valve stenosis and regurgitation requiring reoperation. This option should be considered in small children, pregnant women, and other patients with contraindications to coumarin derivatives.

Pulmonary autografts are not recommended. The role of valve-sparing procedures, in which the aortic valve leaflets are left *in situ*, in patients with Marfan syndrome is controversial. Since the aortic valve leaflets express the same abnormality in fibrillin-1, most Marfan specialists believe that Marfan syndrome is a contraindication for valve-sparing surgery. There has been concern about the possibility of dilatation of the aortic annulus and development of aortic regurgitation after the valve-sparing procedure. Others have reported satisfactory long-term results with the valve-sparing procedure in patients with Marfan syndrome (104-105).

Gott et al. recently published a multicenter review of aortic root replacement in 675 patients with Marfan syndrome, including 604 who underwent composite graft replacements, 21 who underwent placement of a homograft aortic root, and 50 patients who underwent a valve-sparing procedure. The 30-day mortality rate was 1.5 percent among the 455 patients who underwent elective repair, 2.6 percent among the 117 patients who underwent urgent repair, and 11.7 percent among the 103 patients who underwent emergency repair (within 24 hours after a surgical consultation). Thirty percent had aortic dissection involving the ascending aorta. The 30-day mortality rate was 9.1 percent among the 99 patients with acute dissection and 1.9 percent among the 103 patients with chronic dissection. Nearly a third of adult patients with aortic dissection had an aneurysm with a diameter of 6.5 cm or less. There were 114 late deaths (more than 30 days after surgery); dissection or rupture of the residual aorta (22 patients) and arrhythmia (21 patients) were the principal causes of late death. Other causes for late deaths included congestive heart failure, endocarditis, pneumonia, dehiscence of coronary anastomosis, operative encephalopathy, and warfarin-induced hemorrhage. The risk of death was greatest within the first 60 days after surgery, then rapidly decreased to a constant level by the end of the first year. Overall survival rate was 93 percent at 1 year, 91 percent at 2 years, 84 percent at 5 years, 75 percent at 10 years, and 59 percent at 20 years. Major late complications included thromboembolism (n= 27), endocarditis (n=24), and coronary dehiscence (n=8).

Reports of surgical therapy in young children are limited. Gillinov AM et al. reported on 26 patients with Marfan syndrome who were less than 18 years of age and underwent cardiac operations at the Johns Hopkins Medical Institutions. The mean age at the time of operation was 10.3 +/- 1 years (range, 8 months to 17 years); 18 of the patients were male. There were no operative deaths, and there were 4 late deaths, all of presumed cardiac origin. The 10-year survival rate was 79% +/-10%. At a mean follow-up of 67.1 +/- 10.2 months, 8 patients required a second cardiac procedure

(41% +/- 17% 10-year freedom from reoperation). They concluded that (1) aortic root dilatation was the most common surgical indication in children with Marfan syndrome; (2) mitral regurgitation was the second most common; (3) aortic dissection is unusual in children with Marfan syndrome, and (4) careful follow-up is necessary, particularly in younger children, because more than half of all children with Marfan syndrome require repeated cardiac operations within 10 years. Risk factors for a second cardiac procedure included age less than 10 years at the time of the first operation and mitral regurgitation (107). Our experience and that of Tsang et al. (106) who reported on a surgical series of 7 children with Marfan syndrome, have been similar to the results reported by Gillinov et al.

Mitral valve surgery

Some patients require mitral valve surgery alone, or in addition to aortic surgery. In most cases, repair (valvuloplasty) rather than replacement of the mitral valve is possible, with acceptable long-term outcome (87).

Life Expectancy

Based on a natural history study done 30 years ago by Murdoch et al. (11), the mean age of survival for Marfan syndrome was said to be 43 years for men and 46 years for women with Marfan syndrome. In 1995, Finkbohner et al. (15) reported a median cumulative probability of survival of 61 years compared to 47 years in the natural history study of Murdoch et al. Another recent study by Silverman et al. found that life-expectancy has significantly increased overall for individuals affected by Marfan syndrome (13). This increase could be attributed to an overall increase in life expectancy for the general population, advances in aortic surgery such as the composite graft operation, advances in medical treatment including beta-adrenergic blockade, a decrease in the mean age at the time of diagnosis, and a larger proportion of patients diagnosed with a milder form of the disease.

Pregnancy

Women with Marfan syndrome are at further increased risk of aortic dissection during pregnancy. All the contributing factors are not certain, but hormonal changes, increased blood volume, increased cardiac output, and the sudden volume surge of autotransfusion as the uterus contracts postpartum probably contribute. The risk is greatest during the second half of pregnancy and for several months postpartum. However, most women with Marfan syndrome suffer no major complication (108-109). Pyeritz reported on the largest retrospective survey of pregnancy in Marfan syndrome, examining 105 pregnancies in 26 women (108). Only one death occurred, due to endocarditis in a woman with severe mitral valve disease that predated the pregnancy. Rossiter et al. then followed 21 women through 45 pregnancies and thereafter (109). None with minimal aortic dilatation (less than 42 mm) had any vascular complication during pregnancy, and echocardiography every 6 weeks showed no further aortic dilatation. During mean follow-up evaluation of 6 years in these women, none suffered apparent cardiovascular worsening attributable to pregnancy, compared to a group of nulliparous women with Marfan syndrome of similar severity. Two women (one with aortic regurgitation and moderate aortic dilatation and one with a pre-existing dissection) suffered acute dissection of the descending aorta during pregnancy.

Pyeritz described the following risk factors for cardiovascular complications of pregnancy which should be explored in any woman with Marfan syndrome of child-bearing age: aortic root dilatation (aortic roots greater than 40 mm carry increasing risk), aortic regurgitation, aortic dissection, mitral regurgitation, left ventricular dysfunction (especially dilated cardiomyopathy), any other structural cardiovascular abnormality, and family history of aortic dissection.

Echocardiography and cardiovascular assessment is recommended every 6 to 8 weeks during pregnancy. Beta-blockers can be continued during pregnancy, although some practitioners avoid their use during the first trimester. Delivery should be by whatever approaches to anesthesia, volume support, and parturition are least hemodynamically stressful to the mother; however Cesarian section is not indicated for other than standard obstetric reasons (1,108-109).

Ophthalmologic Features and Management

Ectopia lentis, the cardinal ocular feature of Marfan syndrome, is caused by an abnormality of the suspensory ligament of the lens (110). Ectopia lentis is unlikely to develop after age 10 years. Surgical removal of the lens is seldom necessary. Retinal detachment is more common after lens removal. Myopia is common.

Patients with Marfan syndrome should be followed by an ophthalmologist experienced in connective tisssue disorders. Each patient evaluated for the possibility of Marfan syndrome should undergo an initial ophthalmologic examination to include a dilated, slit-lamp examination. Thereafter, follow-up should be on a yearly basis, or more frequently if there is ectopia lentis or retinal detachment. Special attention should be placed on the correction of amblyopia, the direction and degree of lens subluxation, anterior chamber abnormalities, and detection of cataracts, glaucoma, and retinal detachment. The vast majority of patients can be refracted to vision better than 20/40 without lens surgery. Full correction should be pursued as early as possible and amblyopia treated aggressively.

Skeletal Features and Management

The skeletal features in Marfan syndrome show great variability and age-dependency (111-115). Abnormalities of the skeletal system that may necessitate orthopedic intervention include scoliosis which may progress during growth spurts, chest wall deformities including pectus excavatum and pectus carinatum, flat feet, and joint dislocations resulting from excessive hypermobility. Orthopedic concerns should be managed by an orthopedic surgeon familiar with connective tissue disorders. The major indication for repair of anterior chest deformities is cardiopulmonary compromise. Such repairs should be deferred until late adolescence if possible, due to the possibility of recurrence if repaired early in life (115).

Other Systems

The central nervous system (CNS), the skin and integument, and the pulmonary system may also be affected. Dural ectasia (often lumbar) may be seen as a CNS manifestation of Marfan syndrome (116-117). The true incidence and specificity of this feature are unknown. Dural ectasia can sometimes cause pain in the lower abdomen radiating into the legs. If necessary, surgical intervention is possible. Other CNS manifestations include learning disorders and hyperactivity (with or without attention deficit) (118), for which pemoline (Cylert™) and methylphenidate HCl (Ritalin™) have proven beneficial in some cases.

Involvement of the skin and integument includes striae distensae or striae atrophicae (stretch marks not associated with recent weight loss, usually located on hips, shoulders and lumbar area) and herniae (especially inguinal or incisional).

Almost all patients with Marfan syndrome show diminished lung elasticity, usually causing no noticeable problems (119). However, spontaneous pneumothorax may be a finding in 5% of affected individuals (50 times the rate in the general population). Spontaneous pneumothorax, which causes chest pain and sudden breathlessness, is rarely life-threatening but does require prompt attention. Restriction from contact sports and activities with rapid pressure changes, such as scuba-diving and flying in unpressurized aircraft, is indicated for affected individuals. Because Marfan syndrome predisposes to emphysematous changes, all patients should be counseled rigorously against smoking.

Infantile Marfan Syndrome

Infants with the infantile or neonatal Marfan phenotype are diagnosed with Marfan syndrome within the first year of life. The infantile Marfan syndrome is not a separate entity; rather it represents the phenotypic extreme of the classic phenotype. These infants, who represent spontaneous mutations without a positive family history, usually demonstrate severe, multi-system manifestations of the syndrome at a very young age and require intensive treatment and follow-up (69-71,85-86).

Table 1. Marfan Syndrome: "Berlin Criteria" for Diagnosis*

Skeletal System
Anterior chest deformity, especially asymmetric
   pectus excavatum/carinatum
Dolichostenomelia (long arms and legs)
Arachnodactyly (long fingers)
Vertebral column deformity
   Scoliosis
   Thoracic lordosis
   Reduced thoracic kyphosis (straight back)
Tall stature
High, narrowly arched palate and dental crowding
Protrusio acetabuli
Abnormal joint mobility
   Congenital flexion contractures
   Hypermobility

Ocular System
Ectopia lentis (subluxation of the lens)†
Flat cornea
Elongated globe
Retinal detachment (much more common after
   lens removal)
Myopia

Cardiovascular System
Dilatation of the ascending aorta †
Aortic dissection †
Aortic regurgitation
Mitral regurgitation due to mitral valve prolapse
Calcification of the mitral annulus
Mitral valve prolapse
Abdominal aortic aneurysm
Dysrhythmia
Endocarditis

Pulmonary System
Spontaneous pneumothorax
Apical bleb

Skin and Integument
Striae distensae
Inguinal hernia
Other hernia (umbilical, diaphragmatic, incisional)

Central Nervous System
Dural ectasia (lumbosacral meningocele)†
Dilated cisterna magna
Learning disability
Hyperactivity ± attention deficit disorder

Genetics
Autosomal dominant inheritance (15%-30% of
   cases are sporadic, i.e., no family history)

Requirements for Diagnosis
In the absence of an unequivocally affected first-
   degree relative: involvement of the skeleton
   and at least two other systems; at least one
   major manifestation
In the presence of at least one unequivocally affected
   first-degree relative: involvement of at least two
   systems; at least one major manifestation
   preferred, but this will depend somewhat on the
   family's phenotype
Urine amino acid analysis in the absence of
   pyrodoxine supplementation confirms absence
   of homocystinuria

* Listed in approximate order of decreasing specificity.
† Major manifestation.
Adapted from Beighton P, de Paepe A, Danks D, et al: International nosology of
heritable disorders of connective tissue, Berlin, 1986. Am J Med Genet 29:581-594,
1988. Copyright © 1988. Reprinted by permission of Wiley-Liss, a Division of John
Wiley and Sons, Inc.

Table 2. Marfan Syndrome: "Revised Criteria" for Diagnosis

Skeletal System

Major criterion: presence of at least 4 of the following:
  Pectus carinatum
  Pectus excavatum requiring surgery
  Reduced upper:lower segment or arm span:height ratio >1
  Wrist and thumb signs
  Scoliosis of > 20 degrees
  Reduced extension at the elbows (<170 degrees)
  Medial displacement of medial malleolus causing pes planus
  Protrusio acetabuli of any degree (by radiographs)

Minor criteria
  Pectus excavatum of moderate severity
  Joint hypermobility
  Highly arched palate with crowding of teeth
  Facial appearance (dolichocephaly, malar hypoplasia, enophthalmos, retrognathia, down-slanting palpebral fissures)

Skeletal involvement = at least 2 components comprising the major criterion, or one component comprising the major criterion plus 2 of the minor criteria

Ocular System

Major criterion
  Ectopia lentis (subluxation of the lens)

Minor criteria
  Abnormally flat cornea (by keratometry)
  Increased axial length of globe (by ultrasound)
  Hyoplastic iris or hypoplastic ciliary muscle causing decreased miosis

Ocular involvement = at least 2 minor criteria

Cardiovascular System

Major criteria
  Dilatation of the ascending aorta with or without aortic regurgitation and involving at least the sinuses of Valsalva
  Dissection of the ascending aorta

Minor criteria
  Mitral valve prolapse with or without mitral valve regurgitation
  Dilatation of the main pulmonary artery, in the absence of valvular or peripheral pulmonary stenosis or any other obvious cause, in a patient younger than 40 years of age
  Calcification of the mitral annulus in a patient younger than 40 years of age
  Dilatation or dissection of the descending thoracic or abdominal aorta younger than 50 years old

Pulmonary System

Major criteria
  None
Minor criteria
  Spontaneous pneumothorax
  Apical blebs (ascertained by radiography)

Skin and Integument

Major criteria
  None
Minor criteria
  Striae atrophicae not associated with marked weight changes, pregnancy, or stress
  Recurrent or incisional hernia

Dura

Major criterion
  Lumbosacral dural ectasia by CT or MRI
Minor criteria
  None

Family/Genetic History

Major criteria
  Having a parent, child, or sibling who meets these diagnostic criteria independently
  Presence of a mutation in *FBN1*, known to cause the Marfan syndrome
  Presence of a haplotype around the *FBN1*, inherited by descent, known to be associated with unequivocally diagnosed Marfan syndrome in the family

Minor criteria
  None

Requirements of the Diagnosis of Marfan Syndrome

For the Index Case

If the family/genetic history is not contributory, major criteria in at least two different organ systems and involvement of a third organ system.

If a mutation known to cause Marfan syndrome in others is detected, one major criterion in an organ system and involvement of a second organ system.

For the Relative of an Index Case

Presence of a major criterion in the family history, one major criterion in an organ system, and involvement of a second organ system

Table 3. Management of Patients with Marfan Syndrome

Regular examinations (at least annually)
    General medical
    Cardiologic, including echocardiography
    Ophthalmologic (more often for those with ectopia lentis or retinal detachment)
    Scoliosis screening until skeletal maturity
    Orthopedic (if indicated)
Examinations as needed
        Neurologic/behavioral
        Physical/Occupational therapy
   Computed tomographic (CT) scanning or magnetic resonance imaging (MRI) of the aorta or
      the vertebral column (when echocardiographic imaging is inadequate or when aortic
      aneurysm distal to the root, aortic dissection, or dural ectasia is suspected)
Discussion with parents, patient, spouse, or significant other regarding psychosocial concerns, genetic counseling, and any new advances in treatment or research
Activity restriction depending on age and cardiovascular features
Antibiotic prophylaxis for bacterial endocarditis (regardless of evident valve pathology)
Therapy with beta-blockers
Prophylactic composite graft or homograft repair of ascending aorta

REFERENCES

1. Pyeritz RE. 1996. Marfan syndrome and other disorders offibrillin. In Principles and practice of medical genetics, 3rd ed. DL Rimoin, JM Connors, RE Pyeritz, editors. Churchill Livingstone, New York. 1027-1066.
2. Pyeritz RE. 1986. The diagnosis and management of the Marfan syndrome. AmFam Physician 34:83-94.
3. Pyeritz RE, VA McKusick. 1979. The Marfan syndrome diagnosis and management. N Engl J Med 300:772-777.
4. Goodman RM, M Berkenstadt, M Motro, M Frank. 1989. The Marfan syndrome in Israel (abstract). Am J Med Genet 32:242.
5. Gordon AM. 1962. Abraham Lincoln—A medical appraisal. J KentuckyMed Assoc 60:249-253.
6. McKusick VA. 1991. The defect in Marfan syndrome. Nature 325:279-281.
7. Schoenfeld MR. 1978. Nicolo Paganini: Musical magician and Marfan mutant? JAMA 239:40-2.
8. Baer RW, HB Taussig, EH Oppenheimer. 1943. Congenital aneurysmal dilatation of the aorta associated with arachnodactyly. Bull Johns HopkinsHosp 72:309-331.
9. Etter LE, LP Glover. 1943. Arachnodactyly complicated by dislocated lens and death from rupture of dissecting aneurysm of the aorta. JAMA 123:88-89.
10. Brown OR, H DeMots, FE Kloster, A Roberts, VD Menashe, RK Beals. 1975. Aortic root dilatation and mitral valve prolapse in Marfan's syndrome: Circulation 52:651-657.
11. Murdoch JL, BA Walker, BL Halpern, JW Kuzma, VA McKusick. Life expectancy and causes of death in Marfan syndrome. 1972. NEngl J Med 286:804-808.
12. Shores J, KR Berger, EA Murphy, RE Pyeritz. 1994. Progression of aortic dilatation and the benefit of long-term beta-adrenergic blockade in Marfan's syndrome. N Engl J Med 330:1335-41.
13. Silverman DI, KJ Burton, J Gray, MS Bosner, NT Kouchoukos, MJ Roman, M Boxer, RB Devereux, P Tsipouras. 1995. Life expectancy in the Marfan syndrome. Am J Cardiol 75:157-60.
14. Gott, VL, DE Cameron, RE Pyeritz, AM Gillinov, PS Greene, CD Stone, DE Alejo, VA McKusick. 1994. Composite graft repair of Marfan aneurysm of the ascending aorta. J CardSurg 9:482-489.
15. Finkbohner RD Johnston, S0 Crawford, JCoselli, and D. M. Milewicz. 1995. Marfan syndrome. Long-term survival and complications after aortic aneurysm repair. Circulation 91:728-733.
16. Pyeritz RE. 1989. Pleiotropy revisited: Molecular explanations of a classic concept. Am JMed Genet 34:124-134.
17. Dietz HC, RE Pyeritz. 1995. Mutations in the hur.1an gene for fibrillin-1 (*FBN1*) in the Marfan syndrome and related disorders. HumMolec Genet 4:1799-1809.
18. Ramirez F. 1996. Fibrillin mutations in Marfan syndrome and related phenotypes. Curr Opin Genet Dev 6:309-315.
19. Sakai LY, DR Keene, E Engvall. 1986. Fibrillin, a new 350 kD glycoprotein, is a component of extracellular microfibrils. J Cell Biol 103:2499-2509.
20. Lee B, M Godfrey, E Vitale, H Hori, MG Mattei, M Sarfarazi, P Tsipouras, F Ramirez, DW Hollister. 1991. Linkage of Marfan syndrome and a phenotypically related disorder to two different fibrillin genes. Nature 352:330-334.
21. Maslen CL, GM Corson, BK Maddox, RW Glanville, LY Sakai. 1991. Partial sequence of a candidate gene for the Marfan syndrome. Nature 352:334-337.
22. Dietz HC, GR Cutting, RE Pyeritz, CL Maslen, LY Sakai, GM Corson, EG Puffenberger, A Hamosh, SM Curristin, G Stetten, DA Meyers, CA Francomano. 1991. Marfan syndrome caused by a recurrent *de novo* missense mutation in the fibrillin gene. Nature 352:337-9.
23. Dietz HC, I McIntosh, LY Sakai, GM Corson, SC Chalberg, RE Pyeritz, CA Francomano. 1993. Four novel *FBN1* mutations: Significance for mutant transcript level and EGF-like domain calcium binding in the pathogenesis of Marfan syndrome. Genomics 17:468-475.
24. Nijbroek G, S Sood, I McIntosh, CA Francomano, E Bull, L Pereira, F Ramirez, REPyeritz, HC Dietz. 1995. Fifteen novel *FBN1* mutations causing Marfan syndrome detected by heteroduplex analysis of genomic amplicons. Am J Hum Genet 57:8-21.

25. Emanuel R, RA Ng, EC Moores, KE Jefferson, PA MacFaul, R Withers. 1977. Formes frustes of Marfan's syndrome presenting with severe aortic regurgitation. Br Heart J 39:190-197.
26. Savunen T. 1987. Cardiovascular abnormalities in relatives of patients operated on forannulo-aortic ectasia. Eur J Cardiothorac Surg 1:3-10.
27. Nicod P, C Bloor, M Godfrey, D Hollister, RE Pyeritz, H Dittrich, R Polikar, KL Peterson. 1989. Familial aortic dissecting aneurysm. J AmColl Cardiol 13:811-819.
28. Francke U, MA Berg, K Tynan, T Brenn, W Liu, T Aoyama, C Gasner, DC Miller, H Furthmayr. 1995. A Gly1127Ser mutation in an EGF-like domain of the fibrillin-1 gene is a risk factor for ascending aortic aneurysm and dissection. Am J Hum Genet 56:1287-1296.
29. Tsipouras P, R Del Mastro, M Sarfarazi, B Lee, E Vitale, AH Child, M Godfrey, RB Devereux, D Hewett, B Steinmann, D Viljoen, BC Sykes, M Kilpatrick, F Ramirez. 1992. Genetic linkage of the Marfan syndrome, ectopia lentis,and congenital contractural arachnodactyly to the fibrillin genes on chromosomes 15 and 5. NEngl J Med 326:905-909.
30. Edwards MJ, CJ Challinor, PW Colley, J Roberts, MW Partington, GE Hollway, HM Kozman, JC Mulley. 1994. Clinical and linkage study of a large family with simple ectopia lentis linked to *FBN1*. Am J Med Genet 53:65-71.
31. Kainulainen K, L Karttunen, L Puhakka, L Sakai, L Peltonen. 1994. Mutations in the fibrillin gene responsible for dominant ectopia lentis and neonatal Marfan syndrome. Nature Genet64-9.
32. Lönnqvist L, A Child, K Kainulainen, R Davidson, L Puhakka, L Peltonen. 1994. A novel mutation of the fibrillin gene causing ectopia lentis. Genomics 19:573-576.
33. Milewicz DM, J Grossfield, SN Cao, C Kielty, W Covitz, T Jewett. 1995. A mutation in *FBN1* disrupts profibrillin processing and results in isolated skeletal features of the Marfan syndrome. J Clin Invest 95:2373-2378.
34. Shprintzen RJ, RB Goldberg. 1982. A recurrent pattern syndrome ofcraniosynostosis associated with arachnodactyly and abdominal hernias. JCraniofacial Genet Devel Biol 2:65-74.
35. Sood S, ZA Eldadah, WL Krause, I McIntosh, HC Dietz. 1996. Mutations in fibrillin-1 and the Marfanoid craniosynostosis (Shprintzen-Goldberg) syndrome. Nature Genet 12:209-211.
36. Devereux RB, WT Brown, R Kramer-Fox, I Sacks. 1982. Inheritance of mitral valve prolapse Effect of age and sex in gene expression. Ann InternMed 97:826-832.
37. Devereux RB, R Kramer-Fox, WT Brown, MK Shear, N Hartman, P Kligfield, EM Lutas, MC Spitzer, SD Litwin. 1986. Relation between clinical features of "mitral valve prolapse syndrome" and echocardiographically documented mitral valve prolapse. J AmColl Cardiol 8:763-772.
38. Devereux RB, R Kramer-Fox, MK Shear, P Kligfield, R Pini, DD Savage. 1987. Diagnosis and classification of severity of mitral valve prolapse. Am Heart J 113:1265-1280.
39. Roman MJ, RB Devereux, R Kramer-Fox, MC Spitzer. 1989. Comparison of cardiovascular and skeletal features of primary mitral valve prolapse and Marfan syndrome. Am JCardio 63:317-21.
40. Montgomery RA, MT Geraghty, E Bull, BD Gelb, M Johnson, I McIntosh, CA Francomano, HC Dietz. 1998. Multiple molecular mechanisms underlying subdiagnostic variants of Marfan syndrome. Am J Hum Genet 63:1703-1711.
41. Glesby MJ, RE Pyeritz. 1989. Association of mitral valve prolapse and systemic abnormalities of connective tissue. JAMA 262:523-528.
42. Stahl-Hallengren C, T Ukkonen, K Kainulainen, T Saxne, K Tornqvist, L Peltonen. 1994. An extra cysteine in 1 of the non-calcium-binding epidermal growth factor-like motifs of the*FBN1* polypeptide is connected to a novel variant of the Marfan syndrome. J Clin Invest 94:709-13.
43. Hecht F, RK Beals. 1972. "New" syndrome of congenital contractural arachnodactyly originally described by Marfan in 1896. Pediatrics 49:574-579.
44. Viljoen D. 1994. Congenital contractural arachnodactyly. J Med Genet 31:640-643.
45. Putnam EA, H Zhang, F Ramirez, DM Milewicz. 1995. Fibrillin-2 (*FBN2*) mutations result in the Marfan-like disorder, congenital contractural arachnodactyly. Nature Genet 11:456-458.
46. Marfan MA. 1896. Un cas de deformation congenital des quatre membres plus prononcee aux extremities caracterisee. Bull Mem Soc Med Hop (Paris) 13:220-226.
47. Achard C. 1902. Arachnodactylie. Bull Mem Soc Med Hop (Paris) 19:834-840.
48. Börger F. 1914. Uber zwei Falle von Arachnodaktylie.Zschr Kinderheilk 12:161-184.
49. Williams E. 1873-1879. Rare cases, with practical remarks. Trans AmOphthalmol Soc 2:291.

50.   Weve H. 1931. Uber Arachnodaktylie (dystrophia mesodermalis congenita, Typus Marfan). Archiv Augenheilk 104:1-46.
51.   Salle V. 1912. Uber einen Fall von angeborener Abnormalen grosse der Extremitaten mit einem an Akromegalie erinnernden Symptomenkomplex. Jahrb Kinderheilk 75:540-548.
52.   Pyeritz RE, MA Wappel. 1983. Mitral valve dysfunction in the Marfan syndrome. Am JMed 74:797-807.
53.   McKusick VA. 1955. The cardiovascular aspects of Marfan's syndrome A heritable disorder of connective tissue. Circulation 11:321-341.
54.   McKusick VA. 1956. Heritable disorders of connective tissue. Mosby, St. Louis. 68-71.
55.   Ross R, P Bornstein. 1969. The elastic fiber. J CellBiol 40:366-381.
56.   Mecham RP, J Heuser. 1990. Three-dimensional organization of extracellular matrix in elastic cartilage as viewed by quick freeze, deep etch electron microscopy. ConnectTissue Res 24:83-93.
57.   Mecham RP, EC Davis. 1994. Elastic fiber structure and assembly. *In* Extracellular matrix assembly and structure. PD Yurchenco, DE Birk, and RP Mecham, eds. Academic Press, San Diego. 281-314.
58.   Hollister DW, M Godfrey, LY Sakai, RE Pyeritz. 1990. Immunohistologic abnormalities of the microfibrillar-fiber system in the Marfan syndrome. NEngl J Med 323:152-159.
59.   Kainulainen K, L Pulkkinen, A Savolainen, I Kaitila, L Peltonen. 1990. Location on chromosome 15 of the gene defect causing Marfan syndrome. NEngl J Med 323:935-939.
60.   Dietz HC, RE Pyeritz, BD Hall, RG Cadle, A Hamosh, J Schwartz, DA Meyers, CA Francomano. 1991. The Marfan syndrome locus Confirmation of assignment to chromosome 15 and identification of tightly linked markers at 15q15-q21.3. Genomics 9:355-361.
61.   Magenis RE, CL Maslen, L Smith, L Allen, LY Sakai. 1991. Localization of the fibrillin (FBN) gene to chromosome 15, band q21.1. Genomics 11:346-351.
62.   Corson GM, SC Chalberg, HC Dietz, N Charbonneau, LY Sakai. 1993. Fibrillin binds calcium and is encoded by cDNAs that reveal a multidomain structure and alternatively spliced exons at the 5' end. Genomics 17:468-475.
63.   Pereira L, M D'Alessio, F Ramirez, JR. Lynch, B Sykes, T Pangilinan, J Bonadio. 1993. Genomic organization of the sequence coding for fibrillin, the defective gene product in Marfan syndrome. Hum Mol Genet 2:961-968.
64.   Dietz H, U Francke, H Furthmayr, C Francomano, A De Paepe, R Devereux, F Ramirez, R Pyeritz. 1995. The question of heterogeneity in Marfan syndrome. Nature Genet 9:228-231.
65.   Aoyama T, K Tynan, HC Dietz, U Francke, H Furthmayr. 1993. Missense mutations impair intracellular processing of fibrillin and microfibril assembly in Marfan syndrome. Hum Mol Genet 2:2135-2140.
66.   Aoyama T, U Francke, HC Dietz, H Furthmayr. 1994. Quantitative differences in biosynthesis and extracellular deposition of fibrillin in cultured fibroblasts distinguish five groups of Marfan syndrome patients and suggest distinct pathogenetic mechanisms. J Clin Invest 94:130-137.
67.   Dietz HC, RE Pyeritz. 1994. Molecular genetic approaches to investigating cardiovascular disease. Ann Rev Physiol 56:763-796.
68.   McKusick VA. 1999. On-line Mendelian inheritance in man. Johns Hopkins University, Baltimore (onim@gdb.org).
69.   Geva T, SP Sanders, MS Diogenes, S Rockenmacher, R Van Praagh. 1990. Two-dimensional and Doppler echocardiographic and pathologic characteristics of the infantile Marfan syndrome. Am J Cardiol 65:1230-1237.
70.   Milewicz DM, M Duvic. 1994. Severe neonatal Marfan syndrome resulting from a de novo 3-bp insertion into the fibrillin gene on chromosome 15. Am J Hum Genet 54:447-453.
71.   Wang M, C Price, J Han, J Cisler, K Imaizumi, MN Van Thienen, A De Paepe, M Godfrey. 1995. Recurrent mis-splicing of fibrillin exon 32 in two patients with neonatal Marfan syndrome. Hum Mol Genet 4:607-613.
72.   Beighton P, A De Paepe, D Danks, G Finidori, R Goodman, JG Hall, DW Hollister, W Horton, VA McKusick, JM Opitz, FM Pope, RE Pyeritz, I Young. 1988. International nosology of heritable disorders of connective tissue, Berlin, 1986. Am JMed Genet 29:581-594.

73. Pereira L, O Levran, F Ramirez, JR Lynch, B Sykes, RE Pyeritz, HC Dietz. 1994. A molecular approach to the stratification of cardiovascular risk in families with Marfan syndrome. NEngl J Med 331:148-153.

74. De Paepe A, RB Devereux, HC Dietz, RCM Hennekam, RE Pyeritz. 1996. Revised diagnostic criteria for the Marfan syndrome. Am J Med Genet 62:417-426.

75. Hall JG, UG Froster-Iskenius, JE Allanson. 1989. Handbook of normal physical measurements. Oxford University Press, Oxford. 270-275.

76. Mash AJ, JP Hegmann, BE Spivey. 1975. Genetic analysis of indices of corneal power and corneal astigmatism in human populations with varying incidences of strabismus. Invest Ophthalmol 14:826-832.

77. Fledelius H. 1981. The growth of the eye. In Ultrasonography in ophthalmology. J. M. Thijssen and A. M. Verbeek AM, editors. W Junk, Dordrecht. 211.

78. Godfrey M, N Vandemark, M Wang, M Velinov, D Wargowski, P Tsipouras, J Han, J Becker, W Robertson, S Droste, VH Rao. 1993. Prenatal diagnosis and a donor splice site mutation in fibrillin in a family with Marfan syndrome. Am J Hum Genet 53:472-480.

79. Rantamäki T, L Lönnqvist, L Karttunen, A Child, L Peltonen. 1994. DNA diagnostics of the Marfan syndrome: Application of amplifiable polymorphic markers. Eur J Hum Genet 2:66-75.

80. Eldadah ZA, JA Grifo, HC Dietz. 1995. Marfan syndrome as a paradigm for transcript-targeted preimplantation diagnosis of heterozygous mutations. NatureMed 1:798-803.

81. Lacro RV. 1996. Marfan syndrome. In Gellis and Kagan's Current Pediatric Therapy 15. FD Burg, JR Ingelfinger, ER Wald, RA Polin, editors. W. B. Saunders Co., Phildadelphia. 171-173.

82. Anonymous (American Academy of Pediatrics Committee on Genetics). 1996. Health supervision of children with Marfan syndrome. Pediatrics 98:978-982.

83. Roman MJ, RB Devereux, R Kramer-Fox, J O'Loughlin. 1989. Two-dimensional aortic root dimensions in normal children and adults. Am J Cardiol 64:507-512.

84. Roman MJ, SS Rosen, R Kramer-Fox, RB Devereux. 1993. The prognostic significance of the pattern of aortic root dilatation in the Marfan syndrome. J AmColl Cardiol 22:1470-1476.

85. Sisk HE, KG Zahka, RE Pyeritz. 1983. The Marfan syndrome in early childhood Analysis of 15 patients diagnosed at less than 4 years of age. Am J Cardiol 52:353-358.

86. van Karnebeek CDM, K Gauvreau, SD Colan, RV Lacro. 1998. Clinical and echocardiographic predictors of adverse cardiovascular outcome in childhood Marfan syndrome (abstract). J Am Coll Card 31 No 2, Supp A:70A-71A.

87. Gillinov AM, A Hulyalkar, DE Cameron, PW Cho, PS Greene, BAReitz, VL Gott. 1994. Mitral valve operations in patients with the Marfan syndrome. J Thorac Cardiovasc Surg 107:724-731.

88. Bowers D. 1961. The electrocardiogram in Marfan's syndrome. Am J Cardiol 7:661-672.

89. Bowers D. 1969. Primary abnormalities of the mitral valve in Marfan's syndrome. Electrocardiographic findings. Br Heart J 31:676-678.

90. Banerjee AK. 1988. Marfan's syndrome associated with Wolff-Parkinson-White syndrome type B. Jpn Heart J 29:377-380.

91. Kligfield P, P Levy, RB Devereux, DD Savage. 1987. Arrhythmias and sudden death in mitral valve prolapse. Am J Cardiol 113:1298-1307.

92. Chen S, LF Fagan, S Nouri, JL Donahoe. 1985. Ventricular dysrhythmias in children with Marfan's syndrome. Am J Dis Child 139:273-276.

93. Mehta D, S Wafa, A Child, AJ Camm. 1989. Arrhythmia in Marfan syndrome. Am JMed Genet 32:247.

94. Savolainen A, M Kupari, L Toivonen, I Kaitila, M Viitasalo. 1997. Abnormal ambulatory electrocardiographic findings in patients with Marfan syndrome. J Int Med 241:221-226.

95. Halpern BL, F Char, JL Murdoch, WB Horton, VA McKusick. 1971. A prospectus on the prevention of aortic rupture in the Marfan syndrome with data on survivorship without treatment. Johns Hopkins Med Journal 129:123-129.

96. Simpson CF. 1972. Sotalol for the protection of turkeys from the development of beta-aminopropionitrile-induced aortic ruptures. Br JPharmacol 45:385-390.

97. Simpson CF, JM Kling, RF Palmer. 1970. Beta-aminopropionotrile-induced dissecting aneurysms in turkeys: Treatment with propranolol. Toxicol Appl Pharmacol 16:143-153.

98.   Salim MA, BS Alpert, JC Ward, RE Pyeritz. 1994. Effect of beta-adrenergic blockade on aortic root rate of dilation in the Marfan syndrome. Am J Cardiol 74:629-633.
99.   Opie LH, EH Sonnenblick, NM Kaplan, U Thadani. 1987. Beta-blocking agents. In Drugs for the heart, 2nd ed. LH Opie, K Chatterjee, BJ Gersh, , editors. Grune & Stratton, Orlando. 1-16.
100. Phelps SJ, BS Alpert, JL Ward, JA Pieper, JJ Lima. 1995. Absorption pharmacokinetics of atenolol in patients with the Marfan syndrome. J ClinPharmacol 35:268-274.
101. Gott VL, RE Pyeritz, GJ Magovern, DE Cameron, VA McKusick. 1986. Surgical treatment of aneurysms of the ascending aorta in the Marfan syndrome. NEngl J Med 314:1070-1074.
102. Gott VL, PS Greene, DE Alejo, DE Cameron, DC Naftel, DC Miller, AM Gillinov, JC Laschinger, RE Pyeritz. 1999. Replacement of the aortic root in patients with Marfan's syndrome. N Engl J Med 340:1307-1313.
103. Bentall H, A De Bono. 1968. A technique for complete replacement of the ascending aorta. Thorax 23:338-339.
104. David TE, CM Feindel. 1992. An aortic valve-sparing operation for patients with aortic incompetence and aneurysm of the ascending aorta. JThorac Cardiovasc Surg 103:617-622.
105. Yacoub MH, P Gehle, EJ Birks, A Child, R Radley-Smith. 1998. Late results of a valve-preserving operation in patients with aneurysms in the ascending aorta and root. J Thorac Cardiovasc Surg 115:1080-1090.
106. Tsang VT, A Pawade, TR Karl, RB Mee. 1994. Surgical management of Marfan syndrome in children. J Card Surg 9:50-54.
107. Gillinov AM, KJ Zehr, JM Redmond, VL Gott, HC Dietz, BA Reitz, DE Cameron. 1997. Cardiac operations in children with Marfan's syndrome. AnnThorac Surg 64:1140-1145.
108. Pyeritz RE. 1981. Maternal and fetal complications of pregnancy in the Marfan syndrome. Am J Med 71:784-790.
109. Rossiter JP, JT Repke, AJ Morales, EA Murphy, RE Pyeritz. 1995. A prospective longitudinal evaluation of pregnancy in the Marfan syndrome. Am JObstet Gynecol 173:1599-1606.
110. Maumenee IH. 1981. The eye in the Marfan syndrome. Trans AmOphthalmol 79:684-733.
111. Sponseller PD, W Hobbs, LH Riley III, RE Pyeritz. 1995. The thoracolumbar spine in Marfan syndrome. J Bone JointSurg 77-A;867-876.
112. Steinberg I. 1966. A simple screening test for the Marfan syndrome. Am J Roentgen l 97:118.
113. Walker, B. A. and J. L. Murdoch. 1970. The wrist sign A useful physical finding in the Marfan syndrome. Arch Intern Med 71:349.
114. Kuhlman JE, WW Scott Jr, EK Fishman, RE Pyeritz SS Siegleman. 1987. Protrusio acetabuli in Marfan syndrome. Radiology 164:415-417.
115. Arn PH, LR Scherer, JA Haller Jr, RE Pyeritz. 1989. Clinical outcomes of pectus excavatum in the Marfan syndrome and in the general population. JPediatr 115:954-958.
116. Pyeritz RE, EK Fishman, BA Bernhardt, SS Siegelman. 1988. Dural ectasia is a common feature of the Marfan syndrome. Am J Hum Genet 43:726-732.
117. Stern WE. 1988. Dural ectasia and the Marfan syndrome. JNeurosurg 69:221-227.
118. Hofman KJ, BA Bernhardt, RE Pyeritz. 1988. Marfan syndrome Neuropsychologic aspects. Am J Med Genet 31:331-338.
119. Hall J, RE Pyeritz, DL Dudgeon, JA Haller Jr. 1984. Pneumothorax in the Marfan syndrome Prevalence and therapy. AnnThorac Surg 37:500-504.

22
THE MOLECULAR GENETICS OF CONOTRUNCAL DEFECTS

Elizabeth Goldmuntz, M.D.

Division of Cardiology, The Children's Hospital of Philadelphia
Philadelphia, PA 19104

INTRODUCTION

Although conotruncal defects account for approximately 16% of all types of congenital heart disease (1), little is known about the molecular genetics of these malformations. Epidemiologic studies, naturally occurring animal models and animal experimentation support a genetic contribution to this class of disorders. However, identification of specific genetic etiologies has been difficult to accomplish for several reasons. First, unlike many of the disorders discussed previously in this textbook, most probands with severe conotruncal defects have not historically survived to reproduce so that families with many affected members do not exist. Most cases of conotruncal defects appear to be sporadic rather than familial. Therefore, investigators have not been able to perform linkage analyses to identify chromosomal disease loci or genes. Second, until more recently, very little was known of the developmental pathways and specific proteins involved in conotruncal and cardiac development so that candidate genes for human disease could not be proposed. Third, most probands with a conotruncal defect have normal standard karyotypes, so clues as to where disease genes might map are also uncommon. Nonetheless, significant progress has been made recently and more discoveries are likely to be made through the analysis of genetic syndromes in which congenital heart disease is a major feature. Moreover, a multitude of genes that contribute to conotruncal development are now being identified in mammalian models. These genes begin to unravel the developmental pathways that contribute to outflow tract formation and may turn out to be disease-related in some cases. Though much work remains to be done, the prospects of understanding specific genetic etiologies of these malformations are increasing.

Conotruncal defects are defined as malformations of the outflow tract(s) of the heart. They presumably result from abnormal alignment or septation of the embryonic structure, the conotruncus. This class of defects at a minimum includes: truncus arteriosus (TA), tetralogy of Fallot (TOF), interrupted aortic arch (IAA), double outlet right (or left) ventricle (DORV, DOLV), and transposition of the great arteries (TGA). Other anatomically closely related defects, such as coarctation of the aorta with a posterior malalignment type ventricular septal defect, might also be included in this category. As will become clear in the discussion that follows, the pathologic definition of a conotruncal defect may not correlate with the genetic definition in that some non-conotruncal defects may nonetheless share a common genetic etiology with this group of disorders. In addition, the genetic etiology of these malformations is heterogeneous such that some lesions are likely to share a common genetic etiology in certain cases and have entirely different or unique etiologies in other cases. The discussion that follows will highlight the evidence pointing to a genetic contribution to the development of these disorders in humans and outline the present knowledge about specific human disease loci.

EVIDENCE FOR A GENETIC CONTRIBUTION

Familial Cases

A number of reports have described unusual families with multiple affected members. These reports indicate that, in at least some cases, the propensity of having a conotruncal defect is an inherited trait. They also indicate that the genetic etiology is likely to be heterogeneous. Some families most likely demonstrate autosomal dominant inheritance, others most likely demonstrate autosomal recessive inheritance, while multifactorial inheritance must be invoked to explain still other patterns of transmission. In some families, the affected members have nearly identical lesions (such as TOF), while in other families the affected members have concordant but not identical defects (such as different types of conotruncal defects). In yet other families, affected members may seem to have pathologically discordant defects which must nonetheless share a common genetic etiology. Most familial cases of conotruncal defects are those with TOF. A few reports are highlighted below.

Several families with nearly identical lesions in the affected members have been reported. Pankau and colleagues (2) reported a family in which three of five siblings of non-consanguinous parents had TOF, two with a right aortic arch. Wulfsberg and colleagues (3) also described a family where two of three siblings of non-consanguinous parents had TOF with pulmonary atresia, supporting an autosomal recessive inheritance. Pacileo and colleagues (4) described a family where three of four siblings had TOF, as did the daughter of a maternal cousin. Friedberg (5) described a family with three affected generations with TOF and a right aortic arch, though the pulmonary valve anatomy varied. Of note, Brunson and colleagues (6) described a family where three of four siblings had (TA). The father had a patent ductus arteriosus ligated at 5 years of age, but no other syndromic features were described.

Families where affected members have a range of conotruncal defects have also been described. For example, Gobel and colleagues (7) reported a family where two siblings and one half-sibling had conotruncal defects including one with TA/IAA type B (or TA type 4), one with IAA type B, and one with DORV/IAA type B. Although the family was not tested for the 22q11 deletion (see below), other syndromic features were not described. Rein and Sheffer (8) described a family where all four offspring of a consanguinous couple had either TA or TOF. Of interest, a maternal cousin had DORV and a paternal cousin had TGA.

Miller and Smith (9) described two families that illustrate the variety of defects that can be seen in one family. In the first family, three generations were affected, though the lesion of the grandfather was unknown. Five additional members in two nuclear families were affected with pulmonary valvar stenosis, hypoplastic right heart and pulmonary stenosis, and TOF. In the second family, three siblings of third degree cousins had TOF, TGA and complex congenital heart disease (dextrocardia, L-TGA, pulmonary and tricuspid valve atresia, single ventricle and right aortic arch).

Finally, several families have been described with unusual syndromic features and conotruncal defects. Jones and Waldman (10) described six relatives over three generations with a characteristic facial appearance, preauricular pits, fifth finger clinodactyly and TOF. Chen and D'Souza (11) describe another family where three of four offspring of a mother with glaucoma had glaucoma and a conotruncal defect; two had TOF with pulmonary stenosis and one had TOF with absent pulmonary valve syndrome. These two families are suggestive of an autosomal dominant mode of inheritance in association with other defects.

These families illustrate that there is likely to be a genetic component to the development of conotruncal defects. The etiology is undoubtedly heterogeneous. There is also likely to be variable penetrance of genetic traits. These families also illustrate that the specific etiology impacts tremendously on the expected recurrence risk for any one family.

Recurrence Risks
Sibling and offspring recurrence risks for most forms of congenital heart disease have been difficult to estimate given the different study designs, the small number of study subjects, the different methods of pathologic classification, the different methods used for diagnosis, and the historical selection of patients who survived to reproduce. In addition, recurrence risks appear to vary depending upon the specific class of lesion and the specific etiology in each case. However, the overall increased risk of having some form of congenital heart disease in siblings of probands and offspring of parents with conotruncal defects points to a genetic contribution to the development of these disorders in many cases. Each sub-category of conotruncal defects will be discussed below to highlight subtle differences between them. Note that recurrence risk implies recurrence of congenital heart disease in general, which can be a concordant or discordant lesion.

Tetralogy of Fallot: Most studies on recurrence risk have either grouped conotruncal defects together or, more commonly, focused on the recurrence risk if the proband has TOF. In particular, earlier studies reported a recurrence risk in siblings of probands with TOF that ranged from 0% to 2.7% (12-17). Nora and Nora (18) combined their data with that of nine additional studies to arrive at a suggested sibling recurrence risk of 2.5% if one sibling was affected, and 8% if 2 or more siblings were affected. More recently, Burn and colleagues (19) calculated a sibling recurrence risk of 2.2%. Of note, Digilio and colleagues (20) calculated sibling recurrence risks of 3.1% in 102 consecutive patients with TOF and pulmonary stenosis who did not have identifiable genetic syndromes or chromosomal alterations by current standards (no 22q11 deletions, see below). Thus, the sibling recurrence rate appears to range from 2.5-3.0% if only one sibling is affected, but it is likely to increase substantially if more than one sibling is affected. The recurrence risk may also increase if familial disease or syndromic features are present in the affected proband or relatives.

The estimated recurrence risk to offspring of parents with TOF is generally higher than that for siblings and ranges from 1.2 to 8.3% (21,22). Once again, Nora and Nora (23) combined their data with that of other studies and estimated a recurrence risk of 1.4% if the affected parent was male and 2.6% if the affected parent was female. Although several studies have also found that the recurrence risk for CHD in offspring of affected mothers is greater than that in offspring of affected fathers (24-26), several studies do not support that finding. In particular, Whittemore and colleagues (27) found that the recurrence risk to offspring if the father had a conotruncal defect was 20% as opposed to 10% if the mother had a conotruncal defect. Similarly, Zellers and colleagues (17) examined the offspring recurrence risk when one parent had TOF. The offspring recurrence risk if the father was affected was 1.3% as opposed to 0.9% if the mother was affected. Once again, the recurrence risk to offspring of affected parents is likely to vary substantially depending upon the specific genetic and/or environmental etiology of the parent's defect.

Truncus arteriosus and interrupted aortic arch: Very few studies have investigated the specific recurrence risk in siblings or offspring of patients with TA, IAA or DORV given the relative rarity of these defects. Instead, they have reported the recurrence risk for conotruncal defects or "rare defects" altogether. Nora and Nora (23) combined a number of studies and reported a recurrence risk for siblings of probands with TA at 1.2%. They suggested that the risk reported to families should be 1% if one sibling was affected, and 3% if 2 siblings were affected. Pierpont and colleagues (28) specifically investigated the familial recurrence risk for TA and IAA in their patient population. They were able to recruit 49 families with TA and 36 families with IAA for the study (which is a large number of rare lesions but a small sample size from which to estimate recurrence risk). They found a recurrence rate of 6.6% for siblings of patients with TA overall, but found that the rate was only 1.6% in cases with simple TA as compared to a rate of 13.6% in cases with complex TA. The recurrence risk for IAA was 2.1% overall. They concluded that there was a higher than expected rate of recurrence for these defects than previously reported. No specific study on subjects with DORV have been performed.

Transposition of the great arteries: Very few studies provide specific data on the recurrence risk for siblings or offspring of subjects with TGA. Recurrence risk to offspring is particularly difficult to assess given, historically, the very low survival rate of infants with TGA to reproductive ages. Thus, the inheritance pattern for this defect is in many ways unknown. Sanchez-Cascos (14) reported a 1.4% recurrence risk for first degree relatives. Nora and Nora (23) combined data from several published studies and suggested a recurrence risk of 1.5% if one sibling was affected and 5% if two siblings were affected. Becker and colleagues (29) studied the sibling recurrence risk in patients with TGA overall and then divided the study group into four types of TGA, namely d-TGA, l-TGA, complex TGA and asplenia with TGA. Once again, the study is well designed in that it attempts to report on specific sub-categories of defects, but it is limited by the sample size. They reported a recurrence risk of only 0.27% in d-TGA, 2.0% in l-TGA, 1.4% in complex TGA, and 2.0% in asplenia with TGA to give an overall sibling recurrence risk of 0.82%. Most recently, Burn and colleagues (19) found only one case of congenital heart disease among 103 siblings of subjects with TGA and no affected offspring among 20 offspring. Once again, this study is limited by the small sample size.

Summary: The finding of increased sibling and offspring recurrence rates in subjects with conotruncal defects points to a genetic contribution or susceptibility to these defects. The different recurrence risks for each lesion may indicate that the genetic contribution or etiology is quite different depending upon the specific malformation. These studies highlight the utility of grouping defects into mechanistic categories and the subsequent necessity of dividing the lesions into their specific categories as well. They also underscore how little is known about the inheritance pattern of these disorders given that survival to reproductive ages has been so limited, particularly in the group of patients with TGA.

GENETIC SYNDROMES AND CONOTRUNCAL DEFECTS

Conotruncal cardiac defects are common features of numerous genetic syndromes. An online search of the Mendelian Inheritance of Man (OMIM) identifies 12 entries for conotruncal defects overall and 37 entries for TOF alone. Recent molecular investigations on a few of these syndromes have begun to provide insight into the possible genetic etiology of the associated cardiac defects, and will be discussed in detail below.

Of note, different types of conotruncal defects are seen in different genetic syndromes with unequal frequency, once again providing preliminary evidence that the genetic factors operating in one sub-group of conotruncal defects may not be relevant to another. Further evidence comes from the varied frequency of extracardiac anomalies and genetic syndromes in each sub-group of lesions. In particular, the Baltimore Washington Infant Study, a population-based, case-control study, found that non-cardiac anomalies and genetic syndromes rarely occurred in the study population with TGA (10%) but frequently occurred in the study population with conotruncal defects and normally related great arteries (33.7%) (30). Therefore, though both TGA and other conotruncal defects are malformations of the outflow tract, they may or may not share a common genetic etiology in different cases.

The 22q11 Deletion Syndrome
Defining the Syndrome: The recognition that a significant proportion of patients with a conotruncal defect have a 22q11 deletion is one of the more revealing discoveries on the genetic etiology of these malformations to date. DiGeorge syndrome (DGS) was originally considered to be a rare developmental disorder characterized by thymic aplasia or hypoplasia, parathyroid gland aplasia or hypoplasia, conotruncal cardiac defects, and a particular facial appearance (31,32). Infants presented with congenital heart disease, hypocalcemia, distinct facies and occasionally immunodeficiencies. The most common cardiac defects included: IAA type B, TA and TOF (33). Approximately 10-20% of patients with DGS were noted to have chromosomal abnormalities resulting in loss of the proximal long arm of chromosome 22 (34-40). Further molecular studies demonstrated that nearly 90% of patients with the clinical diagnosis of DGS had a deletion of 22q11 (41-45).

Subsequently, it was recognized that velocardiofacial syndrome (VCFS, or Shprintzen's syndrome) shared several clinical features with DGS. The predominant clinical features of VCFS were originally described as cleft palate, speech and learning disabilities, cardiac defects, and typical facies (46), but several patients had hypocalcemia and decreased lymphoid tissue as well (47). The most frequent cardiac defects included TOF, ventricular septal defects and right aortic arch (48). Molecular investigations demonstrated that the vast majority of patients with VCFS had a 22q11 deletion as well (49).

Concurrently, Kinouchi and colleagues (50,51) described patients with a specific facial appearance and conotruncal anomalies which they labeled conotruncal anomaly face syndrome (CTAF). Given the clinical overlap between patients with VCFS and CTAF, patients with this disorder were also screened for a 22q11 deletion. Once again, the vast majority of patients with CTAF were found to have a 22q11 deletion (52).

Together these studies demonstrate that the vast majority of patients with DGS, VCFS and CTAF share a common genetic etiology, namely a 22q11 deletion. Moreover, it is now recognized that the clinical phenotype associated with the 22q11 deletion is highly variable and includes: cardiac malformations, palatal abnormalities, speech and learning disabilities, hypocalcemia, immunodeficiencies, renal anomalies, psychiatric disorders, and distinct facial dysmorphia (53,54). Unrelated patients with a 22q11 deletion can have a very mild phenotype with no more than hypernasal speech and distinct facies, or a very severe phenotype with a complex conotruncal defect, hypocalcemia, palatal abnormality and additional features. In familial cases, the proband frequently has a more severe phenotype than the parent, but this finding most likely reflects the fact that, historically, those with the most severe phenotypes have not survived to reproduce (43,55).

Molecular Findings: Although the clinical phenotype is highly variable in both related and unrelated individuals, two lines of evidence suggests that there is no correlation between the genotype, or the size of the deletion, and phenotype. In particular, the deletion is inherited in 10-25% of cases (53,55). Though the clinical features are highly variable between family members, molecular studies suggest that there is no change in the deletion size between generations or siblings (56). In addition, molecular studies that have compared deletion size and clinical phenotype in unrelated individuals have found no correlation (57). Moreover, unique patients with unusual deletions share the same features as those with the common deletion (58,59). Thus, other factors such as genetic background or environmental exposures are likely to play a role in determining the final phenotype.

The commonly deleted region of 22q11 spans 2-3 megabases of DNA and is estimated to contain numerous genes. Presumably, haploinsufficiency, or a diminished dosage, of one or more genes from the region results in the disease phenotype. As noted above, the genetics of this disorder may be more complicated than originally anticipated. Already, 25 genes have been identified in the region and are under investigation as candidates for the disease-phenotype (60). Several approaches have been used to determine whether a gene is disease-related. First, human tissue and mouse embryo expression studies have been performed to investigate whether the gene is expressed in disease-affected tissues. More convincing evidence is sought from mutation analyses of the candidate gene in patients with the typical phenotype who do not have a deletion. In other words, the identification of mutations in a gene from the deleted region in patients with the typical phenotype and no 22q11 deletion, would provide significant evidence that that gene was disease-related. To date, no single gene has been identified as specifically disease-related given that no mutations in any of the candidate genes have been identified in non-deleted patients.

Other experimental approaches will likely be needed to identify the disease-related gene(s) and the mechanism of disease. In particular, a syntenic region in the mouse has been identified into which many of the human genes map (61). Targeted disruption of expression (so called knock out experiments) of single or contiguous candidate genes in the mouse embryo may lend further insight into the disease mechanism; such experiments are in progress in multiple labs. When the molecular investigations identify the disease-related gene or genes in the 22q11 deletion syndrome, then the syndromic and non-syndromic non-deleted patients with similar forms of heart disease can be screened for sequence alterations in the same gene(s).

Congenital Heart Disease and the 22q11 Deletion Syndrome: Given the frequency of conotruncal defects in patients with the 22q11 deletion syndrome, many investigators have asked how many and which patients with a conotruncal defect have a 22q11 deletion. Numerous studies have demonstrated that the deletion frequency varies substantially with the specific type of conotruncal defect considered. Therefore, estimating the deletion frequency for conotruncal defects overall is infact meaningless.

The highest deletion frequency occurs in patients with IAA type B. Lewin and colleagues (62) found that 50% (11/22) of patients with IAA type B had a 22q11 deletion, while Goldmuntz and colleagues (63) found that 57% (12/21) of prospectively recruited patients with IAA type B had a deletion. In a smaller study, Rauch and colleagues (64) found that 82% (9/11) of their cohort with IAA type B had a deletion. Neither Goldmuntz nor Rauch detected a 22q11 deletion in a patient with IAA type A (0/7 when the studies are combined). Thus, IAA type A and type B would appear to be etiologically and mechanistically different, at least in certain cases.

Patients with TA have also been found to have a high 22q11 deletion frequency. Though most series have studied very few subjects, Momma and colleagues (65) examined 15 patients and found that 5 had a 22q11 deletion. Goldmuntz and colleagues (63) prospectively studied the largest number of patients to date and found that 34.5% (10/29) had a 22q11 deletion. Of note, patients with all four types of TA by the Van Praagh classification were found to have a deletion.

A substantial number of patients with TOF have also been found to have a 22q11 deletion in many studies. If all patients with TOF regardless of pulmonary valve anatomy are considered, the overall frequency ranges between 8-23% (63,66-68). Although some have found no statistical difference in the deletion frequency between those with TOF/pulmonary stenosis (TOF/PS) as compared to TOF/pulmonary atresia (TOF/PA) (63), other investigators have reported a significantly higher frequency of deletions in the sub-group with TOF/PA. For example, Digilio and colleagues (69) found that 32% (7/22) with TOF/PA had a deletion as compared to 6% (9/150) with TOF/PS. Chessa and colleagues (70) reported that 40% (16/40) with TOF/PA had a deletion as compared to 17% (9/54) with TOF/PS. Of note, Johnson and colleagues (71) found that 6 of 8 patients with TOF and an absent pulmonary valve had 22q11 deletion, suggesting that a 22q11 deletion was a very common finding in the absent pulmonary valve syndrome. Goldmuntz and colleagues (63) found that 1 of 4 subjects with TOF and an absent pulmonary valve had a 22q11 deletion. Given that the number of subjects studied in both series is small, it is difficult to conclusively state the frequency for this rare defect.

In contrast, very few patients with TGA or DORV have been found to have a 22q11 deletion. In the largest published series on these lesions, Goldmuntz and colleagues (63) found that only 1 of 20 patients with DORV had a deletion. They did not find any 22q11 deletions in patients with either d-TGA (0/39) or 1-TGA (0/6). The patients with d-TGA included those with and without a ventricular septal defect. Likewise, Takahashi and colleagues (67) did not find a deletion in their patients with DORV (0/8) or TGA (0/16). Additional evidence stems from the reported frequency of different types of congenital heart disease in the deleted population. Ryan and colleagues (53) found that less than 1% (4/545) of patients with a 22q11 deletion had TGA in the European collaborative study, while none of the 181 deleted patients reported by McDonald-McGinn and colleagues (54) had TGA. In contrast, Melchionda and colleagues (72) reported that 4 of 32 patients with d-TGA had a 22q11 deletion; two had d-TGA with an intact ventricular septum while two had a ventricular septal defect. In a case report, Marble and colleagues (73) described one infant with d-TGA, mild dysmorphic features and a 22q11 deletion. Overall, it appears that a 22q11 deletion is an uncommon finding in patients with DORV and d-TGA.

The deletion frequency varies not only with the primary cardiac diagnosis, but also varies independently in the presence or absence of associated vascular anomalies. Momma and colleagues (74,75) observed additional vascular anomalies, such as aorto-pulmonary collaterals, right aortic arch, or aberrant subclavian arteries, more frequently in patients with TOF who had a deletion than in those who did not have a deletion. They also found aortopulmonary collaterals in patients with TA and the deletion more frequently than in those without a deletion (65). Goldmuntz and colleagues (63) performed a logistic regression analysis which demonstrated that the risk of carrying a 22q11 deletion was significantly associated with both the primary intracardiac anatomy and the presence (or absence) of associated vascular features. For example, the predicted risk of having a 22q11 deletion was 0.06 if the patient had TOF and a normal left aortic arch, but increased to 0.40 in the presence of a right aortic arch and an additional vascular anomaly (such as an aberrant subclavian artery or aortopulmonary collateral). The same trend was seen for each of the primary diagnoses, namely TA or IAA. The authors caution that these numbers are derived from a limited study population and should not be used for counseling purposes.

Though the cardiac defects associated with a 22q11 deletion are most commonly conotruncal malformations, other types of congenital heart disease have been reported as well. Goldmuntz and colleagues reported that several patients with posterior malalignment type ventricular septal defects and coarctation of the aorta had a 22q11 deletion (though this lesion could be considered mechanistically similar to IAA). Ryan and colleagues (53) and McDonald-McGinn and colleagues (54) reported patients with ventricular septal defects, atrial septal defects, isolated vascular anomalies or rings, pulmonary stenosis and atrioventricular canal defects in patients with a 22q11 deletion. Yates and colleagues (76) reported one patient with heterotaxy syndrome and a deletion, while Consevage and colleagues (77) reported one patient with hypoplastic left heart syndrome who was mosaic for a 22q11 deletion. Therefore, other types of congenital heart disease are less commonly associated with the 22q11 deletion syndrome. Any patient with congenital heart disease and typical features of the 22q11 deletion syndrome warrants molecular evaluation.

Given the substantial frequency with which 22q11 deletions are found in patients with IAA, TA and TOF, the appropriate screening strategy in this patient population is debated. Several authors advocate testing for the 22q11 deletion in a patient with congenital heart disease only in the presence of additional syndromic features typical of the 22q11 deletion syndrome. Such a strategy minimizes the population that might be unnecessarily tested (78,79). Others advocate screening all neonates with either IAA, TA or TOF given the high frequency of deletions in these diagnostic groups and the utility of identifying those patients with a deletion as an infant (80,81). Although nearly everyone with a 22q11 deletion can be found to have syndromic features at some point, these findings are often unrecognized in the infant and only become apparent in the older child, or they may not even be appreciated until the deletion status is known. Thus, the diagnosis of the 22q11 deletion syndrome might be missed or delayed. However, identifying the patient with the deletion as an infant is important for both clinical and counseling purposes. This debate is likely to continue until further prospective, cost-benefit analyses of the deleted population and the at-risk cardiac population are completed. At this time, each clinician must decide based on their available services and their assessment of the risks and benefits of screening for a 22q11 deletion in the at-risk population.

Other Etiologies of DiGeorge, Velocardiofacial, or Conotruncal Anomaly Facies Syndromes: Although the vast majority of patients with the typical clinical features of either DiGeorge, velocardiofacial, or conotruncal anomaly facies syndromes have a 22q11 deletion, some patients are not found to have a 22q11 deletion. In some cases, the clinical features may result from environmental teratogens such as maternal diabetes or alcohol use. In other cases, mutations in the disease-related genes or undetected chromosomal alterations of the 22q11 critical region might explain the clinical findings in the absence of the common, large deletion. However, in a small number of patients, chromosomal alterations other than that involving chromosome 22 have been identified (82,83).

Several patients with terminal deletions of the short arm of chromosome 10 have been reported (84,85). Daw and colleagues (86) studied 3 DGS patients with terminal deletions of 10p and one VCFS patient with an interstitial deletion of 10p; the patients had overlapping deletions at the boundary of 10p13 and 10p14. They were able to define a smallest region of overlap of approximately 2 megabases of DNA that presumably defines a second DGS locus (DGSII). Subsequently,

Schuffenhauer and colleagues (87) studied 12 patients with 10p deletions, of which 9 had features of DGS, and found a similar smallest region of overlap as Daw. However, Dasouki and colleagues (88) described a patient with the DGS phenotype and a translocation between chromosome 10 and 22 which left the 22q11 region intact but deleted a terminal portion of 10p. However, the 10p deletion in this patient did not overlap with the smallest region of overlap defined by Daw and colleagues. In addition, Gottlieb and colleagues (89) studied 5 patients with 10p deletions and found that there were two non-overlapping deleted regions of 10p in these patients. One of the deleted regions contained the smallest region of overlap defined by Daw's study, but the other did not. Further, when they screened DGS/VCFS patients without a 22q11 deletion for a 10p deletion, none was detected. In summary, the story is more complicated than originally suggested. The terminal region of 10p is likely to be associated with DGS in some cases, but it remains to be defined whether there is one or two disease loci.

Alagille Syndrome
Additional insight into the molecular causes of some conotruncal defects may come from recent discoveries about Alagille syndrome. Alagille syndrome is an autosomal dominant disorder characterized by bile duct paucity in conjunction with cardiac disease, skeletal and ocular abnormalities and a characteristic face. The associated cardiac defects are generally right sided and most commonly include peripheral pulmonic stenosis or hypoplasia. However, a recent review of a large cohort of Alagille patients meeting all of the classic criteria for the disorder showed that 24% (22/92) had more significant congenital heart disease including a substantial number with TOF, with and without pulmonary atresia (90). *Jagged1*, a gene coding for a cell surface protein known to function as a ligand for the Notch transmembrane receptor, has recently been shown to be the Alagille syndrome disease gene (91,92).

Although the diagnosis of Alagille syndrome has previously required bile duct paucity, recent studies have demonstrated that the phenotype associated with Alagille syndrome is highly variable and may include patients with cardiac disease and only subtle syndromic features in the absence of clinically overt liver disease. For example, relatives of patients with Alagille syndrome have been observed to have right sided cardiac disease in the absence of any other visible features of Alagille syndrome. These relatives presumably have a limited manifestation of the Alagille syndrome disease gene (93). Krantz and colleagues (94) studied two cardiac patients for *Jagged1* mutations because they had typical right sided cardiac defects of Alagille syndrome even though they did not technically fulfill the clinical criteria for the syndrome. The investigators identified *Jagged1* mutations in these patients nonetheless. Moreover, a preliminary study of 66 presumably non-syndromic patients with TOF demonstrated that 2 subjects had mutations in the coding region (95). Thus, *Jagged1* appears to be an interesting candidate gene for right sided cardiac defects, and TOF in particular. Further investigations to better define the cardiac disease associated with Alagille syndrome and to determine whether *Jagged1* is a disease-related gene in patients with presumably isolated right sided cardiac defects are underway.

Other Genetic Syndromes

Molecular evaluation of other genetic syndromes which include conotruncal defects are also likely to provide insight into additional molecular mechanisms contributing to outflow tract malformations. In addition to DGS/VCFS and Alagille syndrome, conotruncal cardiac defects are frequently seen in patients with Down syndrome, Kabuki Make Up syndrome, Cat Eye syndrome, CHARGE association, and VATER or VACTERL association. The syndromes where molecular studies have been initiated are noted below.

Down Syndrome: Approximately half of all children with Down syndrome, or trisomy 21, have congenital heart disease. The most common lesions include common atrioventricular canal defects and ventricular septal defects. However, TOF is also relatively commonly seen in this syndrome. Moreover, trisomy 21 is relatively commonly seen in patients with TOF. In the Baltimore Washington Infant study, 6.8% of all patients with TOF had trisomy 21 (30). Molecular investigations of unique patients with partial trisomy 21 have begun to identify disease-loci associated with particular features of Down syndrome. In particular, the chromosomal region defined by D21S55 to MX1 is thought to be critical for development of congenital heart disease (96,97). Identification of the disease-related gene(s) in this region may provide further insight into the molecular mechanisms of syndromic as well as non-syndromic patients with similar cardiac defects.

The San Luis Valley Recombinant Chromosome 8 syndrome [SLV Rec(8)]: The SLV Rec(8) syndrome is characterized by congenital heart disease, facial dysmorphia, failure to thrive, developmental delay, and occasionally other anomalies. The vast majority have a conotruncal defect including 38% with TOF, 16% with DORV, and 2% with TA (98). The disorder occurs in Hispanic families in the southwestern United States and most likely results from a founder effect or a common ancestor. Chromosome analysis of the parents of the probands shows that one parent carries a balanced, pericentric inversion of chromosome 8. However, the proband has an unbalanced recombinant chromosome 8 resulting in duplication of the distal segment of the long arm of chromosome 8 (8q22.1-qter) and deletion of the distal end of the short arm of chromosome 8 (8p23.1-pter). On review of the literature, Gelb and colleagues (98) found that congenital heart disease was frequently present in other cases with isolated duplication of 8q or deletion of 8p, but neither of the isolated chromosomal anomalies were particularly associated with TOF. Therefore, it was unclear which of the resulting chromosomal aberrations seen in SLV Rec(8) was related to the development of conotruncal defects, or TOF in particular. Additional molecular analysis of patients with the SLV Rec(8) abnormality and other patients with chromosome 8 aberrations may identify additional disease loci for conotruncal defects in the future.

Non-Syndromic Genetic Etiologies

Very few studies investigating the genetic etiology of isolated, non-syndromic conotruncal defects have been performed given the rarity of large families with multiple affected members that would be appropriate for linkage analyses, and the lack of cytogenetic clues as to specific chromosomal loci that might be involved. However, one recent report demonstrated that the transcription factor Nkx2.5 (or CSX) was disease-related in four families with atrial septal defects (ASD) and conduction delays (99). Of particular interest was the finding that two of the patients in one family had TOF instead of an ASD. Therefore, Nkx2.5 , or other genes identified in a similar manner, may be shown to be disease-related in the etiology of conotruncal defects in the future.

ANIMAL MODELS AND NEW CANDIDATE GENES FOR CONOTRUNCAL DEFECTS

An increasing number of naturally occurring and experimentally derived animal models with conotruncal malformations are being recognized. Molecular and phenotypic characterization of these models provide insight into the developmental pathways critical to conotruncal development. These experiments also identify new genes or molecular pathways to consider in the etiology of human congenital heart disease. Although beyond the scope of this chapter, a few notable models and candidate genes are noted below.

Naturally Occurring Vertebrate Models

Several naturally occurring vertebrate models for conotruncal defects have been identified. In particular, the *Patch* (*Ph*) mouse has a spontaneous deletion of the platelet-derived growth factor receptor alpha subunit (αPDGFR) (100). The homozygote (*Ph/Ph*) frequently has conotruncal defects including TA and DORV, as well as other non-cardiac malformations (101). The homozygous *Splotch* (*Sp*) mouse has conotruncal defects as well as malformations in other neural crest derived tissues (102). The molecular alterations in the *Splotch* mutants have been identified as mutations or deletions in the *Pax3* gene. Therefore, these genes, their protein products and the developmental pathways in which they participate are now known to be critical to normal conotruncal morphogenesis. Finally, the keeshond dog was recognized to have conotruncal defects. Breeding studies have demonstrated that the malformations result from a single gene defect, although the disease-related gene has yet to be identified (103). Identification of this gene will most likely provide insight into similar human disease as well.

Experimentally Derived Models

The ability to manipulate gene expression in mouse embryos by transgenic technology or targeted disruption of gene expression (so-called knock-out models) has identified an increasing number of gene products that are critical to normal conotruncal development including: endothelin-1, Hoxa3, Pax3, NF-1, Sox4, Nt3, MSX1 HOX7, TGFβ1, TGFβ2, HLX1, RXRα,β,γ, and connexin 43 (104-120). Some of these may prove to be disease-related. Even if they are not the major gene involved in the disease process, they may act as modifying genes and at the very least provide insight into the molecular mechanisms underlying normal and abnormal conotruncal development.

CONCLUSIONS

The molecular genetic alterations involved in conotruncal malformations are just beginning to be investigated. Unlike many other disorders discussed in this text, the ability to study the genetic contributions to this group of disorders has been limited by the rarity of large families for which a parametric linkage analysis can be performed and a disease locus identified. However, reports of unique families with multiple affected members and studies on recurrence risk support the hypothesis that there are genetic factors that contribute to the development of these defects. They also suggest that while in some cases the specific types of conotruncal defects are mechanistically related, in other cases they are likely to be mechanistically distinct. These studies also point to the etiologic heterogeneity of this class of defects. Molecular investigation of genetic syndromes such as DGS/VCFS in which conotruncal defects are a cardinal feature, have already provided much insight into the genetic etiology of some of these malformations and will continue to do so. Likewise, the multitude of genes and developmental pathways now recognized to participate in conotruncal morphogenesis provide an expanding list of candidate genes for these disorders. Animal studies in conjunction with human genetic studies will undoubtedly contribute to our understanding of the molecular genetics of these malformations in the future.

REFERENCES

1.   Perry LW, Neill CA, Ferencz C, Rubin JD, Loffredo CA.. Infants with congenital heart disease: the cases. In Perspectives in Pediatric Cardiology.Epidemiology of Congenital Heart Disease, the Baltimore-Washington Infant Study 1981-1989. C.Ferencz, J. D. Rubin, C. A. Loffredo, and C. A. Magee, editors. Futura, NY. 1993, 33-62.

2.   Pankau R, Siekmeyer W, Stoffregen R. Tetralogy of Fallot in three sibs. *Am J Med Genet* 1990;37:532-533.

3.   Wulfsberg EA, Zintz EJ, Moore JW. The inheritance of conotruncal malformations: a review and report of two siblings with tetralogy of Fallot with pulmonary atresia. *Clin Genet* 1991;40:12-16.

4.   Pacileo G, Musewe NN, Calabro R. Tetralogy of Fallot in three siblings. *Eur J Pediatr* 1992;151:726-727.

5.   Friedberg DZ. Tetralogy of Fallot with right aortic arch in three successive generations.*Am J Dis Child* 1974;127:877-878.

6.   Brunson SC, Nudel DB, Gootman N, Aftalion B. Truncus arteriosus in a family.*Am Heart J* *1978;*96:419-420.

7.   Gobel JW, M. E. M. Pierpont, J. H. Moller, A. Singh, and J. E. Edwards. 1993. Familial interruption of the aortic arch. *Ped. Card.* 14:110-115.

8.   Rein, A. J. J. T. and R. Sheffer. 1994. Genetics of conotruncal malformations: further evidence of autosomal recessive inheritance. *Am. J. Med. Genet.* 50:302-303.

9.   Miller, M. E. and D. W. Smith. 1979. Conotruncal malformation complex: examples of possible monogenic inheritance. *Pediatrics* 63:890-893.

10.   Jones, M. C. and J. D. Waldman. 1985. An autosomal dominant syndrome of characteristic facial appearance, preauricular pits, fifth finger clinodactyly, and tetralogy of Fallot. *Am. J. Med. Genet.* 22:135-141.

11.   Chen, S.-C. and N. D'Souza. 1990. Familial tetralogy of Fallot and glaucoma. *Am. J. Med. Genet.* 37:40-41.

12.   Boon , A. R., M. B. Farmer, and D. F. Roberts. 1972. A family study of Fallot's tetralogy. *J. Med. Genet.* 9:179-192.

13.   Ando, M., A. Takao, and K. Mori. 1977. Genetic and environmental factors in congenital heart disease. In Gene-Environmental Interaction in Common Diseases. E. Inouye and H. Nishimura, editors. Baltimore University Park Press, Baltimore. 71-88.

14.   Sanchez-Cascos, A. 1978. The recurrence risk in congenital heart disease. *Eur. J. Cardiol.* 7/2-3:197-210.

15.   Dennis, N. R., and J. Warren. 1981. Risks to the offspring of patients with some common congenital heart defects. *J. Med. Genet.* 18:8-16.

16.   Nora, J. J. and H. H. Nora. 1976a. Genetics and environmental factors in the etiology of congenital heart disease. *South. Med. J.* 69:919-926.

17.   Zellers, T. M., D. J. Driscoll, and V. V. Michels. 1990. Prevalence of significant congenital heart defects in children of parents with Fallot's tetralogy. *Am. J. Cardiol.* 65:523-526.

18.   Nora, J. J. and A. H. Nora. 1988. Update on counseling the family with a first-degree relative with a congenital heart defect. *Am. J. Med. Genet.* 29:137-142.

19.   Burn , J., P. Brennan, J. Little, et al. 1998. Recurrence risks in offspring of adults with major heart defects: results from first cohort of British collaborative study. *The Lancet* 351:311-316.

20.   Digilio, M. C., B. Marino, A. Giannotti, A. Toscano, and B. Dallapiccola. 1997. Recurrence risk figures for isolated tetralogy of Fallot after screening for 22q11 microdeletion. *J. Med. Genet.* 34:188-190.

21.   Singh, H., P. J. Bolton, and C. M. Oakley. 1982. Pregnancy after surgical correction of tetralogy of Fallot. *Br. Med. J.* 285:168-170.

22.   Nora, J. J. and A. H. Nora. 1976b. Recurrence risks in children having one parent with a congenital heart disease. *Circulation* 53:701-702.

23.   Nora, J. J. and A. H. Nora. 1987. Maternal transmission of congenital heart diseases: new recurrence risk figures and the questions of cytoplasmic inheritance and vulnerability to teratogens. *Am. J. Cardiol.* 59:459-463.

24.   Czeizel, A., A. Pornoi, E. Peterffy, and E. Tarcal. 1982. Study of children of parents operated on for congenital cardiovascular malformations. *Br. Heart J.* 47:290-293.

25.   Emmanuel, R., J. Somerville, A. Inns, and R. Withers R. 1983. Evidence of congenital heart disease in the offspring of parents with atrioventricular defects. *Br. Heart J.* 49:144-147.

26.   Rose, V., R. J. M. Gold, G. Lindsay, and M. Allen. 1985. A possible increase in the incidence of congenital heart defects among offspring of affected parents. *J. Am. Coll. Cardiol.* 6:376-382.

27.   Whittemore, R., J. A. Wells, and X. Castellsague. 1994. A second-generation study of 427 probands with congenital heart defects and their 837 children. *J. Am. Coll. Cardiol.* 23:1459-1467.

28.   Pierpont, M. E. M., J. W. Gobel, J. H. Moller, and J. E. Edwards. 1988. Cardiac malformations in relatives of children with truncus arteriosus or interruption of the aortic arch. *Am. J. Cardiol.* 61:423-427.

29.   Becker, T. A., R. van Amber, J. H. Moller, and M. E. M. Pierpont. 1996. Occurrence of cardiac malformations in relatives of children with transposition of the great arteries.*Am. J. Med. Genet.* 66:28-32.

30.   Ferencz, C., C. A. Loffredo, A. Correa-Villasenor, and P. D. Wilson, editors. 1997. Malformations of the Cardiac Outflow Tract. In Genetic & Environmental Risk Factors of Major Cardiovascular Malformations: The Baltimore-Washington Infant Study 1981-1989. Armonk, NY: Futura Publishing Co., Inc., 59-102.

31.   DiGeorge, A. M. 1965. Discussion on a new concept of the cellular basis of immunology.*J. Pediatr.* 67:907-908.

32.   Conley, M.E., J. B. Beckwith, J. F. K. Mancer, and I. Tenckhoff. 1979. The spectrum of DiGeorge syndrome. *J. Pediatr.* 94:883-890.

33.   Van Mierop, L. H. S. and L. M. Kutsche. 1986. Cardiovascular anomalies in DiGeorge syndrome and importance of neural crest as a possible pathogenetic factor. *Am. J. Cardiol.* 58:133-137.

34.   de la Chapelle, A., R. Herva, M. Koivisto, and P. A. Aula. 1981. Deletion in chromosome 22 can cause Di George syndrome. *Hum. Genet.* 57:253-256.

35.   Kelley, R. I., E. H. Zackai, B. S. Emanuel, M. Kistenmacher, F. Greenberg, and H. H. Punnell. 1982. The association of the DiGeorge anomalad with partial monosomy of chromosome 22. *J. Pediatr.* 101:197-200.

36.   Greenberg, F., W. E. Crowder, V. Paschall, J. Colon-Linares, B. Lubianski, and D. H. Ledbetter. 1984. Familial DiGeorge syndrome and associated partial monosomy of chromosome 22. *Hum. Genet.* 65:317-319.

37.   Greenberg, F., F. F. B. Elder, P. Haffner, H. Northrup, and D. H. Ledbetter. 1988. Cytogenetic findings in a prospective series of patients with DiGeorge anomaly.*Am. J. Hum. Genet.* 43:605-611.

38.   Bowen, P., H. Pabst, D. Berry, R. Collins-Nakai, and J. J. Hoo. 1986. Thymic deficiency in an infant with a chromosome t(18;22) t(q12.2;p11.2) pat rearrangement.*Clin. Genet.* 29:174-177.

39.   Faed, M. J. W., J. Robertson, J. Swanson Beck, J. I. Carter, B. Bose, and M. M. Madlon. 1987. Features of DiGeorge syndrome in a child with 45,XX,-3,-22,+der(3)t(3;22)(p25;q11). *J. Med. Genet.* 24:255-234.

40.   Mascarello, J. T., J. F. Bastian, and M. C. Jones. 1989. Interstitial deletion of chromosome 22 in a patient with the DiGeorge malformation sequence. *Am. J. Med. Genet.* 32:112-114.

41.   Driscoll, D. A., M. L. Budarf, H. McDermid, and B. S. Emanuel. 1990. Molecular analysis of DiGeorge syndrome: 22q11 interstitial deletions. *Am. J. Hum. Genet.* 47(suppl):A215.

42.   Driscoll, D. A., M. L. Budarf, and B. S. Emanuel. 1992a. A genetic etiology for DiGeorge syndrome: consistent deletions and microdeletions of 22q11. *Am. J. Hum. Genet.* 50:924-933.

43.   Driscoll, D. A., J. Salvin, B. Sellinger, M. L. Budarf, D. M. McDonald-McGinn, E. H. Zackai, and B. S. Emanuel. 1993. Prevalence of 22q11 microdeletions in DiGeorge and velocardiofacial syndromes: implications for genetic counseling and prenatal diagnosis. *J. Med. Genet.* 30:813-817

44.   Scambler, P. J., A. H. Carey, R. K. H. Wyse, S. Roach, J. P. Dumanski, M. Nordenskjold, and R. Williamson. 1991. Microdeletions within 22q11 associated with sporadic and familial DiGeorge syndrome. *Genomics* 10:201-206.

45.   Carey, A. H., D. Kelly, S. Halford, R. et al. 1992. Molecular genetic study of the frequency of monosomy 22q11 in DiGeorge syndrome. *Am. J. Hum. Genet.* 51:964-970.

46.   Shprintzen, R. J., R. B. Goldberg, M. L. Lewin, et al. 1978. A new syndrome involving cleft palate, cardiac anomalies, typical facies, and learning disabilities: Velo-Cardio-Facial syndrome. *Cleft Palate J.* 15:56-62.

47.　Stevens, C. A., J. C. Carey, and A. O. Shigeoka. 1990. DiGeorge anomaly and velo-cardio-facial syndrome. *Pediatr.* 85:526-530.

48.　Young, D. , R. J. Shprintzen, and R. B. Goldberg. 1980.Cardiac malformations in the velo-cardio-facial syndrome. *Am. J. Cardiol.* 46:643-647.

49.　Driscoll, D. A., N. B. Spinner, M. L. Budarf, et al. 1992. Deletions and microdeletions of 22q11.2 in velo-cardio-facial syndrome. *Am. J. Med. Genet.* 44:261-268.

50.　Kinouchi, A., K. Mori, M. Ando, and A. Takao. 1976.Facial appearance of patients with conotruncal anomalies. *Pediatr. Jpn.* 17:84.

51.　Kinouchi, A. 1980. A study on specific peculiar facial features of conotruncal anomaly.*J Tokyo Women's Med. Coll.* (in Japanese) 50:396-409.

52.　Burn, J., A. Takao, D. Wilson, I. Cross, K. Momma, R. Wadey, P. Scambler, and J. Goodship. 1993. Conotruncal anomaly face syndrome is associated with a deletion within chromosome 22. *J. Med. Genet.* 30:822-824.

53.　Ryan, A. K., J. A. Goodship, D. I. Wilson, et al. 1997. Spectrum of clinical features associated with interstitial chromosome 22q11 deletions: a European collaborative study.*J. Med. Genet.* 34:798-804.

54.　McDonald-McGinn, D. M., D. LaRossa, E. Goldmuntz et al. 1997. The 22q11.2 deletion: Screening, diagnostic workup, and outcome of results; report on 181 patients.*Genetic Testing* 1:99-108.

55.　Leana-Cox, J., S. Pangkanon, K. R. Eanet, M. S. Curtin, and E. A. Wulfsberg. 1996. Familial DiGeorge/velocardiofacial syndrome with deletions of chromosome area 22q11: report of five families with a review of the literature. *Am. J. Med. Genet.* 65:309-316.

56.　Driscoll, D. A., M. Li, P. Chien, S. et al. 1995. Familial 22q11 deletions: phenotypic variability and determination of deletion boundaries by FISH [Abstract].*Am. J. Hum. Genet.* 57:A33.

57.　Carlson C., H. Sirotkin, R. Pandita, et al. 1997. Molecular definition of 22q11 deletions in 151 velo-cardio-facial syndrome patients. *Am. J. Hum. Genet.* 61:620-629.

58.　Kurahashi, H., E. Tsuda, R. Kohama, et al. 1997. Another critical region for deletion of 22q11: a study of 100 patients. *Am. J. Med. Genet.* 72:180-185.

59.　Rauch, A., R. A. Pfeiffer, G. Leipold, H. Singer, M. Tigges, and M. Hofbeck. 1999. A novel 22q11.2 microdeletion in DiGeorge syndrome. *Am. J. Hum. Genet.* 64:659-667.

60.　Emanuel, B. S. , M. L. Budarf, and P. J. Scambler. 1999. The genetic basis of conotruncal cardiac defects: the chromosome 22q11.2 deletion.In Heart Development. R. P. Harvey and N. Rosenthal, editors. Academic Press, New York. 463-478.

61.　Galili, N., H. S. Baldwin, J. Lund, et al. 1997. A region of mouse chromosome 16 issyntenic to the DiGeorge, velocardiofacial syndrome minimal critical region.*Genome Research* 7:17-26.

62.　Lewin, M. B., E. A. Lindsay, V. Jurecic, V. Goytia, J. A. Towbin, and A. Baldini. 1997. A genetic etiology for interruption of the aortic arch type B. *Am. J. Cardiol.* 80:493-497.

63.　Goldmuntz, E., B. J. Clark, L. E. Mitchell, et al. 1998. Frequency of 22q11 deletionsin patients with conotruncal defects. *J. Am. Coll. Cardiol.* 32:492-498.

64.　Rauch, A., M. Hofbeck, G. Leipold, et al.. 1998. Incidence and significance of 22q11.2 hemizygosity in patients with interrupted aortic arch. *Am. J. Med. Genet.* 78:322-331.

65.　Momma, K., M. Ando, and R. Matsuoka. 1997. Truncus arteriosuscommunis associated with chromosome 22q11 deletion. *J. Am. Coll. Cardiol.* 30:1067-1071.

66.　Amati, F., F. Mari, M. C. Digilio, et al. 1995. 22q11 deletions in isolated and syndromic patients with tetralogy of Fallot. *Hum. Genet.* 95:472-482.

67.　Takahashi, K., S. Kido, K. Hoshino, K. Ogawa, H. Ohashi, and Y. Fukushima. 1995. Frequency of a 22q11 deletion in patients with conotruncal cardiac malformations: a prospective study. *Eur. J. Pediat.* 154:878-881.

68.   Trainer, A.H., N. Morrison, A. Dunlop, N. Wilson, and J.Tolmie. 1996. Chromosome 22q11 microdeletions in tetralogy of Fallot. *Arch. Dis. Child.* 74:62-63.

69.   Digilio, M. C., B. Marino, S. Grazioli, D. Agostino, A. Giannotti, and B. Dallapiccola. 1996. Comparison of occurrence of genetic syndromes in ventricular septal defect with pulmonic stenosis (classic tetralogy of Fallot) versus ventricular septal defect with pulmonic atresia. *Am. J. Cardiol.* 77:1375-1376.

70.   Chessa, M., G. Butera, P. Bonhoeffer, et al. 1998. Relation of genotype 22q11 deletion to phenotype of pulmonary vessels in tetralogy of Fallot and pulmonary atresia-ventricular septal defect. *Heart* 79:186-190.

71.   Johnson, M. C., A. W. Strauss, S. B. Dowton, et al. 1995. Deletion within chromosome 22 is common in patients with absent pulmonary valve syndrome. *Am. J. Cardiol.* 76:66-69.

72.   Melchionda, S., M. C. Diglio, R. Mingarelli et al. 1995. Transposition of the great arteries associated with deletion of chromosome 22q11. *Am. J. Cardiol.* 75:95-98.

73.   Marble, M., E. Morava, R. Lopez, M. Pierce, and R. Pierce. 1998. Report of a new patient with transposition of the great arteries with deletion of 22q11.2.*Am. J. Med. Genet.* 78:317-318.

74.   Momma, K., C. Kondo, M. Ando, R. Matsuoka, and A. Takao. 1995. Tetralogy of Fallot associated with chromosome 22q11 deletion. *Am. J. Cardiol.* 76:618-621.

75.   Momma, K., C. Kondo, and R. Matsuoka. 1996. Tetralogy of Fallot with pulmonary atresia associated with chromosome 22q11 deletion. *J. Am. Coll. Cardiol.* 27:198-202.

76.   Yates, R. W. M., F. L. Raymond, A. Cook, and G. K.Sharland. 1996. Isomerism of the atrial appendages associated with 22q11 deletion in a fetus. *Heart* 76:548-549.

77.   Consevage, M. W., J. R. Seip, D. A. Belchis, A. T. Davis, B. G. Baylen, and P. K. Rogan. 1996. Association of a mosaic chromosomal 22q11 deletion with hypoplastic left heart syndrome. *Am. J. Cardiol.* 77:1023-1025.

78.   Webber, S. A., E. Hatchwell, J. C. K. Barber, et al. 1996. Importance of microdeletions of chromosomal region 22q11 as a cause of selected malformations of the ventricular outflow tracts and aortic arch: a three-year prospective study. *J. Pediatr.* 129:26-32.

79.   Digilio, M. C., B. Marino, A. Giannotti, R. Mingarelli, and B. Dallapiccola. 1999. Guidelines for 22q11 deletion screening of patients with conotruncal defects.*J. Am. Coll. Cardiol.* 33:1746-1747.

80.   Johnson, M. C., M. S. Watson, and A. W. Strauss. 1996. Chromosome 22q11monosomy and the genetic basis of congenital heart disease. *J. Pediatr.* 129:1-3.

81.   Goldmuntz, E., B. J. Clark, L. E. Mitchell, et al. 1999. Guidelines for 22q11 deletion screening of patients with conotruncal defects [Reply]. *J. Am. Coll. Cardiol.* 33:1747-1748.

82.   Van Essen, A. J., C. J. F. Schoots, R. A. van Lingen, M. J. E. Mourits, J. H. A. M. Tuerlings, and B. Leegte. 1993. Isochromosome 18q in a girl with holoprosencephaly, DiGeorge anomaly, and streak ovaries. *Am. J. Med. Genet.* 47:85-88.

83.   Lindgren, V., B. Rosinsky, J. Chin, and E. Berry-Kravis. 1994. Two patients with overlapping de novo duplications of the long arm of chromosome 9, including one case with DiGeorge sequence. *Am. J. Med. Genet.* 49:67-73.

84.   Monaco, G., C. Pignata, E. Rossi, O. Mascellaro, S. Cocozza, and F. Ciccimarra. 1991. DiGeorge anomaly associated with 10p deletion. *Am. J. Med. Genet.* 39:215-216.

85.   Lipson, A., K. Fagan, A. Colley, P. Colley, G. Sholler, D. Isaacs, and R. K. Oates. 1996. Velo-cardio-facial and partial DiGeorge phenotype in a child with interstitial deletion at 10p13-implications for cytogenetics and molecular biology. *Am. J. Med. Genet.* 65:304-308.

86.   Daw, S. C. M., C. Taylor, M. Kraman, et al. 1996. A common region of 10p deleted in DiGeorge and velocardiofacial syndromes. *Nature Genet.* 13:458-460.

87.   Schuffenhauer, S., P. Lichtner, P. Peykar-Derakhshandeh, et al. 1998. Deletion mapping on chromosome 10p and definition of a critical region for the second DiGeorge syndrome locus (DGS2). *Eur. J. Hum. Genet.* 6:213-225.

88.   Dasouki, M., V. Jurecic, J. A. Phillips, III, J. A. Whitlock, and A. Baldini. 1997. DiGeorge anomaly and chromosome 10p deletions: one or two loci? *Am. J. Med. Genet.* 73:72-75.

89.   Gottlieb, S., D. A. Driscoll, H. H. Punnett, B. Sellinger, B. S. Emanuel, and M. L. Budarf. 1998. Characterization of 10p deletions suggests two nonoverlapping regions contribute to the DiGeorge syndrome phenotype. *Am. J. Hum. Genet.* 62:495-498.

90.   Emerick, K. M., E. B. Rand, E. Goldmuntz, I. D. Krantz, N. B. Spinner, and D. A. Piccoli. 1999. Features of Alagille syndrome in 92 patients: frequency and relation to prognosis. *Hepatology* 29:822-829.

91.   Li, L., I. D. Krantz, Y. Deng, et al.. 1997. Alagille syndrome is caused by mutations in human *Jagged1*, which encodes a ligand for Notch1. *Nat. Genet.* 16:243-251.

92.   Oda, T., A. G. Elkahloun, B. L. Pike, et al. 1997. Mutations in the human*Jagged1* gene are responsible for Alagille syndrome. *Nat. Genet.* 16:235-242.

93.   Watson, G. H. and V. Miller. 1973. . Arteriohepatic dysplasia: familial pulmonary arterial stenosis with neonatal liver disease. *Arch. Dis. Child.* 48:459-466.

94.   Krantz, I., R. Smith, R. P. Colliton, H. Tinkel, E. H. Zackai, D. A. Piccoli, E. Goldmuntz, and N. B. Spinner. 1999. *Jagged1* mutations in patients ascertained with isolated congenital heart defects. *Am. J. Med. Genet.* 84:56-60.

95.   Smith, R. E. Goldmuntz, J. Shin, I. D. Krantz, and N. B. Spinner. 1998. Human *Jagged1* mutations in patients presenting with Tetralogy of Fallot [Abstr]. *Am. J. Hum. Genet.* 63(suppl 4):A3.

96.   Korenberg, J. R., C. Bradley, and C. M.Disteche. 1992. Down syndrome: molecular mapping of the congenital heart disease and duodenal stenosis. *Am. J. Hum. Genet.* 50:294-302.

97.   Korenberg, J. R., X.-N. Chen, R. Schipper, Z. Sun, R. Gonsky, S. Gerwehr, N. Carpenter, C. Daumer, P. Dignan, C. Disteche, J. M. Graham, Jr., L. Hugdins, B. McGillivray, K. Miyazaki, N. Ogasawara, J. P. Park, R. Pagon, S. Pueschel, G. Sack, B. Say, S. Schuffenhauer, S. Soukup, and T. Yamanaka. 1994. Down syndrome phenotypes: the consequences of chromosomal imbalance. *Proc. Natl. Acad. Sci. USA.* 91:4997-5001

98.   Gelb, B. D., Towbin, J. A., E. R. B. McCabe, and E. Sujansky. 1991. San Luis Valley recombinant chromosome 8 and tetralogy of Fallot: a review of chromosome 8 anomalies and congenital heart disease. *Am. J. Med. Genet.* 40:471-476.

99.   Schott, J. J. , D. W. Benson, C. T. Basson, W. Pease, G. M. Silberbach, J. P. Moak, B. J. Maron, C. E. Seidman, and J. G. Seidman. 1998. Congenital heart disease caused by mutations in the transcription factor *NKX2-5*. *Science* 281:108-111.

100.   Stephenson, D.A., M. Mercola, E. Anderson, et al. 1991. Platelet-derived growth factor receptor a-subunit gene (Pdgfra) is deleted in the mouse patch (*Ph*) mutation.*Proc. Natl. Acad. Sci. U.S.A.* 88:6-10.

101.   Schatteman, G. C., S. T. Motley, E. L. Effmann, and D. F. Bowen-Pope. 1995. Platelet-derived growth factor receptor alpha subunit deleted *Patch* mouse exhibits severe cardiovascular dysmorphogenesis. *Teratology* 51:351-366.

102.   Tremblay P. and P. Gruss. 1994. Pax: Genes for mice and men. *Pharmac. Ther.* 61:205-225.

103.   Patterson, D. F., T. Pexleder, W. R. Schnarr, T. Navratil, and R. Alaili. 1993. A single major-gene defect underlying cardiac conotruncal malformations interferes with myocardial grown during embryonic development: studies in the CTD line of keeshond dogs. *Am. J. Hum. Genet.* 52:388-397.

104.   Kurihara, Y., H. Kurihara, H. Oda, K. Maemura, R. Nagai, T. Ishikawa, and Y.Yazaki. 1995. Aortic arch malformations and ventricular septal defect in mice deficient in endothelion-1*J. Clin. Invest.* 96:293-300.

105.   Chisaka, I. and Capecchi, M.R. 1991. Regionally restricted developmental defects resulting from targeted disruption of the mouse homeobox gene hox-1.5. *Nature* 350:473-479.

106.   Franz, T. 1989. Persistent truncus arteriosus in the splotch mutant mouse.*Anat. Embryol.* 180:457-464.

107.   Brannan, C. I., A. S. Perkins, K. S. Vogel, et al. 1994. Targeted disruption of the neurofibromatosis type-1 gene leads to developmental abnormalities in heart and various neural crest-derived tissues. *Genes & Dev.* 8:1019-1029.

108.   Schilham, M. W., M. A. Oosterwegel, P. Moerer, et al. 1996. Defects in cardiac outflow tract formation and PRO-B lymphocyte expansion in mice lacking Sox-4. *Nature* 380:711-714.

109.   Donovan, M. J., R. Hahn, L. Tessarollo, and B. L. Hempstead. 1996. Identification of an essential nonneuronal function of neutrophin 3 in mammalian cardiac development. *Nature Genet.* 14:210-213.

110.   Suzuki, H. R., B. J. Padanilam, B. Vitale, F. Ramirez, and M. Solursh. 1991. Repeating developmental expression of G-Hox7, a novel homeobox-containing gene in the chicken.. *Devel. Biol.* 148:375-388.

111.   Pelton, R. W., B. Saxena, M. Jones, H. L. Moses and L. I. Gold. 1991. Immunohistochemical localization of TGFβ1, TGFβ2, and TFGβ3 in the mouse embryo: expression patterns suggest multiple roles during embryonic development. *J. Cell Biol.* 115:1091-1105.

112.   Wall, N. A. and B. L. M. Hogan. 1994. TGF-β related genes in development. *Curr. Opin Genet. Dev.* 4:517-522.

113.   Kingsley, D. M. 1996. The TGF-β superfamily: new members, new receptors, and new genetic tests of function in different organisms. *Genes & Dev.* 8:133-146.

114.   Nishimura, D. Y., A. F. Purchio, and J. C. Murray. 1993. Linkage localization of TGFβ2 and the human homeobox gene HLX1 to chromosome 1q. *Genomics* 15:357-364.

115.   Gruber, P. J., S. W. Kubalak., T. Pexieder., H. M. Suvoc., R. M. Evans, and K. R. Chien. 1996. RXRα deficiency confers genetic susceptibiliy for aortic sac, conotruncal, atrioventricular cushion, and ventricular muscle defects in mice. *J. Clin. Invest.* 98:1332-1343.

116.   Lee, R. Y., R. M. Evans, V. Giguere, and H. M. Sucov. 1997. Compartment-selective sensitivity of cardiovascular morphogenesis to combinations of retinoic acid receptor gene mutations. *Circ. Res.* 80:757-764.

117.   Sucov, H. M., E. Dyson, C. L. Gumeringer, J. Price, K. R. Chien, and R. M. Evans. 1994. RXRα mutant mice establish a genetic basis for vitamin A signaling in heart morphogenesis. *Genes & Dev.* 8:1007-1018.

118.   Mendelsohn, C., M. Mark, P. Dolle, et al. 1994. Retinoic acid receptor beta 2 (RAR beta 2) null mutant mice appear normal. *Dev. Biol.* 166:246-258.

119.   Li, J.-Y., X.-E. Hou, and A. Dahlstrom. 1995. GAP-43 and its relation to autonomic and sensory neurons in sciatic nerve and gastrocnemius muscle in the rat. *J. Auton. Nerv. Sys.* 50:299-309.

120.   Baldini A. Is the genetic basis of DiGeorge syndrome all in the HAND? *Nat Genet* 1999;21:246-247.

INDEX

Cytokines, 210
Cytoskeleton, 206
DCM, See dilated cardiomyopathy
Delta wave, 190
Desmin, 206
Desmosomes, 86
Dextrocardia, 318
DiGeorge syndrome, 360
Dilated cardiomyopathy, 195
Disopyramide, 139
Dispersion, 136, 169
Dispersion of refractoriness, 26
DMAHP, 279
DMPK, 279
Dofetilide, 138, 139
Dogs, 24
Dome of the action potential, 163
Down syndrome. See trisomy 21
Dual AV nodes, 319
Duchenne muscular dystrophy, 251
Dystrophin, 203, 252
Dystrophinopathy, 265
Early afterdepolarizations, 135
Ebstein malformation, 84
Ectopia lentis, 329
Electrophysiology, 1, 3, 23, 45
Electrophysiology study, 33
Embryonic development, 84
End-diastolic pressure, 197
Endocardium, 34
Enzyme deficiency, 219
Epicardial, 33
Epsilon waves, 240
Erythromycin, 139
Familial ASD, 288
Familial atrial fibrillation, 94
Familial hypercholesterolemia, 93
Familial WPW. See Wolff-
    Parkinson-White
Fexofenadine, 140
Fibrillin, 329
Fibrillin-1, 330
Fibrillin-2, 332
Fibrous annulus, 87
Final common pathway, 208
Fluorescence, 45
Fluorescent, 46

Frequency, 55
Gap junction, 109
Gap junctions, 4, 62 (see connexins)
Genotype, 131
Glycogen, 219
Glycogen storage diseases, 219
Haloperidol, 139
Haplotype analysis, 314
Heart block, 101 (see atrioventricular
    block)
HERG, 128, 142
Heterogeneity, 163
Heterotaxy, 318
His-Purkinje, 56, 64
HLA, 107
Holt-Oram syndrome, 288, 297
HOX genes, 324
H-V interval, 164
Hyperlipidemia, 221
Hypertrophic cardiomyopathy, 1, 81,
    181, 223
Hypocalcemia, 360
Ibutilide, 138, 139
ICD. See implantable cardioverter-
    defibrillator
Idiopathic ventricular fibrillation,
    147
Immunodeficiencies, 360
Immuno-electron microscopy, 64
Implantable cardioverter-
    defibrillator, 181, 188, 223
Inborn errors of metabolism, 219
Intercalated disks, 69, 86
Interrupted aortic arch, 355
Ion channels, 3, 120, 268
Isochrones, 57
Isoproterenol, 25
J wave, 164
Jagged1 mutations, 366
Jervell and Lange-Nielsen, 121
Ketoconazole, 139
Kinetics, 13
KVLQT1, 124
Langendorff, 4, 31, 54
Late potentials, 240
Laterality, 318